Cardiology

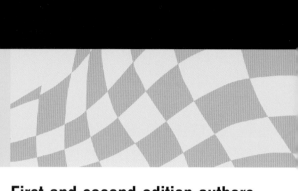

First and second edition authors

Anjana Siva

Mark Noble

Mohamed K Al-Obaidi

Third edition authors

Ajay Jain

Matthew Ginks

4th Edition

CRASH COURSE

SERIES EDITOR

Dan Horton-Szar
BSc(Hons) MBBS(Hons) MRCGP
Northgate Medical Practice,
Canterbury, Kent, UK

FACULTY ADVISOR

Michael Frenneaux
MBBS(Hons) MD FRCP FRACP FACC FESC FMedSci
Regius Professor of Medicine,
School of Medicine and Dentistry,
University of Aberdeen,
Aberdeen, UK

Cardiology

Antonia Churchhouse
BMedSci(Hons) MRCP
Core Medical Trainee,
London Deanery, London, UK

Julian Ormerod
MA PhD MRCP
Cardiology Registrar,
John Radcliffe Hospital,
Oxford, UK

MOSBY

ELSEVIER

Edinburgh London New York Oxford Philadelphia St Louis Sydney Toronto 2015

ELSEVIER
MOSBY

Senior Content Strategist: Jeremy Bowes
Senior Content Development Specialist: Ailsa Laing
Project Manager: Andrew Riley
Designer: Christian Bilbow
Icon illustrations: Geo Parkin
Illustration manager: Jennifer Rose

First edition 1999

Second edition 2004

Third edition 2008

Fourth edition 2013

Updated Fourth edition 2015

ISBN: 978-0-7234-3862-5

British Library Cataloguing in Publication Data
A catalogue record for this book is available from the British Library

Library of Congress Cataloging in Publication Data
A catalog record for this book is available from the Library of Congress

Notices
Knowledge and best practice in this field are constantly changing. As new research and experience broaden our understanding, changes in research methods, professional practices, or medical treatment may become necessary.

Practitioners and researchers must always rely on their own experience and knowledge in evaluating and using any information, methods, compounds, or experiments described herein. In using such information or methods they should be mindful of their own safety and the safety of others, including parties for whom they have a professional responsibility.

With respect to any drug or pharmaceutical products identified, readers are advised to check the most current information provided (i) on procedures featured or (ii) by the manufacturer of each product to be administered, to verify the recommended dose or formula, the method and duration of administration, and contraindications. It is the responsibility of practitioners, relying on their own experience and knowledge of their patients, to make diagnoses, to determine dosages and the best treatment for each individual patient, and to take all appropriate safety precautions.

To the fullest extent of the law, neither the Publisher nor the authors, contributors, or editors, assume any liability for any injury and/or damage to persons or property as a matter of products liability, negligence or otherwise, or from any use or operation of any methods, products, instructions, or ideas contained in the material herein.

ELSEVIER your source for books, journals and multimedia in the health sciences
www.elsevierhealth.com

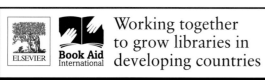

Working together to grow libraries in developing countries

www.elsevier.com • www.bookaid.org

The Publisher's policy is to use **paper manufactured from sustainable forests**

Printed in China

Last digit is the print line: 10 9 8 7 6 5 4 3 2 1

Series editor foreword

The *Crash Course* series first published in 1997 and now, 16 years on, we are still going strong. Medicine never stands still, and the work of keeping this series relevant for today's students is an ongoing process. These fourth editions build on the success of the previous titles and incorporate new and revised material, to keep the series up-to-date with current guidelines for best practice, and recent developments in medical research and pharmacology.

We always listen to feedback from our readers, through focus groups and student reviews of the *Crash Course* titles. For the fourth editions we have completely re-written our self-assessment material to keep up with today's 'single-best answer' and 'extended matching question' formats. The artwork and layout of the titles has also been largely re-worked to make it easier on the eye during long sessions of revision.

Despite fully revising the books with each edition, we hold fast to the principles on which we first developed the series. *Crash Course* will always bring you all the information you need to revise in compact, manageable volumes that integrate basic medical science and clinical practice. The books still maintain the balance between clarity and conciseness, and provide sufficient depth for those aiming at distinction. The authors are medical students and junior doctors who have recent experience of the exams you are now facing, and the accuracy of the material is checked by a team of faculty advisors from across the UK.

I wish you all the best for your future careers!

Dr Dan Horton-Szar

Authors

Cardiology is an exciting and dynamic specialty that combines bedside history taking and clinical examination with a broad range of investigations and interventions. The specialty is constantly growing, and advances in diagnostics, technologies, and therapeutics are reflected in this fully revised 4th Edition.

Having been through the rigours of medical school exams ourselves (some more recently than others!), we are aware that assessments are also changing. Hence we have also developed an up to date self-assessment section, the majority of which is based on the popular "Best of Five" format.

We aim primarily to equip you with the knowledge needed to pass your exams, but hope that this book also gives you the opportunity to further your interest and enjoyment of cardiology.

Best of luck with your studies!

Antonia Churchhouse and Julian Ormerod

Faculty Advisor

Cardiology has seen huge advances over the past three decades and is one of the most popular and competitive specialties. Lives saved by lifestyle modification and treatment of hypertension and lipid disorders together with revascularisation and secondary prevention strategies are reflected in our national statistics which show dramatic reductions in cardiovascular mortality over the last 20 years. Impressive improvements in quality-of-life and prognosis have also resulted from contemporary treatment of systolic heart failure. Nevertheless, cardiovascular disease remains the major cause of premature death and the major challenge to clinical medicine in the 21st century, not only in western societies but increasingly in developing countries as well. There have been some notable areas in which little progress in therapy has been made, particularly in the syndrome of heart failure with normal ejection fraction.

This *Crash Course in Cardiology* is designed to arm the reader with the knowledge base needed for a clinical introduction to this fascinating specialty. The book provides a comprehensive but we hope readable overview. We have aimed to convey the enthusiasm and excitement that the specialty inspires in us. It begins with history taking and physical examination and proceeds to describe investigations commonly used in cardiology. The next few chapters focus on the evaluation of common presenting symptoms in cardiology. Subsequent chapters focus on common presentations of patients with cardiovascular disorders and a summary of common cardiovascular disorders.

Like the other books in this series, the material is contemporary, the content accessible and the coverage comprehensive. We hope that students will enjoy reading this book.

Michael Frenneaux

Contents

Contents

By the end of this chapter you should:
- Be able to take a history from a patient – with specific relevance to symptoms that arise from cardiovascular disease.
- Understand the variety of symptoms that arise from cardiovascular disease.
- Be able to present salient points from a history in a clear and succinct manner.

AIM OF HISTORY TAKING

The aim of history taking is to observe the following points:

- Establish a patient's reasons for seeking medical attention (presenting complaint)
- Highlight important symptoms and present them in a clear and logical manner
- Obtain information about the severity of the symptoms and, therefore, of the underlying disease
- Establish a list of risk factors relevant to the current presentation
- Ask questions relevant to suspected diseases and so narrow the list of suspected differential diagnoses
- Evaluate to what extent the individual's lifestyle has been affected by or has contributed to the underlying disease.

PRESENTING COMPLAINT

The presenting complaint is the patient's reason for seeking medical attention and will usually be one of the following:

- Chest pain or tightness.
- Dyspnoea.
- Syncope or dizziness.
- Ankle swelling.
- Palpitations.

HINTS AND TIPS

The presenting complaint is always in the patient's own words. Thus the presenting complaint will always be 'chest pain' or 'palpitations' and not 'myocardial infarction' or 'arrhythmia'.

It may be an incidental finding of a murmur or hypertension as a reason for referral from a colleague.

The presenting complaint should be documented in a few words at the beginning of the clerking, and is followed by a more in-depth assessment, the history of the presenting complaint.

Chest pain

Ascertain the points in Fig. 1.1 as you would for any type of pain using the mnemonic SOCRATES.

HINTS AND TIPS

Angina means 'choking'. Patients will often deny chest pain and will describe a heavy, aching or crushing sensation instead.

Dyspnoea

This is an uncomfortable awareness of one's breathing. Ascertain the following:

- Precipitating factors, e.g. exercise, how much – compare with peer group.
- Duration of the problem – when did it start and is it getting worse?
- Associated features, such as chest pain, palpitations, sweating, ankle swelling, cough or haemoptysis (Fig. 1.3).
- Is the patient short of breath lying flat (orthopnoea) or do they wake up due to shortness of breath (paroxysmal nocturnal dyspnoea)?

Syncope

This is a loss of consciousness due to inadequate perfusion of the brain. The differential diagnosis is given in Fig. 1.4.

Fig. 1.1	Points to ascertain when asking about chest pain
Site	Location in the chest – is it retrosternal, epigastric, or on the left or right hand side of the chest?
Onset	When did the pain start? Did it come on gradually or suddenly?
Character	Is the pain dull, sharp, or burning?
Radiation	To the neck, jaw or left arm
Associated symptoms	See Fig. 1.2
Timing	Is the pain constant or relapsing and remitting?
Exacerbating/ relieving factors	Any worsening with exercise or improvement with GTN spray?
Severity	Rated on a scale of 1–10

HINTS AND TIPS

Paroxysmal nocturnal dyspnoea may be the first feature of pulmonary oedema. This occurs when fluid accumulates in the lungs when the patient lies flat during sleep. When awake, the respiratory centres are very sensitive and register oedema early with dyspnoea; during sleep sensory awareness is depressed, allowing pulmonary oedema to accumulate. The patient is, therefore, woken by a severe sensation of breathlessness, which is extremely frightening and is relieved by sitting or standing up.

Ask about the following:

- Events leading up to the episode – what was the patient doing at the time?
- The event itself – did the patient drop to the ground, was there any injury, and was there any shaking of limbs?
- Nature of the recovery period.

HINTS AND TIPS

Cardiac syncope often occurs with no warning and is associated with rapid and complete recovery. Be careful, therefore, because the patient will usually be well when you take the history despite having a potentially life-threatening condition.

HINTS AND TIPS

Syncope is often very difficult to differentiate from seizure. Bringing a witness to a first outpatient appointment is often helpful as they will be able to tell the doctor the characteristics of the 'funny turn'.

Palpitations

Ask the following questions:

- Can you describe the palpitations (ask the patient to tap them out)?
- Are there any precipitating or relieving factors?
- How long do they last and how frequent are they?
- Are there any associated features (e.g. shortness of breath, chest pain or loss of consciousness; Fig. 1.5)?

Common manoeuvres used to abolish palpitations include:

- Valsalva manoeuvre (bearing down against a closed glottis), e.g. blowing into a syringe.

Fig. 1.2	Features of different types of chest pain			
Cause	**Angina pectoris**	**Pericarditis**	**Pulmonary embolus or pneumonia**	**Oesophagitis or reflux**
Site	Central	Central or left-sided	Anywhere in chest	Epigastric or retrosternal
Character	Pressure or dull ache	Sharp	Sharp	Dull or burning
Radiation	Left arm, neck, or jaw	No	No	Neck
Associated features	Shortness of breath, sweating, nausea, palpitations	Shortness of breath, sweating, palpitations, fever	Shortness of breath, haemoptysis, cough, fever	Sweating, nausea
Exacerbating features	Exertion, cold weather, stress	Recumbent position, deep inspiration	Deep inspiration, coughing	Recumbent position, presence or lack of food, NSAIDS
Relieving features	Rest, GTN spray, oxygen mask	Sitting forward, NSAIDS	Stopping breathing	Antacids

GTN, glyceryl trinitrate. NSAIDS, non-steroidal anti-inflammatory drugs.

Fig. 1.3   Features of conditions causing dyspnoea

System involved	Disease	Features of dyspnoea
Cardiovascular	Pulmonary oedema	May be acute or chronic, exacerbated by exertion or lying flat (orthopnoea and PND), associated with sweating (and cough with pink frothy sputum)
	Ischaemic heart disease	Exacerbated by exertion or stress, relieved by rest, associated with sweating and angina
Respiratory	COPD	Chronic onset, exacerbated by exertion and respiratory infections, may be associated with cough and sputum, almost always associated with history of smoking
	Interstitial lung disease	Chronic onset, no real exacerbating or relieving factors, may have history of exposure to occupational dusts or allergens
	Pulmonary embolus	Acute onset, associated with pleuritic chest pain and haemoptysis
	Pneumothorax	Acute onset, pleuritic chest pain
	Pneumonia and neoplasms of the lung	Associated with pleuritic pain
Other	Pregnancy	Gradual progression due to splinting of diaphragm or anaemia
	Obesity	Gradual progression due to effort of moving and chest wall restriction
	Anaemia	History of blood loss, peptic ulcer, operations, etc.
	Trauma/musculoskeletal	Shortness of breath due to pain

COPD, chronic obstructive pulmonary disease; PND, paroxysmal nocturnal dyspnoea.

- Carotid sinus massage – remember only one side at a time and listen for carotid bruits beforehand.

Ankle swelling

Cardiac causes of ankle swelling include congestive cardiac failure (fluid retention caused by heart failure).

There are many causes of cardiac failure. Causes of left-heart failure include:

- Ischaemic heart disease.
- Hypertension.
- Mitral and aortic valve disease.
- Cardiomyopathies.
- Congestive cardiac failure.

Causes of right-heart failure include:

- Chronic lung disease (cor pulmonale).
- Pulmonary embolism.
- Tricuspid and pulmonary valve disease.
- Mitral valve disease with pulmonary hypertension.
- Right ventricular infarct.
- Primary pulmonary hypertension.

From the above list it can be seen that a history encompassing all aspects of cardiac disease needs to be taken to identify the possible causes of ankle swelling.

Ankle swelling secondary to cardiac causes is classically worse later in the day after the patient has been walking around. The hydrostatic pressure in the small blood vessels is greater when the legs are held vertical, so increasing the accumulation of fluid in the interstitial spaces. At night, however, the legs are raised, reducing intravascular pressure and allowing flow of fluid back into the venules with reduction of the oedema by morning.

Non-cardiac causes of ankle swelling include:

- Drugs – such as calcium channel blockers, e.g. amlodipine.
- Venous disease – due to decreased venous return.
- Renal – due to proteinuria (nephrotic syndrome).
- Hepatic – due to low serum albumin.
- Protein malnutrition – due to low serum albumin.

Fig. 1.4 Differential diagnosis of syncope

Cause	Speed of onset	Precipitating events	Nature of recovery
Stokes–Adams attack (transient asystole resulting in cerebral hypoxia)	Sudden – patient feels entirely well immediately before syncope	Often none	Rapid, often with no sequelae
Tachycardia – VT or very rapid SVT	Sudden	Often none	Rapid
AS and HCM	Sudden	Exertion, sometimes no warning	Rapid
Vasovagal syncope	Preceded by dizziness	Sudden pain, emotion, micturition. Patient often feels nauseated or vomits	Rapid
Orthostatic hypotension	Rapid onset after standing	Standing up suddenly, prolonged standing, use of antihypertensive or antianginal agents	May feel nauseated
Carotid sinus hypersensitivity	Dizziness or no warning	Movement of the head	May feel nauseated
Seizure – epileptiform or secondary to cerebrovascular event	May have classical aura or focal neurological signs, rapid onset	Often none (certain types of flashing lights or alcohol withdrawal may precipitate epilepsy)	Often drowsy, may have residual neurological deficit
Pulmonary embolus	Chest pain, dyspnoea, or no warning	None (but ask about recent travel, hospitalization, etc.)	May have dyspnoea or pleuritic chest pain
Hypoglycaemia (may be associated with convulsions during the period of unconsciousness)	Slower onset, nausea, sweating, tremor	Exercise, insulin therapy, missing meals	Often drowsy

AS, aortic stenosis; HCM, hypertrophic cardiomyopathy; SVT, supraventricular tachycardia; VT, ventricular tachycardia.

Fig. 1.5 Causes of palpitations

Rhythm	Precipitating factors	Relieving factors
Sinus tachycardia	Anxiety, exertion, thyrotoxicosis, anaemia	Rest or specific treatment of underlying condition
Atrial fibrillation	Ischaemia, thyrotoxicosis, hypertensive heart disease, mitral valve disease, alcoholic heart disease, pulmonary sepsis or embolism, idiopathic	Antiarrhythmic agents or treatment of the underlying disorder
Atrial flutter	Thyrotoxicosis, sepsis, alcohol, caffeine, pulmonary embolus, idiopathic	Antiarrhythmic agents or treatment of the underlying cause
AV and AV nodal re-entry tachycardias	Caffeine, emotion, alcohol, or no obvious cause	Vasovagal stimulation, ablation of re-entry pathway or antiarrhythmic drugs
VT	Ischaemia	Antiarrhythmic agents, treatment of the underlying cause or ablation of focus of arrhythmia
Bradyarrhythmias (AV nodal block or sinus node disease)	Often none (overtreatment of tachycardia with antiarrhythmic agents)	Stop antiarrhythmic agent or insert permanent pacemaker

AV, atrioventricular; VT, ventricular tachycardia.

- Pulmonary – due to hypercapnia and hypoxia in COPD.
- Dependent – mild oedema can occur in the absence of demonstrable disease in the obese or elderly.

SYSTEMS REVIEW

It is very important to learn the skill of taking a rapid, but detailed, systems review. This part of the history consists of direct questions covering the important symptoms of disease affecting systems other than the one covered in the presenting complaint. Learn the questions by heart so that you automatically ask them every time you take a history (note that this is only time-consuming if the doctor has trouble remembering the questions to ask).

Respiratory system

Cough

Cough may suggest the presence of infection; a common cause of arrhythmias. Cough is also a symptom of cardiac failure.

Sputum

Sputum production can indicate infection (green) or pulmonary oedema (pink and frothy).

Haemoptysis

Haemoptysis is a feature of pulmonary embolism, pulmonary hypertension secondary to mitral valve disease and pulmonary infection.

Wheeze

This is classically seen in asthmatics (remember that asthmatics cannot take β-blockers), but is also a feature of cardiac asthma as a sign of pulmonary oedema. Patients who have chronic obstructive airways disease may complain of wheeze; these patients have often been heavy smokers and are, therefore, at risk of cardiac disease.

Gastrointestinal system

Appetite

Appetite is often reduced in cardiac failure; this may be partly because patients are too breathless to eat, but also because they are systemically ill with raised cytokines. Depression also commonly coexists with heart failure and may contribute to reduced appetite.

Weight loss or gain

Oedema can cause marked weight gain. Severe cardiac failure or infective endocarditis can cause weight loss.

Nausea and vomiting

Nausea and vomiting often complicate an acute myocardial infarction (MI), particularly when it affects the inferior wall. They may also occur with vasovagal syncope or drug toxicity (e.g. digoxin toxicity).

Indigestion

This may be confused for ischaemic cardiac pain and vice versa.

Diarrhoea and constipation

Diarrhoea may lead to electrolyte imbalance affecting cardiac rhythm or may be a sign of viral illness leading to myocarditis or pericarditis.

Central nervous system

Headache

Headache may be a side effect of cardiac drugs (e.g. nitrates and calcium channel blockers).

Weakness, sensory loss, visual or speech disturbance

These signs may suggest thromboembolic disease, which may complicate atrial fibrillation or alter the decision to give thrombolysis to a patient who has acute MI.

Skin and joints

Rashes

Rashes are an important sign in the patient who has infective endocarditis or a possible drug side effect. They are also seen in many viral illnesses and autoimmune disease.

Joint pain

Joint pain can occur in infective endocarditis, viral disease, rheumatic fever and autoimmune disease. A history of arthritis will affect the decision to undertake an exercise tolerance test to diagnose angina.

Genitourinary system

Proteinuria

This suggests a renal cause of oedema.

Haematuria

Macroscopic haematuria is sometimes seen in infective endocarditis.

Frequency, hesitancy, nocturia and terminal dribbling

Symptoms of prostatism are common in middle-aged male patients who have heart disease and may affect their compliance with diuretic therapy.

Impotence and failure of ejaculation

These symptoms can be caused by β-blockers and are also quite common in diabetics and arteriopaths, two groups of patients commonly attending cardiology clinics and being treated in coronary care units.

PAST MEDICAL HISTORY

For any patient the past medical history should include all previous illnesses and operations and the dates when they occurred. In particular, in cardiac patients emphasis should be placed on the following aspects of the past medical history:

- Risk factors for ischaemic heart disease – smoking, diabetes mellitus, hypercholesterolaemia, hypertension or family history – it may be easier to ask about this along with the other risk factors rather than in the family history section of the history.
- Past cardiac interventions – cardiac surgery (valve replacement or coronary artery bypass graft – CABG)? How many grafts? Where were they harvested from? Angioplasty? How many stents? What type of stent (bare metal or drug-eluting)?
- History of rheumatic fever.
- History of recent dental work – an important cause of infective endocarditis (others include recent invasive procedures, such as colonoscopy or bladder catheterization).

FAMILY HISTORY

Ischaemic heart disease and sudden cardiac death are recognized as having a genetic component and this should have been ascertained earlier in the history.

Other cardiac conditions that have a genetic component are listed in Fig. 1.6.

SOCIAL HISTORY

The social history aims to identify any areas in the patient's lifestyle that may contribute to or be affected by his or her disease:

Disorder	Inheritance	Cardiac complications
Familial hypercholesterolaemia	AR	Premature ischaemic heart disease
HCM	AD	Sudden death, arrhythmias
Marfan syndrome	AD	Aortic dissection, mitral valve prolapse or incompetence
Haemochromatosis	AR	Cardiomyopathy
Romano–Ward, Jervell Lange-Nielsen syndromes	AR	Long QT syndrome, may lead to sudden death due to ventricular arrhythmias
Homocystinuria	AR	Premature ischaemic heart disease, recurrent venous thrombosis
Brugada Syndrome	AD	Sudden death

Fig. 1.6 Heart conditions that have a genetic component

AD, autosomal dominant; AR, autosomal recessive; HCM, hypertrophic cardiomyopathy.

- Occupation – always ask about the patient's occupation. In cardiac patients this is particularly important because, for example, a history of ischaemic heart disease could result in the loss of a heavy goods vehicle licence. There are many other similar situations where a patient might not be able to continue work, and these need to be identified.
- Smoking – a recognized risk factor in cardiovascular disease.
- Use of illegal drugs – intravenous drug abuse is associated with a high risk of infective endocarditis. The organisms involved are unusual (e.g. *Staphylococcus aureus*, *Candida albicans*, Gram-negative organisms and anaerobes). Cocaine abuse is associated with coronary artery spasm and increased myocardial oxygen demand resulting, in some cases, in myocardial ischaemia and infarction. Long-term use of cocaine may result in dilated cardiomyopathy.
- Alcohol intake – heavy alcohol consumption has many cardiac effects (Fig. 1.7). Alcohol is a potent myocardial depressant when taken in excess over a long period.
- It should also aim to establish the patient's support network – who is at home, does the patient need any

Fig. 1.7 Cardiovascular effects of heavy alcohol consumption

Cardiovascular effect	Comments
Cardiomyopathy	Alcohol is the second most common cause of dilated cardiomyopathy in developed countries (the first most common being ischaemic heart disease). This is due to a direct toxic effect of alcohol on the myocardium and also to a nutritional deficiency of thiamine, which often accompanies alcohol excess and can lead to beriberi; dilated cardiomyopathy is most commonly seen in men aged 35–55 years of age who have been drinking heavily for over 10 years
Arrhythmias	Most commonly atrial arrhythmias (e.g. atrial fibrillation), but also ventricular arrhythmias
Sudden death	Due to ventricular arrhythmias
Hypertension	Alcohol is an independent risk factor for hypertension, possibly due to stimulation of the sympathetic nervous system
Coronary artery disease	In small quantities alcohol has a protective effect on IHD, but heavy alcohol intake is associated with an increased risk of IHD

IHD, ischaemic heart disease.

help with the activities of daily living from friends or family, or are they in need of outside help from social services?

- Exercise capacity – it is useful to gauge how much the patient can do and what limits their activity.

A rare cause of hypertension is excessive liquorice infections. Liquorice inhibits the peripheral metabolism or cortisol, leaving it free to bind to mineralocorticoid receptors and exert its effects.

DRUG HISTORY

For all patients this should include all regular medications with details of doses and times. It should also include details of any over-the-counter and homeopathic medications that they may take. If a patient is on antibiotics, establish why they are taking them and how long they are taking them for. In addition, in the cardiac patient, attention should be paid to the following features:

- Any previous history of thrombolysis, in particular the administration of streptokinase, because this should not be administered again within 2 years of the last dose. Some centres now never administer streptokinase to a patient who has received it before, preferring to use recombinant tissue plasminogen activator instead. This is because it is thought that antibodies develop to the bacterial antigens in streptokinase, so rendering it less effective when administered for a second time because the drug is bound by antibodies and neutralized.
- Nitrates should be taken in such a way as to allow for a drug-free period; therefore if a twice-daily nitrate is being used it is important to establish that it is not being taken at 12-h intervals. For example, isosorbide mononitrate should be taken at 8 a.m. and 2 p.m. so that drug levels fall to very low levels overnight.
- Drugs that have cardiac effects (e.g. anti-asthmatics like salbutamol). Note in particular any drugs that may prolong the QT interval e.g. some antipsychotics (haloperidol, risperidone), antidepressants (amitriptyline, citalopram), antibiotics (clarithromycin, erythromycin), antiarrhythmics (sotalol, amiodarone), and over-the-counter non-sedating antihistamines (loratadine, cetirizine).
- Patients who have had stent implantation will be prescribed aspirin and clopidogrel/prasugrel – it is important to confirm the patients' anti-platelet therapy and the duration of treatment with clopidogrel/prasugrel.
- If a patient is on warfarin, find out why they are on it, how long they are on it for, their target INR and their usual dose.

ALLERGIES

All drug allergies should be carefully documented with information on the precise effects noted.

PRESENTING HISTORY FINDINGS

You will rarely be asked to take a history from a patient without having to present it back to someone. Being able to clearly and succinctly present a history is a vital skill and you should seek out opportunities to do this as much as possible. For example: 'Mr X is a 49-year-old builder who developed sudden onset chest tightness whilst at work this morning which was not relieved by his GTN spray. The tightness was a burning sensation in the centre of his chest and was associated with sweating and nausea but did not radiate down his arm. He has a history of a myocardial infarction, which was treated with an LAD stent last year. He is an ex-smoker with a 20 pack-year history. My differential diagnosis includes unstable angina and GORD. I would like to conduct a full examination and targeted investigations including an ECG and a 12-h troponin to allow me to make a definitive diagnosis.'

Examination 2

Objectives

By the end of this chapter you should:
- Be able to examine the cardiovascular system to elicit signs of cardiovascular disease.
- Be able to differentiate systolic and diastolic murmurs and understand the valve lesions associated with them.
- Understand the clinical manifestations of cardiac disease outside the cardiovascular system.

This chapter provides information on how to examine the cardiovascular system. The method of examination remains the same whether you are sitting for finals or for the membership examination, so you should learn it properly once and for all. Remember that cardiovascular cases are among the most popular used in short-case examinations.

HOW TO BEGIN THE EXAMINATION

COMMUNICATION

Ensure that the patient is comfortable at all times and establish rapport to put them at ease. You need to expose the patient in order to examine them properly but cover the patient to maintain modesty, and as soon as you have finished the examination.

Always start by introducing yourself and shaking hands gently (many elderly patients have painful arthritic joints – never make patients wince when you shake hands with them). Ask if you can examine the patient's chest and heart.

Position the patient correctly. The patient should remove all clothing from the waist upward – it is acceptable for a female patient to cover her breasts when you are not observing or examining the praecordium.

The patient should be sitting comfortably against the pillows with his or her back at 45° with the head supported so that the neck muscles are relaxed – the only three circumstances when you may deviate from this position are:

- If the patient has such bad pulmonary oedema that he or she needs to sit bolt upright.

- If the jugular venous pressure (JVP) is not raised, a more recumbent position will fill the jugular vein and allow examination of the venous pressure waveform.
- Conversely, if the JVP is very high it may be necessary to sit the patient upright to visualise the height of the waveform.

OBSERVATION

As soon as you see the patient, and during your introductions, you should be observing the patient and his or her surroundings. Once the patient has been positioned, expose the chest, step to the end of the bed and observe for a few seconds.

Observation is an art and you will be surprised by how much information you can obtain and remember after only a few seconds. In many cases this part of the examination provides valuable clues about the diagnosis. The secret to this is knowing what to look for.

Look at the patient's face for the following signs:

- Breathlessness, central cyanosis.
- Malar flush of mitral stenosis.
- Corneal arcus or xanthelasma – suggestive of hypercholesterolaemia.
- Any signs of congenital abnormality, such as the classic appearance of Down syndrome or Turner syndrome.

Look at the neck and praecordium:

- Visible pulsation in the neck may be due to a high-volume carotid pulse or giant 'v' waves in the JVP (the JVP usually has a double pulsation).
- Scars and visible pulsation on the chest (it is important to have a working knowledge of the common scars seen; Fig. 2.1) and the apex beat may be visible. Look for peripheral oedema if the patient's feet are visible.

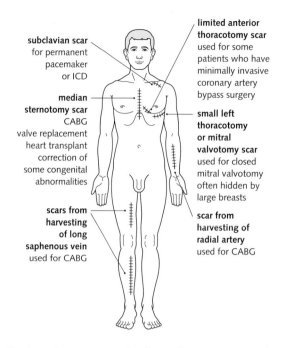

subclavian scar
for permanent
pacemaker
or ICD

limited anterior
thoracotomy scar
used for some
patients who have
minimally invasive
coronary artery
bypass surgery

median
sternotomy scar
CABG
valve replacement
heart transplant
correction of
some congenital
abnormalities

small left
thoracotomy
or mitral
valvotomy scar
used for closed
mitral valvotomy
often hidden by
large breasts

scars from
harvesting
of long
saphenous vein
used for CABG

scar from
harvesting of
radial artery
used for CABG

Fig. 2.1 Common scars related to cardiac surgery. Note that a larger left lateral thoracotomy is used for correction of coarctation and patent ductus arteriosus. CABG, coronary artery bypass grafting; ICD, implantable cardioverter defibrillator.

Look at the patient's surroundings:

- Are there intravenous infusions? If so look at what they contain – high-dose intravenous antibiotics may suggest infective endocarditis.
- Is the patient on oxygen? This suggests heart failure or lung disease.
- Are there any diabetic drinks or food? Diabetics have a high incidence of ischaemic heart disease.
- Is there a GTN spray (often a small red bottle) at the bedside?

All this can be done very rapidly – it tends to irritate examiners if you spend more than about 15–30 s on observation.

EXAMINATION OF THE HANDS

Pick up the patient's right hand gently (alternatively you can ask the patient to lift both hands and look at them one after the other so avoiding the risk of causing any pain). Look for the following:

- Cold peripheries (capillary refill time should be <2 s and gives a good immediate idea of the patient's haemodynamic status.

Fig. 2.2 Common causes of finger clubbing	
System involved	**Pathology**
Respiratory	Carcinoma of the lung (especially squamous cell), suppurative lung conditions (e.g. lung abscess, empyema, bronchiectasis), fibrosing alveolitis
Cardiovascular	Cyanotic heart disease, infective endocarditis (takes several weeks for clubbing to develop)
Gastrointestinal	Inflammatory bowel disease, cirrhosis

- Peripheral cyanosis – suggests peripheral vascular disease or poor cardiac output.
- Nail changes, such as clubbing (Fig. 2.2), splinter haemorrhages or tar staining.
- Janeway lesions on the finger pulps and Osler nodes on the palm of the hand – these suggest infective endocarditis.
- Tendon xanthomata suggest hypercholesterolaemia.

EXAMINATION OF THE PULSE

After examining the pulse you should be able to comment on four things: rate, rhythm, character and volume.

Feel for the radial pulse and time it against your watch for 15–30 s. At the same time, make a mental note of whether it is:

- Regular and sinus rhythm or atrial flutter/re-entry tachycardia if rapid – note that atrial flutter may be slow.
- Irregularly irregular – atrial fibrillation or ventricular ectopic beats.
- Regularly irregular – Wenckebach heart block gives this rhythm because the PR interval progressively lengthens and finally a beat is dropped. You are very unlikely to be asked to diagnose Wenckebach rhythm by feeling the pulse.

HINTS AND TIPS

Don't be confused by occasional ectopic beats that make the pulse seem irregularly irregular for a short time. In these patients it is important to feel the pulse for at least 15 s, and ideally up to a minute, to discover if the basic rhythm is sinus.

Fig. 2.3 Different types of pulse. The first peak of the bisferiens pulse is caused by left-ventricular contraction (the percussion wave); the second peak is the tidal wave due to recoil of the vascular bed. AR, aortic regurgitation; AS, aortic stenosis; HCM, hypertrophic cardiomyopathy.

The character of the pulse is usually best assessed at the carotid pulse, but you may notice a slow rising pulse at the radial pulse (Fig. 2.3).

A collapsing pulse can usually be felt by gently lifting the patient's arm and feeling the pulse with the fingers laid across it. The impulse is felt as it hits the examiner's finger and then rapidly declines.

HINTS AND TIPS

A collapsing (waterhammer) pulse is felt when a strong impulse hits the examiner's fingers and then drops away, rather than the common misconception of there being no pulse felt at all when the patient's arm is lifted up.

The volume of the pulse will give you some idea as to the patient's haemodynamic status; patients who are hypotensive are likely to have a weak pulse.

Finally, check briefly for radio-radial delay by feeling both radial pulses together. This may result from coarctation of the aorta (proximal to the left subclavian artery) or unilateral subclavian artery stenosis. You should then feel for radio-femoral delay.

TAKING THE BLOOD PRESSURE

Always ask whether you can take the blood pressure yourself and be sure that you know how to do this properly using a manual sphygmomanometer.

Strictly speaking, the blood pressure should be measured in both arms, but examiners will probably not ask you to do this unless it is likely to be abnormal (suggesting coarctation of the aorta).

HINTS AND TIPS

Postural hypotension describes a drop in blood pressure in a person who has been standing for more than 2 min of more than 20 mmHg compared with when he or she is lying down. Pulsus paradoxus describes an exaggeration of the normal (not actually a paradox) blood pressure on inspiration (>10 mmHg less than on expiration) – causes are cardiac tamponade, constrictive pericarditis and severe asthma.

EXAMINATION OF THE FACE

Keep this brief because you should have observed the face earlier.

Additional information can be obtained by looking at the conjunctivae. The presence of conjunctival haemorrhages suggests infective endocarditis; the presence of conjunctival pallor suggests anaemia.

Look briefly in the mouth for:

- Tar staining of the teeth – seen in heavy smokers.
- Central cyanosis.

EXAMINATION OF THE JUGULAR VENOUS PRESSURE

This is sometimes difficult, so make things easier by ensuring the patient is in the correct position (at 45° with the head supported and the neck muscles relaxed). It is often easier to find the JVP by looking across the patient rather than directly at them: get them to turn their head to the right and look at their left JVP.

The internal jugular vein is used because it has no valves and is not subject to as much muscular compression as the external jugular vein. The JVP gives an indication of the right atrial pressure (Fig. 2.4). The normal JVP is less than 3 cm H_2O (measured as the vertical distance above the angle of Louis or the sternal angle). This rests at the level of the clavicle so the normal JVP waveform is not usually visible or, if it is seen, the pulsation is just above the clavicle. It can be visualized by lying the patient flat. If the JVP is significantly raised, it may be necessary to sit the patient more upright to quantify the JVP e.g. +6 cm with the patient lying at 60°. In sinus rhythm, there are two waves:

1. The 'a' wave just preceding the carotid pulse – this is absent in atrial asystole and AF.
2. The 'v' wave, which occurs in late ventricular systole.

Occasional 'cannon' waves are seen in heart block when the right atrium contracts against a closed tricuspid valve. In AV nodal re-entrant tachycardia (AVNRT) there may be regular cannon waves with each beat. In tricuspid regurgitation prominent 'cV' (or 'giant v') waves may be seen (which are unobstructed waves from the ventricle and coincide with the carotid pulse).

The differences between the JVP and carotid pulse are highlighted in Fig. 2.5.

HINTS AND TIPS

When you examine the JVP, look for two positive waves (a and v). These can be distinguished by feeling the carotid pulse on the opposite side – the v wave occurs after the carotid upstroke.

Kussmaul sign

Normally, the JVP falls with inspiration because the pressure in the thoracic cavity is negative. In constrictive pericarditis or cardiac tamponade the JVP increases with inspiration; this is known as Kussmaul sign.

EXAMINATION OF THE PRAECORDIUM

Inspection

Although previously observed from the end of the bed, it is worthwhile taking a few seconds to examine the chest closely, particularly with relevance to scars.

HINTS AND TIPS

When you see a midline sternotomy scar, ALWAYS look at the legs and arms for vein harvesting sites. If you don't see any, it is much more likely that you will hear an artificial valve on auscultation.

Palpation

The following sequence of palpation should be observed:

• Palpate the apex beat, defined as the lowest and most lateral point at which the cardiac impulse can be felt. Always start palpating in the axilla and move anteriorly until you feel the apex beat. If you start palpating anteriorly it is possible to miss a grossly displaced apex. Define the character of the apex beat (Fig. 2.6). If you can't feel it, make sure it isn't on the other side (dextrocardia)!

• Palpate the left lower sternal edge to feel for a right ventricular heave (a sign of pulmonary hypertension or pulmonary stenosis) – use the flat of the hand pressing firmly to feel this.

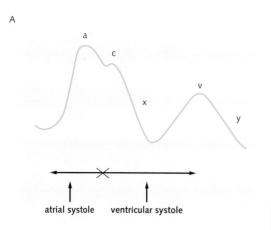

A

atrial systole   ventricular systole

Fig. 2.4B	Causes of the waves and descents in the JVP
Wave or descent	**Cause**
a wave	Right atrial systole, which results in venous distension
c wave	Increasing right ventricular pressure just before the tricuspid valve closes producing an interruption in the x descent
x descent	Atrial relaxation and pulling down of the base of the atrium caused by right ventricular contraction
v wave	Right atrial filling during right ventricular systole
y descent	Fall in right atrial pressure as the tricuspid valve opens

Fig. 2.4 (A) Jugular venous pressure (JVP) waveform. (B) Causes of the waves and descents in the JVP.

Fig. 2.5 Differences between the jugular venous pressure (JVP) and carotid pulse

Feature	JVP	Carotid pulse
Character of pulse	Double pulsation: a wave occurs at end of diastole, v wave in late systole	Single systolic pulse
Potential for obliteration	Can be obliterated by pressing on vein just above the clavicle	Cannot be obliterated
Effect of position	If the patient sits upright it falls	No effect
Effect of pressure on the liver or abdomen	Rises (the hepatojugular reflex)	No effect
Palpable pulsation	Usually not palpable (but may be with pulmonary hypertension and severe TR)	Palpable

Fig. 2.6 Causes of different types of apex beat

Character	Causes
Tapping	Mitral stenosis
Thrusting	Mitral regurgitation, aortic regurgitation
Heaving	Aortic stenosis
Diffuse (the normal apex beat should be discrete and localized to an area no bigger than a 10-pence piece)	Left ventricular failure, cardiomyopathy, pericardial effusion
Double	Hypertrophic obstructive cardiomyopathy, left ventricular aneurysm
Impalpable	Adiposity, emphysema

- Palpate the second left intercostal space where a palpable pulmonary component of the second heart sound (P_2) may be felt (a sign of pulmonary hypertension). This is felt with the fingertips.
- Palpate the second right intercostal space where a palpable thrill of aortic stenosis may be felt – this is also felt with the fingertips.

Auscultation

When listening to the heart every murmur should be systematically excluded. You should at all times be able to explain exactly which sounds you are expecting to hear at any stage during auscultation.

Learn a systematic approach, not necessarily the one described in this chapter, but always listen to the heart in the same way.

The order for auscultation is as follows:

- Using the diaphragm of the stethoscope listen quickly at the mitral, tricuspid, pulmonary and aortic areas in that order – you should already know where these are; if not then learn it now (Fig. 2.7). This enables you to hear any loud murmurs and possibly begin to approach the diagnosis.
- Listen at the apex: first with the bell of the stethoscope to hear any extra heart sounds (i.e. third and fourth heart sounds); listen for mid-diastolic murmur of mitral stenosis by asking the patient to lie on his or her left side and breathe out fully. Again the bell of the stethoscope should be used for this. Listen for the pansystolic murmur of mitral regurgitation at the apex with the diaphragm of the stethoscope. If this is heard listen at the axilla for radiation of the murmur. In some cases, where the regurgitant jet of blood is directed anteriorly, the murmur may be best heard at the left sternal edge.
- Listen at the pulmonary area – using the diaphragm to hear a pulmonary flow murmur and loud P_2 if present. Both are accentuated in inspiration. Splitting of the second heart sound ($S2 – A_2P_2$) is best heard in the pulmonary area. Normally the aortic and pulmonary components of S2 will split in deep inspiration ($A_2 P_2$ – more blood is sucked into the right ventricle, which delays closure of the pulmonary valve). In certain circumstances (LBBB, severe AS) aortic valve closure is late, occuring after that of the pulmonary valve (P_2A_2), and deep inspiration instead brings the two together. This is called paradoxical (or reverse) splitting. This effect is overwhelmed where there is flow between the two atria (a shunt), leading to the fixed wide splitting heard with an atrial septal defect.
- Listen in the aortic area for the ejection systolic murmur of aortic stenosis using the diaphragm. This murmur is usually loud, but if there is any doubt ask the patient to exhale, because left-sided murmurs are loudest in expiration. Take this opportunity to listen over the carotid arteries for radiation of an aortic stenotic murmur if one is present or for evidence

Fig. 2.7 Sequence of auscultation of the heart. AR, aortic regurgitation; AS, aortic stenosis; ICS, intercostal space; MR, mitral regurgitation; MS, mitral stenosis; TR, tricuspid regurgitation.

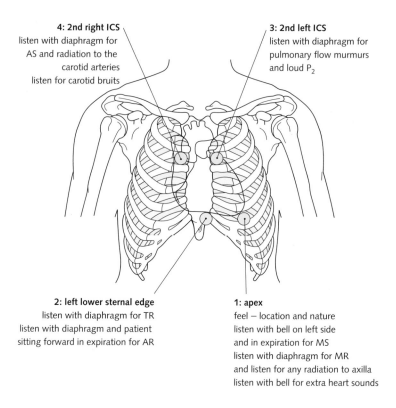

4: 2nd right ICS
listen with diaphragm for AS and radiation to the carotid arteries
listen for carotid bruits

3: 2nd left ICS
listen with diaphragm for pulmonary flow murmurs and loud P_2

2: left lower sternal edge
listen with diaphragm for TR
listen with diaphragm and patient sitting forward in expiration for AR

1: apex
feel – location and nature
listen with bell on left side and in expiration for MS
listen with diaphragm for MR and listen for any radiation to axilla
listen with bell for extra heart sounds

of carotid artery stenosis. In some cases (particularly in the elderly) the ejection systolic murmur of AS may be best heard at the lower left sternal edge or even the apex – assessing the character of any murmur is vital!

- Finally, listen over the tricuspid area for a pansystolic murmur of tricuspid regurgitation. Then ask the patient to sit forward and listen in expiration for the murmur of aortic regurgitation (this murmur is often soft and requires accentuation by asking the patient to exhale). Both murmurs are heard best with the diaphragm of the stethoscope.

HINTS AND TIPS

You cannot say that mitral stenosis has been excluded unless you have listened with the bell of the stethoscope at the apex with the patient lying on his or her left side in full expiration.

HINTS AND TIPS

Knowing when systole and diastole are is fundamental. Know this at all times during auscultation by keeping a finger or thumb on the carotid pulse.

HINTS AND TIPS

Holding breath in fixed expiration exaggerates left-sided murmurs whereas holding breath in fixed inspiration exaggerates right-sided murmurs.

FINISHING OFF THE EXAMINATION

The rest of the examination must be completed efficiently and thoroughly with just as much care as the first part of the cardiovascular examination. The aim of this part of the examination is to look for signs of cardiac failure and for any peripheral signs to confirm the diagnosis, which by now you may suspect:

- At this stage the patient is sitting forwards so start with auscultation of the lung bases. Listen for fine end-inspiratory crepitations and assess how far up the chest these extend (an evaluation of the severity of pulmonary oedema).
- Pleural effusions occur in heart failure and are detected by finding dullness to percussion at one or both lung bases.
- With the patient still sitting forwards check for sacral oedema by gently pressing over the sacrum. Then ask the patient to sit back against the pillows.

- Look for ankle oedema, again very gently, and assess how far up the leg the oedema extends (a guide to its severity). Remember oedema is often tender.

At this stage, in the short cases, it is reasonable to step back and conclude verbally by stating that you would like to go on to do the following:

- Examine the abdomen for ascites and hepatomegaly (signs of congestive cardiac failure) and for an abdominal aortic aneurysm (an expansile mass).
- Examine all peripheral pulses by palpation and listen for bruits to look for evidence of peripheral vascular disease.
- Examine the fundi.
- Look at the temperature chart for all patients who have a valve lesion to look for a fever, which may be due to infective endocarditis.
- Dipstick the patient's urine – haematuria is a very sensitive test for infective endocarditis and proteinuria is associated with renal disease.

If you suspect that the patient has coarctation of the aorta then it is mandatory to examine the peripheral pulses and look for radio-femoral delay as part of the examination, and not just to say you would like to do it at the end.

It can be seen, therefore, that the conclusion of the examination depends upon what you think the diagnosis might be. If in doubt, do the complete cardiovascular examination until you are told to stop.

When you are not in the short-case situation (i.e. if you are clerking a patient 'for real' or in the long-case section of finals), always complete the whole examination.

COMMUNICATION

Always remember to thank the patient when you have finished examining them.

PRESENTING YOUR FINDINGS

As with history taking, it is extremely important that you can communicate your examination findings (including relevant negatives) effectively. For example, 'On examination of Mr Y's cardiovascular system his JVP was raised at 6 cm. This was associated with bibasal crepitations and pitting oedema up to the knees. The first and second heart sounds were normal but I did not hear a third heart sound or any murmurs. My findings would be consistent with a diagnosis of congestive cardiac failure.

How to write a clerking

Objectives

By the end of this chapter you should:
- Understand the importance of clear and accurate note keeping.
- Understand that all entries in the notes should be labelled with the date, time, your name and your grade.
- Have a framework for writing the clerking into the medical notes.

There is no single correct way to write a medical clerking, but there are several incorrect ways! Most hospitals have their own clerking forms. Irrespective of whether you are using one of these or simply a continuation sheet in the notes, remember that doctors, nurses, physiotherapists and many other health professionals use the medical notes during the course of a patient's medical care. The notes need to last for years and your entries in them may provide valuable information to doctors looking after the patient in several years' time. It is also worth remembering that the medical notes are legal documents that might one day be used as evidence in a court of law.

The basic principles when making entries into the notes are as follows:

- Always write legibly – this sounds obvious, but notes are often illegible. Remember, if no one else can read your entry you might as well not write anything.
- A date and time should precede every entry, no matter how brief. At the end of the entry you should sign your name and, if your signature does not clearly show your name, your surname and initials should be written in capitals below it. There are no exceptions to this rule ever!
- Always be courteous to your patients and colleagues when writing in the notes. Rude or angry entries may give a certain degree of satisfaction when they are made, but serve only to make you look unprofessional when read at a later date.
- Write everything down – every time you see a patient an entry should be made in the notes, stating accurately the content and outcome of the consultation. This may sometimes seem pedantic, but most qualified doctors will be able to recall situations when careful documentation resolved a difficult situation.

DOCUMENTATION OF THE HISTORY

The history should always have the following information at the top of the first page:

- Name of patient in full plus at least one other unique identifier (e.g. date of birth or hospital number) – loose sheets often fall out of the notes so all pages of the history should have this information so they are not replaced in the notes of another patient who has the same name.
- Date and time of entry.
- Route of admission – if the patient is being admitted to hospital it is useful to state the route by which the admission came about (i.e. via general practitioner or accident and emergency).

The history should be documented under these main headings:

- Presenting complaint (PC).
- History of presenting complaint (HPC).
- Systems review (SR).
- Past medical history (PMH).
- Family history (FH).
- Social history (SH).
- Drug history (DH).
- Allergies.

Systems review

A full systems review of the other organ systems should be entered here (Fig. 3.1). It is not necessary to document negatives unless they are particularly relevant.

Once you have memorized the questions they will become second nature and the systems review will be very quick to do. It is worth the initial time-consuming

Fig. 3.1 Important questions to ask on systems review

System	Symptoms and signs to ask about
Cardiovascular (CVS)	Chest pain, shortness of breath, orthopnoea, paroxysmal nocturnal dyspnoea, ankle oedema, palpitations, syncope
Respiratory (RS)	Cough, sputum, haemoptysis, shortness of breath, wheeze
Gastrointestinal (GIT)	Appetite, vomiting, haematemesis, weight loss, indigestion, abdominal pain, change in bowel habit, description and frequency of stools, blood and/or mucus per rectum
Genitourinary (GUS)	Frequency, dysuria, hesitancy, urgency, poor stream, terminal dribbling, impotence, haematuria, menstrual cycle, menorrhagia, oligomenorrhoea, dyspareunia
Neurological (CNS)	Headache, photophobia, neck stiffness, visual problems, any other focal symptoms (e.g. weakness, numbness; don't forget olfactory problems), tremor, memory, loss of consciousness
Other	For example muscle pain, joint pain, rashes, depression

effort to do this properly; after all, you will be taking histories for the rest of your career.

Risk calculation

With certain presentations it is helpful to calculate relevant risk scores. A person presenting with cardiac-sounding chest pain would have a TIMI score calculated and a person with a possible diagnosis of PE should have their Wells score calculated.

DOCUMENTATION OF THE EXAMINATION FINDINGS

Writing a clear and logical clerking will help you to organize your thoughts in order to formulate a differential diagnosis and plan for further investigations and management. Leave yourself plenty of room as trying to fit things into a certain space may interfere with this.

There are many ways of documenting the findings on examination and it does not really matter how you do this provided a few rules are obeyed:

- The patient's name and another unique identifier are written on every sheet of paper – this should come as second nature to you.
- Any positive findings are represented in writing – diagrams can be used to aid the description, but should never be used alone to document findings because they are likely to be interpreted differently by different people (Fig. 3.2).

An example of how to write down examination findings is detailed in the sample clerking at the end of this chapter.

AT THE END OF THE CLERKING

The last section is important because it brings together all the information from the clerking. The following should be seen at the end of every clerking:

- A statement summarising the patient's presentation, e.g. 'A 78-year-old female admitted with a 'funny turn'. Denies chest pain or loss of consciousness'.

A   B   fine, end-inspiratory bilateral basal crepitations

Fig. 3.2 Potential confusion caused by lack of annotation. (A) This diagram is usually used to represent bilateral basal crepitations secondary to pulmonary oedema. However, the same diagram can be used to represent coarse inspiratory crepitations due to bronchiectasis. (B) This diagram is unequivocal and confirms the finding of pulmonary oedema.

- An 'impression' and a list of differential diagnoses – with the most likely at the top of the list.
- A list of differential diagnoses with the most likely diagnosis at the top of the list.
- A list of investigations performed and to be performed – it is good practice to tick those tests that have been done already.
- A plan of action including initial drugs to be given, any intravenous fluids, physiotherapy, specific observations needed (e.g. fluid balance chart or daily weights) and any consultant referrals to be made.

This reads like a long list, but you do not need to learn it. The only thing you need to remember is that if you do something that concerns a patient then write it down.

Further reading

Antman, E.M., Cohen, M., Bernink, P.J., et al., 2000. The TIMI risk score for unstable angina/non-ST elevation MI: A method for prognostication and therapeutic decision making. JAMA 284, 835–842.

Wells, P.S., Anderson, D.R., Rodger, M., et al., 2001. Excluding pulmonary embolism at the bedside without diagnostic imaging: management of patients with suspected pulmonary embolism presenting to the emergency department by using a simple clinical model and d-dimer. Ann. Intern. Med. 135, 98–107.

SAMPLE MEDICAL CLERKING

Hospital No: X349182

BLOGGS, Joe

11/06/35

20/06/05 19:30   63 yr old man   Referred by GP — seen in GOPD

PC   Shortness of breath

> 1. Presenting complaint should be brief, but it is necessary to include duration of symptoms.

HPC   Gradual onset of shortness of breath approximately
                6 months ago. Initially only on exertion, but
                breathlessness has deteriorated and now patient
                is breathless on minimal exertion
                (e.g. when dressing in the morning)

> 2. Mention only the relevant negatives. In this case it is important to mention the absence of haemoptysis and weight loss because of the history of cancer. It is always wise to document whether or not there is chest pain.

Associated features

                Orthopnoea
                Ankle swelling
                Cough with clear sputum and occasional flecks of blood
                Palpitations - feels heart beating rapidly and irregularly
                from time to time
                No chest pain
                No known risk factors for coronary heart disease
                NB patient unaware of his cholesterol level

Systems review

GIT: Recent loss of appetite
                No weight loss or vomiting
                No abdominal pain
                No change in bowel habit
CNS: No abnormalities on questioning
EMS: No abnormalities on questioning

PMH   Rheumatic fever when 10 years old
                Cholecystectomy 1989, no complications

DH   frusemide 40mg mane -
                started by GP last week

> 3. Always record the dose and frequency of any drugs.

Allergies   None known Smoking - never smoked
                              Alcohol - approx 10 units/week

Fam Hx   Mother died aged 68 - stroke   SHx   Married with 2 children
                Father still alive - hypertensive   (family fit and well)
                                                                Retired accountant

O/E Looks short of breath at rest.
Temperature 36.5°C
No central or peripheral cyanosis

> 4. Record your initial observations — they are important. 'Alert and chatty' or 'Distressed and looks unwell' tell you a lot about the patient.

CVS Pulse 80, regular
BP 120/80 mmHg
JVP - elevated 6cm
Ankle oedema to knees
Apex not displaced
Soft low-pitched mid-diastolic murmer at apex

Hs $\quad$ P2 $\quad$ S1 $\quad$ S2 $\quad$ S1

> 5. Always use diagrams to clarify your examination findings.

Loud P₂ Marked right ventricular heave

RS: Respiratory rate 30 breaths/min
Percussion and expansion normal
Fine inspiratory bilateral basal crepitations
to mid-zones

GIT: 2cm hepatomegaly

Ascites detected
No palpable kidneys or spleen
PR not performed

CNS: No abnormalities detected on full
neurological examination

> 6. If there is no abnormality of the CNS, simply include a one-line summary.

Summary Progressive dyspnoea in a man who has
a history of rheumatic fever and
clinical signs of mitral stenosis

Impression Pulmonary oedema and congestive heart failure
secondary to rheumatic mitral stenosis

Differential
diagnosis Mitral stenosis of another aitiology
Paroxysmal atrial fibrillation leading to
congestive heart failure

Investigations Blood tests: FBC, V+E, LFT, TFT
Chest radiography
ECG and 24-hour ECG to rule out
paroxysmal atrial fibrilation
Echocardiography

> 7. Always include a management plan— even when you are still a student. It might not be right but you need to start training yourself to think like a doctor.

Plan intravenous diuretics, initially Frusemide
80mg b.d.
Daily V&E to check effect of diuretics on
electrolytes and renal function
Daily weights and fluid input and output chart
Fluid restriction to 1500ml/24 hours
Referral to consultant cardiologist

Al-Obaidi FY1, #4370

> 8. Sign your notes, including printed surname, grade and bleep number.

Objectives

By the end of this chapter you should:
- Understand how to perform an electrocardiogram (ECG).
- Understand the role of non-invasive investigations in the investigation of patients with suspected cardiovascular disease.
- Understand the role of cardiac catheterization in the investigation of coronary artery disease, and assessment of ventricular and valvular function.

ELECTROCARDIOGRAPHY

This investigation records the electrical activity of the heart.

Lead placement

You will be expected to be able to position the electrodes correctly (Fig. 4.1) and perform an ECG by yourself, so be sure to learn this before finals.

Limb leads

There are four limb leads, one attached to each extremity. Many people use the mnemonic 'Ride your green bike', moving clockwise from the patient's right hand, to remember the correct placement (see Fig. 4.1).

HINTS AND TIPS

Remember the limb leads like this:
1. Right arm (RA) 'Ride' = Red
2. Left arm (LA) 'Your' = Yellow
3. Left foot (LF) 'Green' = Green
4. Right foot (RF) 'Bike' = Black

Chest leads

There are six chest leads:

1. V1 – fourth right intercostal space.
2. V2 – fourth left intercostal space.
3. V3 – between V2 and V4.
4. V4 – cardiac apex – you need to feel for it before placing the lead.
5. V5 – anterior axillary line at same level as V4.
6. V6 – mid-axillary line at same level.

12-lead electrocardiogram

The standard 12-lead ECG is derived from information given by the 10 ECG electrodes placed on the patient. It is important to know how this information is obtained when interpreting ECG findings and also when the lead positioning is incorrect.

Leads I, II and III

These are bipolar leads and were first used by Einthoven. They record the differences in potential between pairs of limb leads:

- I records the difference in potential between LA and RA.
- II records the difference in potential between LF and RA.
- III records the difference in potential between LF and LA.

These three leads form Einthoven's triangle (Fig. 4.2).

AVR, AVL and AVF

With regard to these leads:

- The letter V indicates that the lead is unipolar.
- The information is obtained by connecting the electrode to a central point, which is said to have zero voltage (the reference electrode).
- AVR records the difference between RA and zero.
- AVL records the difference between LA and zero.
- AVF records the difference between LF and zero.

Chest leads

The chest leads:

- Are the precordial leads V1 to V6 and are unipolar (as seen by the prefix V).
- They each record the difference between the voltage at their location and zero.

Common investigations

Fig. 4.1 Lead positions for electrocardiography. LA, left arm; LF, left foot; RA, right arm; RF, right foot.

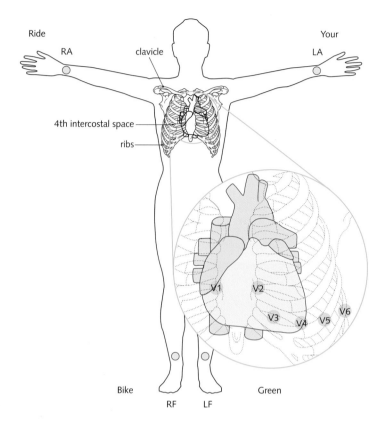

Ride

Your

RA

clavicle

LA

4th intercostal space

ribs

V1 V2
V3 V4 V5 V6

Bike

Green

RF LF

QRS axis

The normal axis is between −30° and +90° (Fig. 4.3).

The most accurate way to calculate the axis is shown in (Fig. 4.4). With a little practice, you can estimate the angle in your head, without the need for pen and paper.

Causes of right and left axis deviation are given in Fig. 4.5.

> **HINTS AND TIPS**
>
> A simple way to estimate the axis very roughly is:
> - The normal axis is in the same direction as I and II; therefore, both should be positive.
> - In right axis deviation the axis swings to the right and lead I becomes negative and III more positive.
> - In left axis deviation the axis swings to the left so lead III and lead II become negative and lead I remains positive.

Paper speed

The standard ECG paper speed is 25 mm/s:
- One large square (5 mm) is 0.2 s.
- One small square (1 mm) is 0.04 s.

Fig. 4.2 Leads I, II and III. (A) Lead I is 0° to the horizontal, II is +60° to the horizontal and lead III is +120° to the horizontal – Einthoven's triangle. (B) Leads I, II and III are often drawn as shown here.

24

Fig. 4.3 Hexaxial reference system.

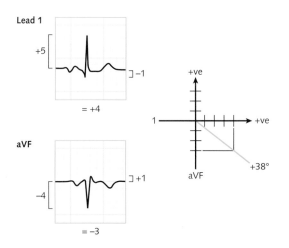

Fig. 4.4 Calculation of the axis. The net positive displacement of the QRS in leads I and aVF is measured (A) and plotted on a graph (B). The angle (θ) subtended by a line between this point and the origin is equal to the mean QRS axis. Note that positive displacement in aVF is plotted **down** the y-axis.

Fig. 4.5	Causes of right and left axis deviation
Left axis deviation	LBBB, left anterior hemiblock, LVH, septum primum ASD
Right axis deviation	RBBB, RVH, cor pulmonale, septum secundum ASD

ASD, atrial septal defect; LBBB, left bundle branch block; LVH, left ventricular hypertrophy; RBBB, right bundle branch block; RVH, right ventricular hypertrophy.

The rate is calculated by counting the number of large squares between each QRS and dividing into 300 (e.g. if there are five large squares the rate is 60 beats/min).

P wave

The P wave represents atrial depolarization, which originates in the SA node on the right atrium and spreads across the right and then the left atrium.

The amplitude of the P wave should be less than two small squares (0.2 mv) and the width should be less than three small squares (0.12 s). A tall P wave is a feature of right atrial enlargement whereas left atrial enlargement is associated with broad and often bifid P waves.

The PR interval represents the time taken for conduction of the impulse to pass through the AV node and bundle of His. This is normally no greater than five small squares (0.2 s).

QRS complex

The QRS represents the depolarization of the ventricles, which begins at the septum. The septum is depolarized from left to right, and the left and right ventricles are then depolarized. The left ventricle has a larger muscle mass and, therefore, more current flows across it. The left ventricle, therefore, exerts more influence on the ECG pattern than the right.

The maximum normal duration of the QRS is 0.12 s (three small squares) and the QRS is abnormally wide in bundle branch block (left and right bundle branch block, Ch. 00). It is also wide when the ventricles are paced (Fig. 4.6).

Fig. 4.6 Ventricular pacing. The sharp spikes are the artificial stimuli from the pacemaker. Each is followed by a wide QRS complex indicating the left-ventricular response. Whenever the impulse is generated in one ventricle, because of either a pacing wire or a ventricular ectopic focus, the QRS is widened. This mimics the electrical disturbances seen in bundle branch block, because the two ventricles are not depolarized in the normal sequence.

ST segment

This segment is normally isoelectric (i.e. it shows no deflection from the baseline).

T wave

The T wave represents ventricular repolarization. Normally the only leads that show negative T waves are AVR and V1; the rest are positive. (A negative QRS should, however, be accompanied by a negative T wave.) Certain T wave abnormalities suggest particular non-cardiac disorders (Fig. 4.7).

QT interval

The QT interval extends from the beginning of the QRS complex to the end of the T wave and, therefore, represents time from depolarization to repolarization of the ventricles (i.e. the action potential duration).

The duration of the QT interval is dependent upon cycle length and the corrected QT interval (QTc) is normalized according to heart rate (QTc = QT/square root of the RR interval in seconds). The upper limit of normal is 0.40 s in women and 0.44 s in men.

Q waves

A Q wave is a negative deflection at the beginning of the ventricular depolarization. Small, non-significant Q waves are often seen in the left-sided leads due to the depolarization of the septum from left to right. Significant (pathological) Q waves:

- Are more than 0.04 s (one small square) in duration and more than 25% of the following R wave in depth.

Fig. 4.7 Electrocardiographic abnormalities in non-cardiac disease

Cause	ECG abnormalities
Hypothermia	J waves, baseline shiver artefact, bradycardia; watch out for arrhythmias as the patient is warmed up
Hyperkalaemia	Tall peaked T waves, small P wave, gradual widening of the QRS, if serum potassium very high – ventricular fibrillation
Hypokalaemia	Decreased T wave amplitude. Long QT interval, U waves
Hypocalcaemia	Long QT interval, U waves
Hypercalcaemia	Short QT interval, ST segment depression
Digoxin	Downsloping ST segment (reverse tick shape), T wave inversion
Digoxin toxicity	AV block, atrial tachycardia with block, ventricular arrhythmias

AV, atrioventricular.

- Occur after transmural myocardial infarction (MI) where the myocardium on one side of the heart dies. This myocardium has no electrical activity and, therefore, the leads facing it are able to pick up the electrical activity from the opposite side of the heart. (The myocardium depolarizes from the inside out; therefore, the opposite side of the heart depolarizes away from these leads, resulting in a negative deflection or Q wave.)

- May also occur in patients with hypertrophic cardio-myopathy (HCM) due to depolarisation of the thickened septum. This may lead to an erroneous diagnosis of previous MI.

U wave

This is an abnormal wave in some patients, but can appear in the chest leads of normal ECGs. It is an upright wave that appears after the T wave (Fig. 4.8); causes include:

- Hypokalaemia.
- Hypocalcaemia.

Reporting an electrocardiogram

You will often be asked to comment on an ECG and it is difficult to remember to include everything. This exercise should be treated like the history or the examination in that you should always follow a strict routine. After a short time this will become second nature to you.

The order of examination of an ECG is as follows:

- Name of the patient and date of the ECG.
- Rate (i.e. the number of large squares between the QRS complexes divided into 300).
- Rhythm (e.g. regular, irregular or irregularly irregular).
- Look at each part of the complex-P waves, PR interval, QRS complexes and QRS duration, ST segment

and T waves – comment on these either out loud when you are starting to do this or in your head when you are more experienced, and comment on any abnormalities.

If there are abnormalities look to see whether they are global or territorial. Remember the territories:

- Anterior – V1–V4.
- Inferior – II, III and AVF.
- Lateral – I, AVL, V4–V6.

Exercise electrocardiography

This investigation is important in the management of ischaemic heart disease. In addition it provides prognostic information.

Fig. 4.8 U waves, J waves and ST segment depression.

Indications for exercise testing

Current NICE guidelines do not recommend exercise testing for the evaluation of recent onset chest pain (see discussion in Ch. 5), which was formerly the most common use of this investigation. Indications now are:

- After MI to evaluate prognosis and the need for further investigation or treatment.
- After MI to aid rehabilitation – this gives the patient and doctor an idea of exercise capabilities.
- To detect exercise-induced arrhythmias – the increased catecholamine levels and metabolic acidosis caused by exercise potentiate arrhythmias in those patients vulnerable to this. This gives an indication of prognosis and whether treatment is required or not.
- DVLA requirements, e.g. for holders of an HGV licence.
- Risk assessment in hypertrophic cardiomyopathy.

Methods of exercise

The aim of the exercise test is to stress the cardiovascular system, hence it is often referred to as an exercise stress test (EST) or exercise tolerance test (ETT). All exercise protocols have a warm-up period, a period of exercise with increasing grades of intensity and a cool-down period.

The best method is treadmill exercise. Other methods, such as bicycle testing, are often less effective because many patients are not used to the cycling action and, therefore leg fatigue may set in before cardiovascular fatigue, resulting in early termination of the test. However, bicycle testing has the advantage that the workload can be controlled and recorded in watts.

The Bruce protocol is often used in conjunction with treadmill testing. This involves 3-min stages starting with 3 min at a speed of 1.7 miles/h and a slope of 10°. Subsequent stages are at incrementally higher speeds and steeper gradients. The final stage (stage 6) is at a rate of 5.5 miles/h and a gradient of 20°.

The modified Bruce protocol is sometimes used for patients likely to have poor exercise tolerance. An additional two stages are added to the beginning of the standard Bruce protocol. Again they are 3 min in duration and at a speed of 1.7 miles/h, but the gradient starts at 0° and increases to 5° in the first and second stage, respectively.

Patient preparation

The following should be completed before testing:

- All patients should have been seen and examined by a physician to ensure there are no contraindications to testing (see below).
- The test and its indications and risks should have been fully explained to the patient.

Certain patients are advised to stop all antihypertensive and antianginal medication before the test. The operator should be aware of patients still taking their medication (especially drugs affecting the heart rate such as β-blockers), because this affects the response to exercise.

Variables measured

12-lead electrocardiogram
The patient is fitted with the standard 12-lead ECG equipment. Poor electrode contact is avoided by shaving hair.

Blood pressure
Normal response to exercise involves an increase in blood pressure. An inadequate response or a fall in blood pressure with exercise indicates the likelihood of the following disorders:

- Coronary artery disease – the most common cause.
- Cardiomyopathy.
- Left-ventricular outflow tract obstruction.
- Hypotensive medication.

Heart rate response
Heart rate normally increases with exercise. If the increase is inadequate ischaemic heart disease or sinus node disease must be suspected (also ingestion of β-blockers and calcium channel antagonists).

An excessive increase in heart rate indicates reduced cardiac reserve as in left-ventricular failure (LVF) or anaemia.

These variables are measured before, during and after exercise. Measurements are stopped once all variables have returned to their pre-exercise levels.

Test end-points

The following are appropriate indications for terminating an exercise test:

- Attainment of maximal heart rate (maximal heart rate is 220 minus age in years; in a modified Bruce protocol the submaximal heart rate is used, which is 85% of maximal heart rate).
- Completion of all stages of the test with no untoward symptoms and without attaining maximum heart rate.

Premature termination of the exercise test is indicated if any of the following occur:

- Excessive dyspnoea or fatigue.
- Chest pain.
- Dizziness or faintness.
- Any form of arrhythmia.
- Failure of blood pressure to increase or an excessive increase in blood pressure (e.g. systolic 220 mmHg).
- Failure of heart rate to increase.
- ST segment depression greater than 1 mm.
- ST segment elevation.

Positive exercise test

The following are indications of a positive exercise test (i.e. highly suggestive of coronary artery disease):

- ST segment depression of more than 1 mm – this should occur in more than one lead and the ST segments should preferably not be upsloping (Fig. 4.9).
- ST segment elevation.
- Chest pain – provided that the pain has the characteristics of angina pain.
- Ventricular arrhythmias.
- Abnormal blood pressure response.

Causes of ST segment depression are listed in Fig. 4.10.

Contraindications to exercise testing

This list includes conditions in which additional stress on the heart may be very hazardous:

- Marked aortic stenosis – gradient greater than 50 mmHg with normal left-ventricular function.
- Acute pyrexial or flu-like illness.
- Cardiac failure.
- Unstable angina.
- Second- or third-degree atrioventricular block.
- Patients unable to walk effectively (e.g. due to severe arthritis or peripheral vascular disease).

Despite adhering to these rules, exercise testing does have a mortality rate of approximately 0.5–1/10 000.

In all cases there should be a defibrillator at hand and all the necessary equipment for advanced cardiopulmonary resuscitation.

Fig. 4.10   Causes of ST segment depression

Source	Pathology
Cardiac	Ischaemia, AS, LVH, intraventricular conduction defect (e.g. LBBB)
Non-cardiac	Hypokalaemia, digoxin, hypertension

AS, aortic stenosis; LBBB, left bundle branch block; LVH, left ventricular hypertrophy.

ECHOCARDIOGRAPHY

Echocardiography is the use of ultrasound to investigate the structure and function of the heart. The frequency of the ultrasound waves used is between 1 and 10 MHz (1 MHz = 1 000 000 Hz). The upper limit of audible sound is 20 kHz (1 kHz = 1000 Hz).

The ultrasound waves are generated by a piezoelectric element within the transducer. They travel through certain structures (e.g. blood) and are reflected off others (e.g. muscle and bone). The reflected waves are picked up by the transducer and, by knowing the time taken for the sound to return and the speed of the waves through the medium, the distance of the reflecting object from the transducer can be calculated.

By rapidly generating waves and detecting reflected waves a picture of the heart can be built up.

Fig. 4.9   Computer-averaged exercise ECG report showing ST depression after exercise (right-hand trace) compared with resting ECG (left-hand trace) in each of the ECG leads. There is a good tachycardia in response to exercise and the blood pressure rises to 166/84 mmHg. The ST depression is in the lateral leads V3–V6 and the inferior leads II, III and AVF. ETT, exercise tolerance test.

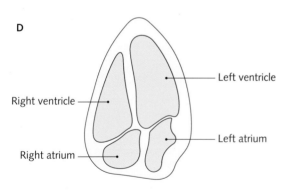

M mode echocardiography

The transducer is stationary and records only a single cut through the heart producing an image on a moving page. The result is the activity along that line seen changing with time. This accurate mode of echocardiography is useful for:

- Visualizing the movement of the mitral and aortic valve leaflets.
- Assessing left-ventricular dimensions and function.
- Assessing aortic root size.
- Assessing left atrial size.

Two-dimensional echocardiography

The ultrasound generator moves from side to side so a sector of the heart is visualized.

In the echocardiographic examination standard views of the heart are taken (Fig. 4.11) to provide information on:

- Valve structure and function.
- Left-ventricular contractility.
- Size of the chambers.
- Congenital cardiac malformations.
- Pericardial disease.

The inadequacies of this approach are:

- The presence of lung between the heart and chest wall precludes ultrasound travel – 'poor windows'.
- The posterior part of the heart is furthest from the transducer and may not be viewed adequately, particularly when searching for thrombi and vegetations.

Doppler echocardiography

This uses the principle of the Doppler effect to record blood flow within the heart and great vessels. The Doppler effect is the phenomenon where the change in frequency of ultrasound reflected off moving objects (e.g. blood cells) varies according to the speed and direction of movement. Colour Doppler echocardiography uses different colours, depending on the direction of blood flow, to enable the operator to assess both the speed and the direction of blood flow.

Doppler echocardiography is used for assessment of:

- Valve stenosis and regurgitation.

Fig. 4.11 Two-dimensional echocardiography. The top illustration (A) shows a long axis view of the heart taken from the left parasternal position with the transducer placed at the left sternal edge. Rotating the probe 90° gives the parasternal short axis view. (B) Shows the mitral valve (MV), looking like the mouth of a fish. Tilting the probe upwards from this point shows the three-pointed star of the aortic valve (C), and downwards shows the apex of the left ventricle. Placing the probe over the apex of the heart gives the apical four-chamber view (D). Tilting the probe anteriorly to include the left ventricular outflow tract and aortic valve gives a five-chamber view. IVS, interventricular septum; LA, left atrium; LV, left ventricle; RA, right atrium; RV, right ventricle.

- Atrial and ventricular septal defects, patent ductus arteriosus and other congenital anomalies.
- Pulmonary hypertension.

A relatively new modality called tissue Doppler imaging uses the same principles to assess the motion of the myocardium, rather than blood. This can give enhanced information about left ventricular systolic function and, in particular, diastolic relaxation of the heart.

Other echocardiography modalities

Three-dimensional (3D) echo can produce detailed anatomical recordings, which can then be manipulated in a similar way to MRI images. Real-time 3D echo can be used to guide intervention. Miniaturised echo probes can also be deployed through catheters, to produce intra-cardiac echo (ICE) images. These modalities will undoubtedly become more common in the future.

Transoesophageal echocardiography

Transoesophageal echocardiography (TOE) uses a flexible probe with a two-dimensional transducer incorporated into the tip. Images are obtained by introducing the transducer into the distal oesophagus. The advantage of TOE is that images are much clearer because the transducer is in close apposition to the heart. Because of this, TOE is the investigation of choice for assessment of:

- Intracardiac thrombus – transthoracic echocardiography (TTE) is unreliable.
- Prosthetic valve function – the planes used in TTE result in a great deal of artefact generated by the prosthesis.
- Valve vegetations.
- Congenital heart lesions (e.g. atrial and ventricular septal defects).

TOE imaging can be performed in multiple planes, whereas TTE is restricted to a few planes. TOE can also be used intraoperatively during cardiac surgery to provide information on valve function and left-ventricular function.

Stress echocardiography

When myocardium is ischaemic it contracts less strongly and efficiently.

The patient's heart is stressed with a drug such as dobutamine, which increases the rate and force of contraction and causes peripheral vasodilatation, so mimicking exercise. With a skilled operator echocardiography images are obtained before, during and after dobutamine and areas of ischaemia are seen as areas of regional wall motion abnormality, which recover at rest.

MYOCARDIAL PERFUSION IMAGING

This investigation uses radiolabelled agents, which are taken up by the myocardium proportional to local myocardial blood flow. It is more sensitive and specific than exercise testing alone, but much more expensive. A number of radiolabelled agents are used:

- Technetium-99m-labelled agents (e.g. ^{99m}T-sestamibi). ^{99m}T-sestamibi has a half-life of 6 h and is taken up by perfused myocardium. It remains in the myocardium for several hours and imaging of the heart provides an accurate picture of regional myocardial perfusion. Because of this phenomenon, resting and exercise images are obtained on two different days with an injection of ^{99m}T-sestamibi for each day.
- Thallium-201 is also taken up by the myocardium only in perfused areas. Unlike ^{99m}T-sestamibi, thallium is continually being passed across the cell membrane (i.e. it is extruded by one cell and taken up by another). This redistribution allows for early and late images to be taken after exercise using only a single injection. The image early after exercise (or drug stimulation) shows any areas of reduced uptake and the second image a few hours later will show whether these areas have normal uptake, suggesting the presence of reversible ischaemia.

Methods of stressing the heart

There are a number of ways to stress the heart. Wherever possible, physical exercise should be used, because this is actual physiological stress.

For those patients who are unable to exercise due to poor mobility, peripheral vascular disease, or respiratory disease, pharmacological stress may be used. (Patients who have severe aortic stenosis or cardiac failure should in general not have stress testing.)

The following are commonly used agents for pharmacological stress:

- Dipyridamole – this blocks the reabsorption of adenosine into the cells, so increasing intravascular adenosine concentrations. Adenosine is a powerful vasodilator and vasodilates normal coronary arteries, but not diseased coronary arteries. It, therefore, redistributes blood flow away from diseased vessels. This relative hypoperfusion of diseased areas is picked up by radionucleotide myocardial imaging.
- Adenosine – a direct infusion of adenosine may be used.
- Dobutamine – this drug mimics exercise by increasing myocardial rate and contractility.

Note that both dipyridimole and adenosine are contra-indicated in patients who have bronchospasm.

Myocardial perfusion imaging or stress echocardiography are useful in the following situations:

- If the exercise ECG is equivocal and confirmation of reversible ischaemia is required before coronary angiography.
- If the patient cannot perform an exercise ECG due to poor mobility – in this situation a perfusion scan is performed using drugs to stress the heart.
- In the UK, exercise ECG will be used less in future, as per recent NICE guidance.

Multigated acquisition scanning

Multigated acquisition (MUGA) scanning is a radionuclide technique for evaluating cardiac function.

Technetium-99 m label is used to label the patient's red blood cells.

The amount of radioactivity detected within the left ventricle is proportional to its volume and its degree of contraction during systole will affect this.

The imaging of the cardiac blood pool is synchronized to the ECG trace and each image is identified by its position within the cardiac cycle.

Hundreds of cycles are recorded and an overall assessment of the left-ventricular ejection fraction can be made using the averaged values for end-systolic and end-diastolic volume. This method is used less often than in the past, but it remains superior to echocardiography for the accurate assessment of ejection fraction.

CARDIAC MAGNETIC RESONANCE

Cardiac magnetic resonance (CMR) is increasingly common. It has a number of advantages:

- It is non-invasive.
- It can be gated by an ECG trace, so producing still images from each stage of the cardiac cycle.
- It does not expose the patient to ionizing radiation.

Depending on which imaging mode is used, MRI has a number of uses:

- In ischaemic heart disease, myocardial perfusion and scar (infarcted) tissue can be assessed using contrast techniques. The coronary arteries can be directly visualized, although, at present, the resolution of this is limited by cardiac and respiratory motion. Also myocardial function before and after pharmacological stress can be assessed.
- It is the gold standard for assessment of cardiomyopathy.

- In structural heart disease MRI can provide a very good spatial resolution and, therefore, detailed structural information.

POSITRON EMISSION TOMOGRAPHY

Positron emission tomography provides images of the metabolic processes of the myocardium. It is used to assess myocardial viability in patients when conventional techniques (radionucleotide perfusion scanning and coronary angiography) have given equivocal results.

CARDIAC CATHETERIZATION

This invasive investigation is the gold standard for the assessment of coronary disease.

Technique

Access to the right side of the heart (right heart catheter) is gained by one of the great veins (e.g. femoral vein).

Access to the left side of the heart is gained by a peripheral artery (e.g. femoral or radial artery).

In either case the vessel is punctured using a Seldinger needle (a large hollow needle) and a guide-wire is passed through the centre of the needle and into the heart using X-ray guidance. A sheath can then be passed over the wire through which hollow catheters can be placed in the desired chamber or vessel, where a number of investigations may be carried out:

- The pressure in the chamber or vessel can be recorded.
- Oxygen saturation of the blood at that location can be measured.
- Radio-opaque dye can be injected via the catheter to provide information, depending on the location of the catheter – if in the ostia of the coronary arteries the anatomy and patency of the coronary arteries can be assessed (coronary angiography); if in the left ventricle the contractility of the ventricle can be assessed by visualizing the manner in which the dye is expelled from the ventricular cavity; if in the aortic root the size and tortuosity of the aortic root can be seen by the outline of the dye within it.

Left heart catheterization and coronary angiography

Indications

This is indicated for patients who:

- Have a positive exercise test or myocardial perfusion scan.

- Give a good history of and have multiple risk factors for ischaemic heart disease.
- Have had a cardiac arrest.
- Have had a heart transplant – there is a high incidence of atherosclerosis after transplant and yearly angiograms are performed.
- Occupational reasons – for patients who have chest pain even if non-invasive tests are negative (e.g. airline pilots).

Note that the list of indications is much more complicated than this, but you only need to have a general idea of the common indications.

Patient preparation

The following must be completed before the procedure:

- A detailed history to ensure that the indications are appropriate and that the patient has no other serious diseases that may affect the decision to proceed. Any history of allergy to iodine must be noted.
- Examination of the patient to ensure that he or she is well. Peripheral pulses must all be felt for and their absence or presence noted. If the femoral approach is to be used the groin area will need to be shaved just before the procedure.
- The procedure must be carefully explained to the patient.
- The risks must be explained.
- Informed consent is obtained.

Left ventriculography

This is performed to assess left-ventricular function. Contrast is injected rapidly to fill the left ventricle and X-ray images are obtained of ventricular contraction.

Coronary angiography

The left and right coronary ostia are located in turn and contrast is gently injected into the arteries. Several images are obtained of each artery from different angles so a detailed picture of the anatomy of the arteries can be obtained. Images are recorded using X-ray video recording or cine camera.

Complications of coronary angiography

The average mortality or serious complication rate of coronary angiography is 1/1000 cases. The following complications may occur:

- Haemorrhage from the arterial puncture site – this is more common at the femoral site than if the procedure is performed via the radial artery. Firm pressure should be applied to the site of bleeding and a clotting screen performed; rarely operative repair is necessary.

- Formation of a pseudoaneurysm – this results from weakening of the femoral artery wall and may require surgical repair.
- Infection of the puncture site or rarely septicaemia may occur. Blood cultures and intravenous antibiotics may be required.
- Contrast reaction – which may range from mild urticaria and a pyrexia, to full-blown anaphylactic shock.
- Thrombosis of the artery used – this results in a cold blue foot or hand and necessitates peripheral angiography and a referral to the vascular surgeons.
- Arrhythmias – these may occur during the angiography due to coronary arterial spasm or occlusion by the catheter. Any form of arrhythmia may occur (ventricular arrhythmias are more common).
- Pericardial tamponade – this is rare and occurs as a result of coronary artery tear or left-ventricular tear. The patient becomes acutely cyanosed and hypotensive. Pericardial aspiration is required urgently.
- Displacement of atherosclerotic fragments, which then embolize more distally, resulting in MI, cerebrovascular emboli, ischaemic toes, etc.

HINTS AND TIPS

Coronary angiography is mandatory before a patient can undergo a coronary artery bypass operation. It provides detailed information on the severity and location of coronary atherosclerotic lesions, without which surgery cannot be undertaken. Older patients undergoing valve replacement surgery also have coronary angiography before surgery to exclude coexistent coronary artery disease. If this is found, coronary artery bypass may be undertaken at the same time as valve replacement.

CARDIAC COMPUTED TOMOGRAPHY

The advent of rapid-acquisition of images has led to the use of computed tomography (CT) as a non-invasive alternative for imaging the coronary arteries. Modern scanners give ever-higher resolution at a lower dose of radiation, but are still not as sensitive or specific as coronary angiography, which remains the gold standard. The option to intervene with angioplasty at the time of angiography remains a significant further advantage. CT calcium scoring, which uses a single beam of electrons and multiple detectors, gives an even lower-dose of radiation but does not provide information on specific lesions. Instead it gives a risk score, which can guide further investigations. The current NICE recommendations (discussed in Ch. 5) recommend the use of calcium scoring to rule out coronary disease in low-risk patients.

COMMUNICATION

You need to have a working knowledge of the common cardiac investigations so that you can explain to patients what is involved and how the findings may guide further treatment.

Chest pain (5)

Objectives

By the end of this chapter you should:
- Be able to take a clear history from a patient presenting with chest pain.
- Be aware of the differential diagnosis of chest pain.
- Be able to examine the patient with chest pain.
- Understand the appropriate investigations for a patient presenting with chest pain.

DIFFERENTIAL DIAGNOSIS OF CHEST PAIN

Chest pain is one of the most common presenting complaints seen by cardiologists. It is important to remember that:

- There are many causes of chest pain.
- Some causes of chest pain are life-threatening and require prompt diagnosis and treatment; other causes are more benign.

The first differentiation to be made is between cardiac and non-cardiac chest pain (Fig. 5.1).

HISTORY TO FOCUS ON THE DIFFERENTIAL DIAGNOSIS OF CHEST PAIN

The differential diagnosis of chest pain is very diverse; a thorough history is, therefore, very important.

PRESENTING COMPLAINT

Differentiation depends on a detailed history of the pain, with particular emphasis on the following characteristics of the pain (Fig. 5.2):

- Whether the pain is continuous or intermittent.
- Duration of the pain.
- Position of the pain – central or lateral/posterior.
- Exacerbating factors – exertion, emotion, food, posture, movement, breathing.
- Radiation of the pain – to neck, arms, head.
- Quality of pain – crushing, burning, stabbing.

COMMUNICATION

To get an idea of the severity of a patient's symptoms ask them about their 'exercise tolerance' – how far can they walk on the flat? Do they have stairs at home, and does walking up them cause chest pain? Pain at a reproducible distance or effort is typical of angina.

Past medical history

This can provide important clues:

- A history of ischaemic heart disease.
- A history of peptic ulcer disease, or of frequent ingestion of non-steroidal anti-inflammatory drugs.
- Recent operations – cardiothoracic surgery can be complicated by Dressler syndrome, mediastinitis, ischaemic heart disease or pulmonary embolus (PE).
- Pericarditis might be preceded by a prodromal viral illness.
- PE can be preceded by a period of inactivity (e.g. a recent operation, illness or long journey).
- Hypertension is a risk factor for both ischaemic heart disease and dissection of the thoracic aorta.

Drug history, family history and social history

Other risk factors for ischaemic heart disease, such as a positive family history and smoking, should be excluded. A history of heavy alcohol intake is a risk factor for gastritis and peptic ulcer disease.

Fig. 5.1 Differential diagnosis of chest pain

System involved	Pathology
Cardiac	Myocardial infarction Angina pectoris Pericarditis Prolapse of the mitral valve
Vascular	Aortic dissection
Respiratory (all tend to give rise to pleuritic pain)	Pulmonary embolus Pneumonia Pneumothorax Pulmonary neoplasm
Gastrointestinal	Oesophagitis due to gastric reflux Oesophageal tear Peptic ulcer Biliary disease
Musculoskeletal	Cervical nerve root compression by cervical disc Costochondritis Fractured rib
Neurological	Herpes zoster

EXAMINATION OF PATIENTS WHO HAVE CHEST PAIN

Points to note on examination of the patient who has chest pain are shown in Fig. 5.3.

Inspection

On inspection, look for:

- Signs of shock (e.g. pallor, sweating) – may indicate myocardial infarction (MI), dissecting aorta, PE.
- Laboured breathing – may indicate MI leading to left ventricular failure (LVF) or a pulmonary cause.
- Signs of vomiting – suggests MI or an oesophageal cause.
- Coughing – suggests LVF, pneumonia.

Cardiovascular system

Note the following:

- Pulse and blood pressure – is there any abnormal rhythm, tachycardia, bradycardia, hypotension,

Fig. 5.2 Characteristics of different types of chest pain

Characteristic	Myocardial ischaemia	Pericarditis	Pleuritic pain	Gastrointestinal pain	Musculoskeletal	Aortic dissection
Quality of pain	Crushing, tight or bandlike	Sharp (may be crushing)	Sharp	Burning	Usually sharp, although can be a dull ache	Sharp, stabbing, tearing
Site of pain	Central anterior chest	Central anterior	Anywhere (usually very localized pain)	Central	Can be anywhere	Retrosternal, interscapular
Radiation	To throat, jaw or arms	Usually no radiation	Usually no radiation	To throat	To arms or around chest to back	Usually no radiation
Exacerbating and relieving factors	Exacerbated by exertion, anxiety, cold; relieved by rest and by glyceryl trinitrate	Exacerbated when lying back; relieved by sitting forward	Exacerbated by breathing, coughing or moving; relieved when breathing stops	Peptic ulcer pain often relieved by food and antacids; cholecystitis and oesophageal pain are exacerbated by food	Can be exacerbated by pressing on chest wall or moving neck	Constant with no exacerbating or relieving factors
Associated features	Patient often sweaty, breathless and shocked; might feel nauseated	Fever, recent viral illness (e.g. rash, arthralgia)	Cough, haemoptysis, breathlessness; shock with pulmonary embolus	Excessive wind	Other affected joints; patient otherwise looks very well	Unequal radial and femoral pulse and blood pressure; aortic regurgitant murmur may be heard on auscultation

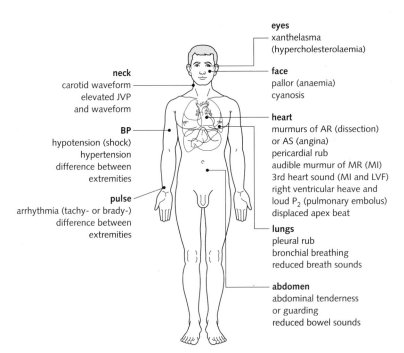

eyes
xanthelasma
(hypercholesterolaemia)

face
pallor (anaemia)
cyanosis

heart
murmurs of AR (dissection)
or AS (angina)
pericardial rub
audible murmur of MR (MI)
3rd heart sound (MI and LVF)
right ventricular heave and
loud P_2 (pulmonary embolus)
displaced apex beat

lungs
pleural rub
bronchial breathing
reduced breath sounds

abdomen
abdominal tenderness
or guarding
reduced bowel sounds

neck
carotid waveform
elevated JVP
and waveform

BP
hypotension (shock)
hypertension
difference between
extremities

pulse
arrhythmia (tachy- or brady-)
difference between
extremities

Fig. 5.3 Points to note when examining a patient who has chest pain. AR, aortic regurgitation; AS, aortic stenosis; BP, blood pressure; JVP, jugular venous pressure; LVF, left ventricular failure; MI, myocardial infarction; MR, mitral regurgitation; P2, pulmonary component of the second heart sound.

hypertension? Inequalities in the pulses or blood pressure between different extremities are seen in aortic dissection.

- Mucous membranes – pallor could suggest angina due to anaemia; cyanosis suggests hypoxia.
- Any increase in jugular venous pressure – a sign of right ventricular infarction or pulmonary embolus.
- Carotid pulse waveform – a collapsing pulse is seen with aortic regurgitation, which can complicate aortic dissection. It is slow rising if angina is due to aortic stenosis.
- Displaced apex beat, abnormal cardiac impulses (e.g. paradoxical movement in anterior MI).
- Auscultation – listen for a pericardial rub, third heart sound (a feature of LVF), mitral or aortic regurgitation (features of MI or dissection respectively), aortic stenosis (causes angina).

Respiratory system

Note the following signs:

- Breathlessness or cyanosis.
- Unequal hemithorax expansion – a sign of pneumonia and pneumothorax.
- Abnormal dullness over lung fields – a sign of pneumonia.
- Any bronchial breathing or pleural rub – signs of pneumonia and pleurisy.

Gastrointestinal system

Specifically look for:

- Abdominal tenderness or guarding.
- Scanty or absent bowel sounds – suggests an ileus (e.g. due to perforated peptic ulcer and peritonitis).

INVESTIGATION OF PATIENTS WHO HAVE CHEST PAIN

A summary of tests used to investigate chest pain is shown in Fig. 5.4; an algorithm is given in Fig. 5.5.

Blood tests

These include:

- Cardiac biomarkers including cardiac troponin and creatine kinase – cardiac troponin T and I are now commonly used to risk stratify patients presenting with acute coronary syndrome (Fig. 5.6).
- Full blood count – anaemia may exacerbate angina.
- Renal function and electrolytes – may be abnormal if the patient has been vomiting, leading to dehydration and hypokalaemia, or due to diuretic therapy.
- Arterial blood gases – hypoxia is a sign of PE and LVF, hypocapnoea is seen with hyperventilation.
- Liver function tests and serum amylase – deranged in cholecystitis and peptic ulcer disease.

Fig. 5.4 First-line tests to exclude a chest pain emergency

Test	Diagnosis
ECG	If normal excludes MI, although evidence for this may emerge upon observation
CXR	Widened mediastinum suggests aortic dissection; may show pleural effusion or pulmonary consolidation
Biochemical markers	May be normal in first 4 h after MI, but CK-MB, cardiac troponins will then increase
Arterial blood gases	In the dyspnoeic patient severe hypoxaemia suggests pulmonary embolus, LVF or pneumonia
CT scan	Carry out urgently for suspected aortic dissection

CK-MB, creatine kinase composed of M (muscle) and B (brain) subunits, which is found primarily in cardiac muscle; CT, computed tomography; CXR, chest radiography; ECG, electrocardiography; LVF, left ventricular failure; MI, myocardial infarction.

Electrocardiography

Findings may include:

- ST elevation in absence of bundle branch block (BBB) – indicates acute MI (occasionally it is due to Prinzmetal's angina).
- ST depression in absence of BBB – indicates myocardial ischaemia. At rest this equates with unstable angina or non-ST elevation MI (NSTEMI); on exertion this equates with effort-induced angina pectoris or tachyarrhythmias.
- BBB – if new LBBB occurs with chest pain this may be due to MI; if it is old, MI cannot be diagnosed from the electrocardiogram (ECG) alone.
- Fully developed Q waves – indicate old MI (i.e. over 24 h old).
- Atrial fibrillation secondary to any pulmonary disease or myocardial ischaemia.

In the event of a large PE the classic changes are:

- Sinus tachycardia (the most commonly seen change).
- Atrial fibrillation.
- Tall P waves in lead II (right atrial dilatation).

Fig. 5.5 Algorithm for investigation of chest pain.

Fig. 5.6 Percentage of people estimated to have coronary artery disease according to typicality of symptoms, age, sex and risk factors

Age (years)	Non-anginal chest pain				Atypical angina				Typical angina			
	Men		Women		Men		Women		Men		Women	
	Lo	Hi	Lo	Hi	Lo	Hi	Lo	Hi	Lo	Hi	Lo	Hi
35	3	35	1	19	8	59	2	39	30	88	10	78
45	9	47	2	22	21	70	5	43	51	92	20	79
55	23	59	4	25	45	79	10	47	80	95	38	82
65	49	69	9	29	71	86	20	51	93	97	56	84

For men older than 70 with atypical or typical symptoms, assume an estimate >90%.
For women older than 70, assume an estimate of 61-90% EXCEPT women at high risk AND with typical symptoms where a risk >90% should be assumed.

Values are per cent of people at each mid-decade age with significant coronary artery disease (CAD).
Hi = high risk = diabetes, smoking and hyperlipidemia (total cholesterol >6.47 mmol/litre).
Lo = low risk = none of these three.
The shaded area represents people with symptoms of non-anginal chest pain, who would not be investigated for stable angina routinely.
Note:
These results are likely to overestimate CAD in primary care populations.
If there are resting ECG ST-T changes or Q waves, the likelihood of CAD is higher in each cell of the table.

From NICE 2010 Clinical Guidelines 95 Chest Pain of Recent Onset: Assessment and diagnosis of recent onset chest pain or discomfort of suspected cardiac origin, with permission.

- Right axis deviation and right BBB.
- S wave in lead I, Q wave in lead III, and inverted T wave in lead III (the classic, though rare, SI QIII TIII pattern).

Chest radiography

The following signs may be seen:

- Cardiomegaly.
- Widening of the mediastinum in aortic dissection.
- Lung lesions.
- Pleural and pericardial effusions.
- Oligaemic lung fields in PE.

Echocardiography

This may reveal:

- Pericardial effusion – suggests pericarditis or dissection.
- Regional myocardial dysfunction – a feature of MI or ischaemia.
- Aortic dissection with false lumen.
- Aortic or mitral valve abnormalities.

Computed tomography and magnetic resonance imaging

Computed tomography (CT) should be performed urgently if aortic dissection is suspected. CT pulmonary angiography (CTPA) is a sensitive and specific test for PE. It is rapid and can also give information about the lung tissue.

Ventilation/perfusion (V/Q) scan

V/Q scanning is a sensitive test for PE in selected patients, but is generally only performed in patients with otherwise normal lungs (e.g. not in those with asthma/ COPD).

Angiography, myocardial perfusion imaging or stress echocardiography

Current NICE guidelines recommend risk scoring in stable patients who present with possible cardiac chest pain. The important factors are age, gender, risk factors and the nature of their symptoms (typical angina is central chest pain, brought on by exertion and relieved by rest) (Fig. 5.6). In summary, in patients with a high risk of coronary disease (>60%) the first-line investigation is coronary angiography. For medium risk patients (30–60%), functional imaging (commonly myocardial perfusion imaging, sometimes stress echocardiography, but the choice depends upon availability) is recommended. For patients with a low risk of coronary disease (<30%), NICE recommends CT calcium scoring where this is available.

NEW ONSET CENTRAL CHEST PAIN AT REST IN AN ILL PATIENT

The importance of this subject is that this situation represents a medical emergency requiring rapid diagnosis and treatment.

It is necessary in this situation to distinguish between the following:

- MI (see Ch. 14).
- Unstable angina (see Ch. 13).
- Pericarditis (see Ch. 21).
- Dissection of thoracic aorta.
- Mediastinitis secondary to oesophageal tear.
- Pulmonary embolus.
- Non-cardiac chest pain.

HINTS AND TIPS

In the context of cardiac chest pain, ST elevation on the ECG is usually indicative of proximal occlusion of a major epicardial coronary artery. If untreated myocardial necrosis begins within 30 min. Urgent restoration of coronary blood flow (reperfusion) prevents further left-ventricular damage and improves prognosis. Two strategies are available: primary angioplasty and thrombolysis. The management will be discussed in Ch. 14.

Dissection of the thoracic aorta

The pain is typically sharp and tearing. There is often radiation of the pain to the back. There might be a previous history of hypertension.

On examination, the patient might be shocked and there could be delays between the major pulses (e.g. right brachial versus left brachial, brachial versus femoral).

Chest radiography might show a widened mediastinum. The ECG will not show ST elevation unless the coronary ostia are dissected. Confirmation might require high-resolution spiral CT, echocardiography, or magnetic resonance imaging (which is the best investigation when available; Fig. 5.7).

Thrombolysis is contraindicated because it causes massive bleeding from the aorta (Fig. 5.8).

Mediastinitis

This is unusual but should be considered where there is a possibility of an oesophageal leak (e.g. after endoscopy or oesophageal surgery). Rupture of the oesophagus does occasionally occur due to vomiting, this is known as Boerhaave syndrome.

Pulmonary embolus

Pulmonary emboli can present as acute chest pain in an ill patient or as intermittent chest pain in a relatively well patient. For this reason it is crucial to suspect PE in all patients who have chest pain that is not typically anginal.

Fig. 5.7 Overview of dissection of the thoracic aorta

Predisposing factors	Hypertension
	Bicuspid aortic valve Pregnancy Marfan, Turner, Noonan syndromes Connective tissue diseases – SLE, Ehlers–Danlos syndrome Men > women Middle age
Pathophysiology	Damage to the media and high intraluminal pressure causing an intimal tear Blood enters and dissects the luminal plane of the media creating a false lumen
Classification	Stanford classification: type A – all dissections involving the ascending aorta; type B – all dissections not involving the ascending aorta
Symptoms	Central tearing chest pain radiating to the back Further complications as the dissection involves branches of the aorta: coronary ostia – myocardial infarction; carotid or spinal arteries – hemiplegia, dysphasia, or paraplegia; mesenteric arteries – abdominal pain
Signs	Shocked, cyanosed, sweating Blood pressure and pulses differ between extremities Aortic regurgitation Cardiac tamponade Cardiac failure

Fig. 5.7 Overview of dissection of the thoracic aorta—cont'd

Predisposing factors	Hypertension
Investigation	CXR – widened mediastinum ± fluid in costophrenic angle ECG – may be ST elevation CT/MRI – best investigations, show aortic false lumen Transoesophageal echo if available is also very sensitive Echocardiography – may show pericardial effusion if dissection extends proximally; tamponade may occur
Management	Pain relief – morphine Intravenous access – central and arterial line Fluid replacement – initially colloid then blood when available – crossmatch at least 10 units Blood pressure control – intravenous nitroprusside infusion or labetalol infusion if no cardiac failure – keep blood pressure 120/80 mmHg Surgery for all type A dissections Medical management and possibly surgery or percutaneous treatment for type B

CT, computed tomography; CXR, chest radiography; ECG, electrocardiography; MRI, magnetic resonance imaging; SLE, systemic lupus erythematosus.

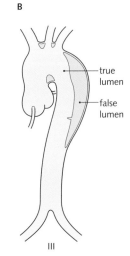

Fig. 5.8 Classification of aortic dissection.

The pain of a PE can be pleuritic or tight in nature and might be located anywhere in the chest. It can be accompanied by the following symptoms and signs:

- Dyspnoea.
- Dry cough or haemoptysis.
- Hypotension and sweating.
- Sudden collapse with syncope.

Massive PE can cause collapse with cardiac arrest. The ECG will show ventricular tachyarrhythmias or sinus rhythm with electromechanical dissociation. Patients will often experience a sense of 'impending doom' or profound anxiety. Thrombolysis may be attempted as a life-saving therapy in massive PE where there is haemodynamic compromise.

Conditions predisposing to clot formation in the deep veins of the leg are associated with a high incidence of PE (Fig. 5.9).

As the mortality rate resulting from PE is approximately 10%, appropriate investigations to exclude PE should be carried out promptly and anticoagulation commenced using either intravenous heparin as an infusion or an appropriate low-molecular-weight heparin preparation subcutaneously. Warfarin therapy should be commenced if PE is confirmed.

Fig. 5.9 Conditions predisposing to deep venous thrombosis

Condition	Examples
Immobility	Prolonged bed rest for any reason, long air journeys
Postoperative	Abdominal and pelvic surgery, leg and hip surgery
Haemoconcentration	Diuretic therapy, polycythaemia
Hypercoagulable states	Malignancy, oral contraceptive pill, protein C/protein S deficiency, etc.
Venous stasis (poor flow of venous blood)	Congestive cardiac failure, atrial fibrillation (formation of thrombus in the right ventricle can result in PE)
Pregnancy	Hypercoagulable state with possible immobility, venous stasis, haemoconcentration or surgery (caesarean section)

● Objectives

By the end of this chapter you should:
- Be able to take a history and examine a patient presenting with breathlessness.
- Understand the appropriate investigations for a patient presenting with breathlessness.
- Understand the differential diagnosis of a patient presenting with breathlessness.

Dyspnoea is an uncomfortable awareness of one's own breathing. It is considered abnormal only when it occurs at a level of physical activity not normally expected to cause any problem. For example, a 32-year-old man can expect to be dyspnoeic after running a marathon, but not when he is getting out of bed in the morning.

DIFFERENTIAL DIAGNOSIS OF DYSPNOEA

Dyspnoea is the main symptom of many cardiac and pulmonary diseases. A working knowledge of the differential diagnosis is required to be able to differentiate acute life-threatening conditions from those that do not require immediate treatment. Revise the list of differential diagnoses in Ch. 1 (see Fig. 1.3).

HISTORY TO FOCUS ON THE DIFFERENTIAL DIAGNOSIS OF DYSPNOEA

Differentiation depends upon a detailed history of the dyspnoea (Fig. 6.1) with particular emphasis on whether:

- The dyspnoea is acute or chronic.
- It is continuous or intermittent.
- There are exacerbating and relieving factors – such as exertion, lying flat (suggests orthopnoea in pulmonary oedema), sleep (suggests paroxysmal nocturnal dyspnoea (PND), i.e. waking from sleep gasping for breath in left ventricular failure (LVF)).
- There are associated features, such as cough – ask for details of sputum production. Yellow-green sputum suggests pneumonia or exacerbation of chronic obstructive pulmonary disease (COPD); pink frothy sputum suggests LVF; haemoptysis can be a feature

of pulmonary embolism (PE) and carcinoma of the lung.
- There is chest pain – ask for details of location, nature of pain, radiation, etc. (see Ch. 5).
- There are palpitations – ask about rate and rhythm.
- There is ankle oedema – suggestive of congestive cardiac failure, swelling usually worse at the end of the day and best first thing in the morning.
- There is a wheeze – suggestive of airways obstruction (i.e. asthma, COPD, or neoplasm of the lung causing airway obstruction). Wheeze can also occur during LVF.

HINTS AND TIPS

In the investigation of patients with breathlessness it is important to exclude a cardiac source of their symptoms. These include valvular heart disease and left ventricular failure (LVF) – both may be detected by echocardiography. Some patients may have breathlessness as their only symptom of ischaemic heart disease, this is called 'angina equivalent'.

EXAMINATION OF DYSPNOEIC PATIENTS

A thorough examination will be needed because the differential diagnosis is potentially wide (Fig. 6.2).

Inspection

Note the following:

- Signs of shock, e.g. pallor, sweating – suggest acute LVF, pneumonia, PE.
- Inspect for laboured or obstructed breathing (any intercostal recession?), tachypnoea or cyanosis. One or more usually present with resting dyspnoea.

Fig. 6.1 Presenting history for different diseases causing dyspnoea

	Cardiac failure	Coronary artery disease	Pulmonary embolus	Pneumothorax	COPD and asthma
Acute or chronic	May be acute or chronic	Acute	Acute (less commonly recurrent small PEs may present as chronic dyspnoea)	Acute	Acute or chronic
Continuous or intermittent	May be continuous or intermittent	Usually intermittent, but an acute MI may lead to continuous and severe LVF	Continuous	Continuous	Continuous or intermittent; these disorders range from the acute, life-threatening exacerbations to chronic, relatively mild episodes
Exacerbating and relieving factors	Exacerbated by exertion and lying flat (orthopnoea and PND may occur) and occasionally by food; relieved by rest, sitting up, oxygen and GTN	Exacerbated by exertion, cold; may be relieved by oxygen			Exacerbated by exertion, pulmonary infections, allergens (e.g. pollen, animal danders); relieved by bronchodilator inhalers
Associated features	May be chest pain (ischaemia may cause LVF); palpitations-arrhythmias may precipitate LVF; cough with pink frothy sputum	Chest pain (central crushing pain radiating to the left arm or throat) and sweating; occasionally palpitations – atrial fibrillation may be precipitated by ischaemia	Pleuritic chest pain (sharp, localized pain worse on breathing and coughing) and bright red haemoptysis; atrial fibrillation may occur	Pleuritic chest pain; there may be a history of chest trauma	Cough with sputum; pleuritic chest pain if associated infection; wheeze

COPD, chronic obstructive pulmonary disease; GTN, glyceryl trinitrate; LVF, left ventricular failure; MI, myocardial infarction; PE, pulmonary embolus; PND, paroxysmal noctumal dyspnoea.

- Cough – suggests acute LVF, pneumonia; note the appearance of the sputum (always ask to look in the sputum pot if it is present).
- Appearance of hands and fingers – such as clubbing, carbon dioxide retention flap.
- Appearance of chest – a barrel-shaped chest (hyper-expanded) is a feature of emphysema; kyphoscoliosis causes distortion.
- Pyrexia – suggests infection (PE or myocardial infarction may be associated with a low-grade pyrexia).

Cardiovascular system

Check the following:

- Pulse and blood pressure – any abnormal rhythm, tachycardia, bradycardia, hypotension, hypertension?
- Mucous membranes – pallor suggests dyspnoea in anaemia; cyanosis suggests hypoxia in LVF, COPD, PE, pneumonia and lung collapse.
- Carotid pulse waveform and jugular venous pressure (JVP) – JVP is elevated in cardiac failure and conditions causing pulmonary hypertension with associated right heart failure (e.g. PE, COPD).
- Apex beat – displacement suggests cardiac enlargement and a right ventricular heave suggests pulmonary hypertension.
- Heart sounds – note any audible murmurs or added heart sounds (third heart sound in LVF); mitral regurgitation or aortic valve lesions can cause LVF.
- Peripheral oedema.

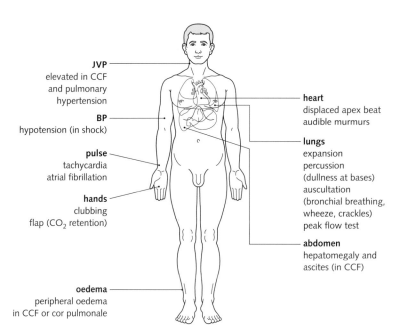

JVP
elevated in CCF and pulmonary hypertension

BP
hypotension (in shock)

pulse
tachycardia
atrial fibrillation

hands
clubbing
flap (CO_2 retention)

oedema
peripheral oedema
in CCF or cor pulmonale

heart
displaced apex beat
audible murmurs

lungs
expansion
percussion
(dullness at bases)
auscultation
(bronchial breathing,
wheeze, crackles)
peak flow test

abdomen
hepatomegaly and
ascites (in CCF)

Respiratory system

Check the following:

- Expansion – unequal thorax expansion is a sign of pneumonia or pneumothorax.
- Vocal fremitus – enhanced vocal fremitus is a sign of consolidation; reduced vocal fremitus is a sign of effusion and pneumothorax.
- Abnormal dullness over hemithorax with reduced expansion – suggests pneumonia.
- Stony dullness at one or both lung bases – suggests pleural effusion.
- Hyperresonance over hemithorax with less expansion – suggests pneumothorax.
- Bilateral hyperresonance with loss of cardiac dullness – suggests emphysema.
- Bronchial breathing – suggests pneumonia.
- Crepitations – suggests pneumonia, pulmonary oedema, pulmonary fibrosis.
- Wheeze – asthma, COPD, cardiac asthma in LVF.
- Peak flow test – this is part of every examination of the respiratory system and you should always ask to do this. Explain the technique to the patient clearly and then perform three attempts and take the best out of three. Peak flow will be reduced in active asthma and COPD.

Gastrointestinal system

Examine for hepatomegaly and ascites – seen in congestive cardiac failure or isolated right-sided failure.

INVESTIGATION OF DYSPNOEIC PATIENTS

A summary of first-line tests to exclude emergencies is shown in Fig. 6.3.

Fig. 6.3 First-line tests to exclude a dyspnoeic emergency

Test	Diagnosis
CXR	Acute LVF – pulmonary oedema ± large heart shadow
	Acute asthma – clear over-expanded lungs
	Pneumothorax – absence of lung markings between lung edge and chest wall
	Pneumonia – consolidation
ECG	Look for evidence of MI, ischaemia, pulmonary embolus
Arterial blood gases	Hypoxia suggests LVF or significant lung disease (use the level of hypoxia to guide the need for oxygen therapy or artificial ventilation)
Peak flow	Reduced in airway obstruction (asthma, COPD), but may also be reduced in sick patients because of weakness (it is an effort-dependent test)

COPD, chronic obstructive pulmonary disease; CXR, chest radiography; ECG, electrocardiography; LVF, left ventricular failure; MI, myocardial infarction.

Blood tests

These include:

- Full blood count – might reveal anaemia or leucocytosis (in pneumonia).
- Urea and electrolytes – deranged due to diuretic treatment of cardiac failure, possible syndrome of inappropriate antidiuretic hormone secretion in pneumonia.
- Cardiac enzymes – elevated if dyspnoea secondary to myocardial infarction.
- Liver function tests – deranged in hepatic congestion secondary to congestive cardiac failure.
- Arterial blood gases (Fig. 6.4).
- D-dimer – a fibrin degradation product (elevated in pulmonary embolus).
- CRP – elevated in inflammatory processes such as pneumonia.

HINTS AND TIPS

Assays for D-dimer have a high sensitivity but low specificity, generating a lot of false positive results (D-dimer is also raised in inflammatory processes or malignancy, for example). It is therefore important to test D-dimer only in appropriate patients. Many hospitals now require clinicians to calculate pre-test probability of a pulmonary embolus using the Wells score (Ch. 3).

Electrocardiography

This might show:

- Ischaemic changes may be seen in patients with coronary artery disease.

- Sinus tachycardia with SI, QIII, TIII or RBBB in patients who have had a PE.
- Atrial fibrillation – may be seen secondary to any lung pathology or ischaemia.

Chest radiography

Note the following:

- Cardiomegaly in cardiac failure – pulmonary oedema may also be seen (Fig. 6.5).
- Focal lung consolidation in pneumonia (shadowing of a lung segment with an air bronchogram).
- Pleural effusion – suggests PE, infection or cardiac failure.
- Hyperexpanded lung fields in emphysema (ability to count more than six rib spaces over the lung fields); bullae may be seen in emphysema.
- Presence of a pneumothorax – ask for a film in full expiration if this is suspected.
- Oligaemic lung fields in PE.

HINTS AND TIPS

Notes on blood gases:
- Hypoxia and hypocapnoea are seen in LVF and pulmonary embolus (this shows a drop in PCO, due to hyperventilation as a response to hypoxia).
- Hypoxia and hypercapnoea can occur in COPD and severe asthma – in the former condition this is because the respiratory centre has readjusted to the chronic low oxygen levels.

Fig. 6.4 Examples of arterial blood gas results in dyspnoeic patients. The low pH in ventilatory failure is secondary to an acute retention of carbon dioxide. The high pH in acute hyperventilation results from an acute loss of carbon dioxide (respiratory alkalosis). The case of hypoxia shown here has led to hyperventilation and a fall of carbon dioxide and must have been present for some time because the pH is compensated to normal by renal excretion of bicarbonate

	Po_2 (kPa)	PCo_2 (kPa)	pH
Normal range	10.5–13.5	5.0–6.0	7.36–7.44
Ventilatory failure (e.g. chronic obstructive airways disease, severe asthma with exhaustion)	↓	↑	↓
Acute hyperventilation	-	↓	↑
Hypoxia (e.g. left ventricular failure, pulmonary embolism)	↓	↓	-

Upper lobe blood diversion Peri-hilar shadowing

Diffuse interstitial shadowing Enlarged heart

Fig. 6.5 Chest X-ray with features of pulmonary oedema.

- Hypoxia and oxygen therapy causes the blood PO_2 to rise and the respiratory drive to fall, so ventilation is reduced and the blood PCO_2 rises. In asthma, exhaustion causes the ventilatory drive to fall off and the PCO_2 to rise; this precedes respiratory arrest and is an indication for artificial ventilation of the patient.
- Arterial pH – in acute conditions, such as acute LVF, pulmonary embolus, pneumothorax and early asthma-a respiratory alkalosis occurs (i.e. a low PCO_2 and a high pH of 7.4). The kidneys have not yet compensated by excreting bicarbonate.
- COPD with chronic CO_2 retention – the pH is normal because metabolic compensation has occurred and bicarbonate levels rise as a result of renal retention of bicarbonate (this takes a few days to occur).
- Severe asthma with acute CO_2 retention – the pH falls as the PCO_2 rises as there has been insufficient time for metabolic compensation to occur.

Echocardiography

This may reveal:

- LV systolic dysfunction.
- Valve lesions.
- Left atrial myxoma.
- Right ventricular hypertrophy and pulmonary hypertension.

Computed tomography

This is used to obtain detailed visualization of pulmonary fibrosis or small peripheral tumours that cannot be reached with a bronchoscope. CT pulmonary angiography (CTPA) is used to analyse blood flow in the pulmonary system and is the gold standard for identifying pulmonary emboli.

Pulmonary function tests

These tests are used to investigate:

- Lung volumes – increased in COPD, reduced in restrictive lung disease.
- Flow-volume loop – scalloped in COPD.
- Carbon monoxide transfer – reduced in the presence of normal airway function in restrictive lung diseases.

> **HINTS AND TIPS**
>
> Notes on dyspnoea and arterial blood gases:
> - The life-threatening cardiopulmonary conditions of respiratory failure and carbon monoxide poisoning might not cause prominent dyspnoea, but could present as coma or semi-coma.
> - Severe hypoxia or tissue underperfusion causes metabolic acidosis (low pH) with normal or low PCO_2
> - Most importantly, arterial blood gases must be performed for all dyspnoeic patients at presentation.

DYSPNOEA AT REST OF RECENT ONSET IN AN ILL PATIENT

This situation is important because it represents a cardiopulmonary emergency requiring rapid diagnosis and treatment. It is necessary to distinguish between the following life-threatening causes:

- Tension pneumothorax.
- Life-threatening asthma.
- Acute LVF.
- PE.
- Fulminant pneumonia.
- Pneumothorax.

Pneumothorax

Pneumothorax (air in the pleural space) can cause acute or chronic dyspnoea. A number of possible causes all create a connection between the pleural space and the atmosphere (via either the chest wall or the airways):

- Trauma (e.g. a blow to the chest resulting in fracture of the ribs or insertion of a central venous cannula).
- Rupture of bullae on the surface of the lung – this occurs in some otherwise healthy young patients (more commonly in men than in women) or in patients who have emphysema.

Tension pneumothorax can occur if the air continues to accumulate in the pleural cavity, resulting in a progressive increase in pressure and displacement of the mediastinum away from the side of the lesion. This is characterized by the following clinical signs:

- Severe and worsening dyspnoea.
- Displaced trachea and apex beat.
- Hyperresonance on the affected side with reduced breath sounds and vocal fremitus.
- Progressive hypotension due to reduced venous return and therefore reduced filling of the right ventricle.
- Eventual collapse and cardiac arrest and possibly electromechanical dissociation.

Treatment should be immediate, with insertion of a needle into the second intercostal space in the midclavicular line to allow gas to escape spontaneously from the pleural cavity. A chest drain should then be inserted and connected to an underwater seal.

Acute asthma

This is another medical emergency requiring prompt diagnosis and treatment. Signs suggestive of a severe asthma attack include:

- The patient being unable to talk in full sentences due to dyspnoea.
- The patient sitting forwards and using accessory muscles of respiration – prominent diaphragmatic movements and pursing of the lips on expiration.
- Tachycardia.
- Peak flow 30% of normal or less.
- Pulsus paradoxus – a drop in systolic blood pressure of more than 10 mmHg on inspiration.
- Silent chest due to severe airflow limitation.

Hypercapnoea on blood gas analysis suggests that the patient is becoming exhausted and respiratory arrest could be imminent – this might occur before there is severe hypoxia. The patient should be considered for intubation and artificial ventilation.

Appropriate treatment with intravenous hydrocortisone, oxygen therapy, nebulized bronchodilators and intravenous fluids should be commenced immediately.

Acute left ventricular failure

The detailed management of acute LVF is discussed in more detail in Ch. 19. The patient needs urgent treatment or will die from asphyxiation. Classic signs of LVF can be seen and include:

- Severe dyspnoea.
- Central cyanosis.
- Patient sits upright.
- Bilateral basal fine end-respiratory crepitations (in severe LVF the crepitations extend upwards to fill both lung fields).

- Hypotension secondary to poor left ventricular output (common).
- Blood gases show hypoxia and often hypocapnoea due to hyperventilation. There is usually a metabolic acidosis as a result of poor tissue perfusion.

Treatment includes high-concentration inhaled oxygen via a mask and intravenous diuretic (frusemide) and diamorphine injections.

Pulmonary embolus

This can present in a number of ways, for example:

- Severe dyspnoea.
- Collapse and syncope.
- Hypotension.
- Cardiorespiratory arrest (often with electromechanical dissociation or ventricular fibrillation).

If PE is suspected, anticoagulation should be commenced immediately with an intravenous heparin infusion or subcutaneous low-molecular-weight heparin (LMWH).

If the patient is cardiovascularly unstable, suggesting a massive PE, thrombolysis can be administered or emergency pulmonary angiography carried out in an attempt to disrupt the embolus.

Pneumonia

The patient may be pyrexial or even show signs of septic shock (e.g. hypotension, renal failure). Blood gases may reveal hypoxia, which can be extremely severe in pneumonia caused by *Pneumocystis carinii*.

The chest radiograph might show lobar or patchy consolidation. Radiographic changes can be deceptively mild in mycoplasma or legionella infections.

The most common community-acquired organisms are streptococci and atypical organisms such as mycoplasma, so appropriate antibiotic therapy should be commenced immediately after blood (and sputum if possible) cultures have been taken.

By the end of this chapter you should:
- Be able to take a history and examine a patient who presents with syncope.
- Understand the differential diagnoses of a patient who presents with syncope.
- Understand the appropriate investigations for a patient presenting with syncope.

Syncope is a loss of consciousness usually due to a reduction in perfusion of the brain.

DIFFERENTIAL DIAGNOSIS OF SYNCOPE

Many conditions can give rise to loss of consciousness – these can be divided into: cardiac, vasovagal, circulatory, cerebrovascular, neurological and metabolic (Fig. 7.1).

HISTORY TO FOCUS ON THE DIFFERENTIAL DIAGNOSIS OF SYNCOPE

The first differentiation to be made is between cardiac and non-cardiac (usually neurological) syncope.

Differentiation depends upon a detailed history of the syncopal episode with particular emphasis on the features outlined below.

- The events preceding the syncope should be elucidated:
  - exertion – can precipitate syncope in hypertrophic cardiomyopathy (HCM) or aortic stenosis
  - pain or anxiety, or prolonged standing – in vasovagal syncope
  - soon after standing – postural hypotension
  - neck movements – aggravate vertebrobasilar attacks.
- Speed of onset of syncope might be:
  - immediate with no warning – classic presentation of Stokes–Adams attacks
  - rapid with warning – preceded either by lightheadedness (vasovagal) or by an aura (epilepsy)
  - gradual with warning – hypoglycaemia preceded by lightheadedness, nausea and sweating.
- A witness account of the syncope itself; this is very important; indeed, no history is complete without one:
  - patient lies still, breathing regularly – Stokes–Adams attack (a prolonged Stokes–Adams attack can cause epileptiform movements secondary to cerebral hypoxia)
  - patient shakes limbs or has facial twitching, possibly associated with urinary incontinence and tongue biting – suggestive of epilepsy but myoclonus can occur with vasovagal syncope
  - patient becomes very pale and grey immediately before collapsing – vasovagal (patients who have cardiac syncope become very pale after collapse before regaining consciousness).
- The recovery of consciousness can also be characteristic. If the patient:
  - feels normal soon after episode – a cardiac cause is likely
  - feels washed out and nauseated and takes a few minutes to return to normal – the cause is probably vasovagal
  - is very drowsy and falls asleep soon after regaining consciousness – epilepsy (post-ictal state) is probable.

Past medical history

As always a thorough history is needed:
- Any cardiac history is important – ischaemia may precipitate arrhythmias.
- A history of stroke or TIA may suggest a cerebrovascular cause.
- Diabetes mellitus may cause autonomic neuropathy and postural hypotension, whereas good control of diabetes mellitus puts the patient at risk of hypoglycaemia.
- A history of head injury may suggest epilepsy secondary to cortical scarring.

Drug history

Important points include the following:
- Antihypertensives and diuretic agents predispose to postural hypotension.

Fig. 7.1 Differential diagnosis of syncope (see also Fig. 7.3)

System involved	Pathology
Cardiac	Tachyarrhythmia – supraventricular or ventricular Bradyarrhythmia – sinus bradycardia, complete or second-degree heart block, sinus arrest Stokes–Adams attack – syncope due to transient asystole Left ventricular outflow tract obstruction – aortic stenosis, HCM Right ventricular outflow tract obstruction – pulmonary stenosis Pulmonary hypertension
Vasovagal (simple faint)	After carotid sinus massage and also precipitated by pain, micturition, anxiety; these result in hyperstimulation by the vagus nerve leading to AV node block (and therefore bradycardia, hypotension and syncope)
Vascular	Postural hypotension – usually due to antihypertensive drugs or diuretics; also caused by autonomic neuropathy as in diabetes mellitus Pulmonary embolus – may or may not be preceded by chest pain Septic shock – severe peripheral vasodilatation results in hypotension
Cerebrovascular	Transient ischaemic attack Vertebrobasilar attack
Neurological	Epilepsy
Metabolic	Hypoglycaemia

AV, atrioventricular; HCM, hypertrophic cardiomyopathy.

- Class I and class III antiarrhythmics may cause long QT syndrome and predispose to torsades de pointes – all antiarrhythmic agents may cause bradycardia leading to syncope.
- Some other drugs may also predispose to long QT syndrome.
- Vasodilators precipitate syncope in pulmonary hypertension.

Family history

A family history of sudden death or recurrent syncope may occur in patients who have hypertrophic cardiomyopathy and also in those rare cases of familial long QT syndrome (Romano–Ward and Jervell Lange–Nielson syndromes).

A few patients who have epilepsy have a family history.

Social history

Note that:

- Alcohol excess is a risk factor for withdrawal fits.
- Smoking is a risk factor for ischaemic heart disease.

EXAMINATION OF PATIENTS WHO PRESENT WITH SYNCOPE

The points to note on examination of the patient who has syncope are summarized in Fig. 7.2 and discussed in turn below. On inspection, look for any:

- Neurological deficit suggestive of a cerebrovascular cause.
- Signs of shock – such as pallor or sweating.

HINTS AND TIPS

Notes on syncope:
- Cardiovascular syncope is always accompanied by hypotension.
- Syncope with normal blood pressure is likely to have a neurological, cerebrovascular or metabolic cause.
- Stokes–Adams attacks are episodes of syncope due to cardiac rhythm disturbance.
- Fitting while unconscious is not always caused by epilepsy – it can occur in any patient who has cerebral hypoperfusion or a metabolic disorder (e.g. a patient with vasovagal syncope alone may convulse if held up by a well-meaning bystander – don't let this catch you out!).

Cardiovascular system

On examination note the following:

- Pulse – any tachy- or bradyarrhythmia and character of pulse (slow rising in aortic stenosis, jerky in HCM).
- Blood pressure lying and standing to detect postural hypotension (>20 mmHg drop in blood pressure from lying to standing).

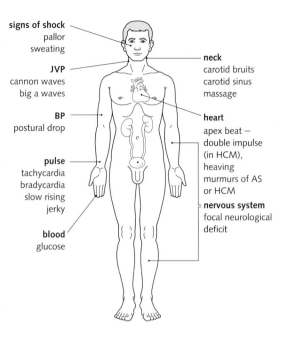

Fig. 7.2 Points to note on examination of a patient presenting with syncope. AS, aortic stenosis; BP, blood pressure; HCM, hypertrophic cardiomyopathy; JVP, jugular venous pressure.

- Jugular venous pulse – cannon waves in complete heart block (due to the atrium contracting against a closed tricuspid valve); prominent 'a' wave in pulmonary hypertension.
- Apex beat – double impulse (HCM), heaving (aortic stenosis).
- Any murmurs.
- Carotid bruits – indicating carotid artery stenosis and cerebrovascular disease.
- Response to carotid sinus massage – apply unilateral firm pressure over the carotid sinus with the patient in bed and attached to a cardiac monitor. Full resuscitative equipment should be easily accessible. Patients who have carotid sinus hypersensitivity will become very bradycardic or asystolic (sinus arrest).

Neurological system

This system should be fully examined to detect any residual deficit.

Fingerprick test for blood glucose

This is an easy test and, if positive, may provide valuable diagnostic information.

INVESTIGATION OF PATIENTS WHO PRESENT WITH SYNCOPE

An algorithm for the investigation of syncope is given in Fig. 7.3.

First-line tests to exclude emergencies are shown in Fig. 7.4.

Blood tests

The following tests should be performed:

- Full blood count – anaemia may be secondary to haemorrhage, which will cause postural hypotension; leucocytosis in sepsis and in the postictal period.
- Electrolytes and renal function – hypokalaemia predisposes towards arrhythmias.
- Calcium – hypocalcaemia is a cause of long QT syndrome.
- Cardiac enzymes – a myocardial infarction may cause sudden arrhythmia.
- Blood glucose.

Electrocardiography

This may show:

- A brady- or tachyarrhythmia.
- Heart block.
- A long QT interval.
- Evidence of ischaemia.
- Evidence of a pulmonary embolus.

Holter monitor

This is used to provide a 24- or 48-h ECG trace to detect arrhythmias and bradycardias (e.g. sick sinus syndrome, intermittent heart block). Longer cardiac monitoring can be performed using implantable event recorders.

Tilt test

This may aid diagnosis:

- Simple tilt produces hypotension and possibly syncope in autonomic denervation.
- Prolonged tilt may provoke vasovagal syncope with bradycardia and hypotension.

Chest radiography

On the chest radiograph:

- There may be cardiomegaly.
- The lung fields may be oligaemic due to a PE.

Fig. 7.3   Algorithm for syncope.

Fig. 7.4   First-line tests to exclude an emergency syncope

Test	Diagnosis
ECG	To look for rhythm disturbance or signs of pulmonary embolus
ECG monitoring on CCU	If suspected cardiac arrhythmia
Temperature, Hb, WBC	To look for septic or haemorrhagic cause
Blood sugar	To look for hypoglycaemia
CT scan	For possible cerebral infarct or TIA, or intracranial bleed causing fits in a patient who has a recent head injury

CCU, coronary care unit; CT, computed tomography; CXR, chest radiography; ECG, electrocardiography; Hb haemoglobin; TIA, transient ischaemic attack; WBC, white blood cell count.

Echocardiography

This may reveal:

- Aortic stenosis.
- Hypertrophic cardiomyopathy.
- Left atrial enlargement in supraventricular tachycardia.
- Left-ventricular abnormalities in ventricular tachycardia or ventricular fibrillation.
- Right-ventricular abnormalities in pulmonary hypertension.

Electrophysiological study of the heart

Consider this if cardiac arrhythmia strongly suspected, but not revealed by Holter monitoring.

Electroencephalography

This will assist in the diagnosis of epilepsy in selected patients.

SYNCOPE OF RECENT ONSET IN AN ILL PATIENT

The importance of this subject is that this situation represents a medical emergency requiring rapid diagnosis and treatment.

It is necessary in this situation to distinguish between the life-threatening causes:

- Intermittent ventricular tachycardia or fibrillation.
- Intermittent asystole ('pauses').
- Pulmonary embolus.
- Shock.
- Hypoglycaemia.

Differentiating features of syncope

The method is to differentiate between cardiac, circulatory and neurological causes. Various diagnoses may disqualify the patient from driving for a period of time (Fig. 7.5).

Cardiac causes

Aortic stenosis

Syncope is effort-induced as the left ventricular output is restricted by the outflow obstruction. The murmur is ejection systolic (a 'seagull murmur' when critically stenosed) and the diagnosis of severe aortic stenosis is supported by the finding of a slow-rising carotid pulse and a heaving apex beat.

Electrocardiography may show left-ventricular hypertrophy. Echocardiography reveals the stenotic valve and assessment by Doppler velocity change through the valve may give an indication of the severity.

Tachyarrhythmias

Syncope tends to be due to a supraventricular tachyarrhythmia only if the heart rate is extremely fast. Ventricular tachycardia is more likely to cause syncope because it is accompanied by asynchronous ventricular contraction. If these arrhythmias are not prominent on Holter monitoring, they may be induced during electrophysiological testing.

Bradyarrhythmias

Syncope may occur secondary to a bradyarrhythmia if the cardiac output falls markedly as a consequence of the drop in rate. An ongoing bradyarrhythmia is easily detected on ECG (e.g. sinus bradycardia and second-degree complete heart block). Some conditions, however, occur intermittently and the ECG may be normal after the syncopal episode; for example, heart block may occur intermittently with normal sinus rhythm between episodes.

Ambulatory ECG monitoring is, therefore, needed to capture these episodes. This may be difficult, if they are separated by long periods of time.

Cardiomyopathies

Hypertrophic obstructive cardiomyopathy can give rise to syncope by obstructing left-ventricular outflow on exercise or as a result of ventricular tachycardia or fibrillation. This arrhythmic 'sudden death syndrome' can also commonly occur in patients who have non-hypertrophic myocardial dysplasias, or patients with severe heart failure (dilated cardiomyopathy).

Prolonged QT interval

This may be congenital or drug-induced, usually by psychiatric or class III antiarrhythmic drugs (see Ch. 16). The syncope is caused by a self-limiting ventricular tachycardia characterized by a systematically rotating QRS vector (torsades de pointes). The tachycardia and syncope are relieved by rapid ('overdrive') pacing or pharmacological sinus tachycardia (e.g. using isoprenaline). The resting non-arrhythmic ECG shows QT prolongation.

Brugada syndrome

This syndrome was first described in 1992 and general awareness of it is still limited. The typical finding is ST elevation at rest in leads V1–V3 of the ECG. The patient presents with episodes of syncope caused by polymorphic VT, which may progress to VF and death if not terminated. It is inherited in an autosomal dominant fashion so there may be a family history of syncope or sudden death.

Circulatory causes

Hypovolaemia

This can present as postural hypotension (i.e. loss of consciousness on standing, relieved by lying flat). This occurs because the blood volume is inadequate, even with an intact baroreflex, to maintain arterial blood pressure in the face of gravity-dependent blood pooling. If this is due to acute haemorrhage there are usually other obvious manifestations such as trauma or haematemesis and melaena. However, internal bleeding can sometimes be difficult to detect. With acute blood loss, the haemoglobin may be normal because there may not have been time for haemodilution to occur.

Septic shock

This causes similar effects by excessive vasodilatation, which prevents baroreflex compensation for postural-dependent blood pooling. However, the patient is usually obviously septic and febrile.

Fig. 7.5 Overview of current DVLA guidelines on driving after syncope

	Group 1 (cars, motorcycles)	Group 2 (HGVs)
Cardiac arrhythmia (atrial or ventricular)	Driving may recommence after condition is diagnosed and has been adequately treated for 1 month	Ejection fraction >40% and condition controlled for 3 months
SA node disease, AV conduction defect	As above	As above
Congenital complete heart block	No restriction if asymptomatic	Permanently bars from driving group 2 vehicles
Pacemaker implantation	1 week off driving	6 weeks off driving
Implantable defibrillator	6 months off driving after implantation and after any shock	Permanently bars from driving group 2 vehicles
First seizure/fit	6 months off driving (unless further seizure is medically likely, see below)	5 years off driving (unless further seizure is medically likely, see below)
Epilepsy	Must be fit-free for 1 year	Must be fit-free for 10 years off anti-epileptic medication

Overview only. See http://www.dft.gov.uk/dvla/medical/medical_professionals.aspx for full guidelines.

Classic postural hypotension

This is due to inadequate baroreflex control. As well as a drop in blood pressure on standing, there may be very little compensatory tachycardia (part of the baroreflex efferent mechanism is to increase heart rate). This can be formally tested by a simple tilt test, during which there is an excessive blood pressure drop and an inadequate tachycardic response.

Obstruction of pulmonary arteries

Obstruction of pulmonary arteries by embolus enters into the differential diagnosis of all cardiovascular emergencies in which syncope is a feature. Chronic thromboembolism or primary pulmonary hypertension can also lead to postural hypotension because the resistance to right ventricular ejection is too high to allow adequate cardiac output when the filling pressure drops on standing.

Cerebrovascular causes

For full explanation of these syndromes, consult *Crash course: Neurology*.

Stroke and transient cerebral ischaemia

TIA very rarely causes loss of consciousness, while the patient is unlikely to regain consciousness quickly after a sufficiently large major territory infarct or haemorrhage. You should be cautious about offering TIA as part of your differential diagnosis for syncope.

Vertebrobasilar syndrome

This is caused by obstruction of the arteries to the posterior part of the brain (brain stem and cerebellum). The syncope may be preceded by vertigo or dizziness. This syndrome is often associated with cervical spondylosis. The vertebral artery becomes kinked on head movement as it travels through the distorted cervical vertebra, causing ischaemia.

Other neurological causes

Neurological causes without any cardiac or arterial aetiology should be studied in *Crash course: Neurology*, but epilepsy should always be borne in mind during history taking.

Metabolic causes

For rare causes see *Crash course: Metabolism and nutrition*.

In the common situation of insulin-dependent diabetes mellitus, most patients are inadequately controlled, which leads to more rapid development of heart disease and autonomic neuropathy. Fear of this drives some patients to control their diabetes mellitus very obsessively and tightly. These patients tend to experience episodes of loss of consciousness due to hypoglycaemia. However, hypoglycaemia can occur in any treated diabetic patient and may be precipitated by exercise or a reduction in food intake.

Palpitations

Objectives

By the end of this chapter you should:
- Be able to take a history and examine a patient who presents with palpitation.
- Understand the differential diagnosis of the causes of palpitation.
- Understand the appropriate investigations for a patient who presents with palpitation.

Palpitation is the abnormal awareness of the heartbeat. Palpitations (multiple episodes of palipitation) may be rapid, slow or just very forceful beats at a normal rate.

DIFFERENTIAL DIAGNOSIS OF PALPITATION

Palpitation may be caused by any disorder producing a change in cardiac rhythm or rate and any disorder causing increased stroke volume.

Rapid palpitations

These may be regular or irregular. Regular palpitation may be a sign of:

- Sinus tachycardia.
- Atrial flutter.
- Atrial tachycardia.
- Supraventricular re-entry tachycardia.

Irregularly irregular palpitation may indicate:

- Atrial fibrillation.
- Multiple atrial or ventricular ectopic beats.

Slow palpitations

Patients often describe these as missed beats or forceful beats (after a pause the next beat is often more forceful due to a long filling time and, therefore, a higher stroke volume). The following may be causes of slow palpitation:

- Sick sinus syndrome.
- Atrioventricular block.
- Occasional ectopics with compensatory pauses.

Disorders causing increased stroke volume

Increased stroke volume may result from:

- Valvular lesions (e.g. mitral or aortic regurgitation).
- High-output states (e.g. pregnancy, thyrotoxicosis or anaemia).

HISTORY TO FOCUS ON THE DIFFERENTIAL DIAGNOSIS OF PALPITATION

When taking a history from a patient complaining of palpitation, aim to find answers to the following three questions:

1. What is the nature of the palpitation?
2. How severe or life-threatening is it?
3. What is the likely underlying cause?

Nature of the palpitation

Ask the patient to describe the palpitation by tapping it out (fast, slow, regular or irregular). Are the episodes continuous or intermittent (paroxysmal is the term used for intermittent tachycardias), is the onset sudden or progressive?

Severity of palpitation

Determine the severity of the palpitation (i.e. is it in the context of cardiac failure, exacerbation of ischaemic heart disease or thromboembolic events?).

Is the palpitation associated with:

- Syncope, dizziness or shortness of breath – suggesting that cardiac output is compromised?
- Angina – suggesting it is causing or being caused by underlying ischaemic heart disease?
- A history of stroke or transient ischaemic attack or limb ischaemia – suggesting thromboembolic complications of arrhythmia?

Likely underlying causes of palpitation

Are there any features in the history suggestive of the recognized causes of arrhythmias shown in Fig. 8.1.

Fig. 8.1 Features in the history that might suggest the cause of an arrhythmia

Features in the history	Cause of arrhythmia
Chest pain, breathlessness on exertion, history of myocardial infarction, history of bypass surgery	Ischaemic heart disease
Tremor, excessive sweating, unexplained weight loss, lethargy, obesity, history of thyroid surgery	Thyroid disease
History of rheumatic fever	Heart valve disease
Peptic ulcer disease, menorrhagia, recent operation	Anaemia
Alcohol, caffeine, amphetamine, antiarrhythmic agents	Proarrhythmic drugs
Anxiety	Anxiety

EXAMINATION OF PATIENTS WHO HAVE PALPITATION

HINTS AND TIPS

Remember, when examining any patient who has a supposedly cardiac problem you must perform a thorough examination of all systems. Cardiac disease

can both cause and be caused by disease in other systems, so don't get caught out.

Fig. 8.2 summarizes the important points in the examination of a patient who has palpitation, which are outlined below.

General observation

Look for:
- Cyanosis – suggestive of cardiac failure or lung disease (remember that pulmonary embolus is a well-recognized cause of tachyarrhythmia).
- Dyspnoea – suggestive of cardiac failure or lung disease.
- Pallor – suggestive of anaemia.
- Thyrotoxic or myxoedematous facies.

Cardiovascular system

Pulse

Note the rate, rhythm and character of the pulse at the radial artery (time it for at least 15 s). Information on the character of the pulse is often more clearly elicited from the carotid pulse, especially features such as a:
- Slow rising pulse – due to aortic stenosis.
- Collapsing pulse – due to aortic regurgitation.

Fig. 8.2 Important points to note when examining a patient who has palpitation. CVA, cerebrovascular accident; JVP, jugular venous pressure.

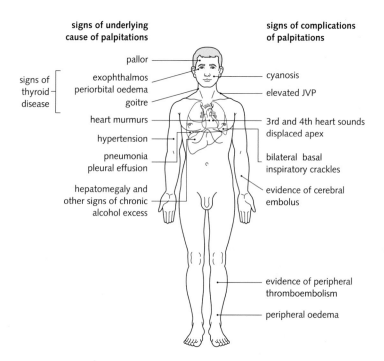

A high-volume pulse (due to high-output states and aortic or mitral regurgitation) is often most easily felt at the radial pulse, where it is felt as an abnormally strong pulsation.

Blood pressure

Hypertension is a cause of atrial fibrillation. A wide pulse pressure is a sign of aortic regurgitation.

Jugular venous pressure

The jugular venous pressure may be elevated if the patient has congestive cardiac failure as a consequence of an uncontrolled tachycardia or has atrial flutter or fibrillation secondary to pulmonary embolism.

Apex beat

This may be displaced in a patient who has left-ventricular failure.

Heart sounds

A third or fourth heart sound may be heard. Murmurs of mitral or aortic regurgitation are possible causes of high-output state. The murmur of mitral stenosis may be heard in patients who have atrial fibrillation.

Respiratory system

Bilateral basal inspiratory crepitations are heard in a patient who has left-ventricular failure. There may be signs of an underlying chest infection (consolidation or effusion), a common cause of palpitations.

Gastrointestinal system

Hepatomegaly and ascites may be signs of congestive cardiac failure or alcoholic liver disease – alcohol is one of the most common causes of tachyarrhythmias. Look for other signs of liver disease if this is suspected.

Limbs

On examining the limbs note the following points:
- Peripheral oedema may be a sign of congestive cardiac failure.
- Tremor may be a sign of thyrotoxicosis or alcohol withdrawal.
- Brisk reflexes seen in thyrotoxicosis.
- Weakness – may be a sign of previous cerebral embolus.

INVESTIGATION OF PATIENTS WHO HAVE PALPITATION

An algorithm for the investigation of palpitation is given in Fig. 8.3.

Biochemical tests

The following blood tests may aid diagnosis:
- Electrolytes – hypokalaemia is an aggravating factor for most tachyarrhythmias.
- Full blood count – anaemia or a leucocytosis suggesting sepsis may be evident.
- Thyroid function tests.
- Liver function tests – deranged in congestive cardiac failure or alcoholic liver disease.
- 24-h urinary catecholamines – to exclude phaeochromocytoma.

Electrocardiography

12-lead electrocardiography

This may enable the diagnosis to be made instantly. However, if the palpitation is intermittent or paroxysmal the ECG may be normal.

There may be signs of the cause of the palpitation on the ECG, for example ischaemia, hypertension or presence of a delta wave or short PR interval as seen in some congenital causes of paroxysmal tachyarrhythmias, such as Wolff–Parkinson–White syndrome (pre-excitation).

24-h electrocardiography

Monitoring of the ECG for 24 h may reveal paroxysmal arrhythmias. Patients press an alert button when they have symptoms, and this section of the ECG is then marked for review. Longer-term monitors (external or implantable) may be necessary to document infrequent episodes.

> **COMMUNICATION**
>
> Ask about frequency of episodes; remember, a normal 24-h tape doesn't exclude arrhythmia if they haven't had any symptoms

Exercise electrocardiography

This test can be used to reveal exercise-induced arrhythmias. Examples of ECGs illustrating atrial fibrillation, atrial flutter and supraventricular re-entry tachycardia (SVT) are shown in Fig. 8.4.

Vagotonic manoeuvres

Such manoeuvres include:
- Valsalva manoeuvre.
- Carotid sinus massage.
- Diving reflex.
- Painful stimuli.

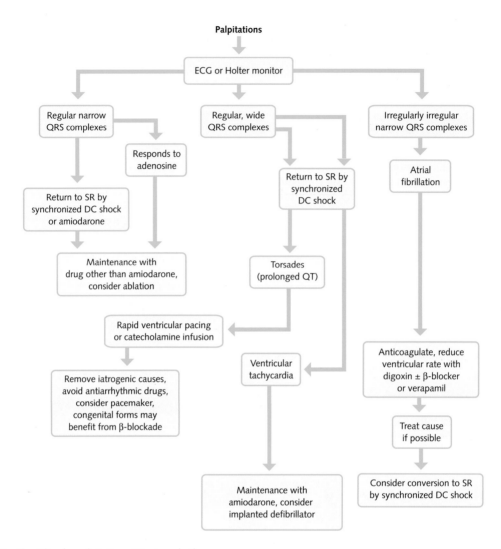

Fig. 8.3 Algorithm for palpitations. SR, sinus rhythm.

These manoeuvres all act by increasing vagal tone, which in turn increases the refractory period of the atrio-ventricular (AV) node and increases AV node conduction time. By doing this it is possible to differentiate between three common tachyarrhythmias that are sometimes indistinguishable on ECG recording:

1. Atrial flutter.
2. Atrial fibrillation.
3. Supraventricular re-entry tachycardia.

HINTS AND TIPS

The first thing to do when you see a fast heart rhythm is to establish the clinical status of the patient. Following this, determine if it is narrow complex (atrial flutter, SVT) or broad complex tachycardia (ventricular tachycardia).

You also need to determine whether the rhythm is regular (atrial flutter, SVT or VT) or irregular (atrial fibrillation).

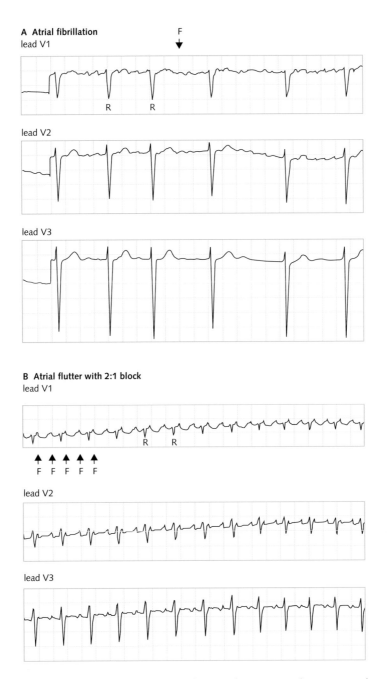

Fig. 8.4 Electrocardiograms illustrating atrial fibrillation, atrial flutter and supraventricular re-entry tachycardia. **(A)** Note the narrow QRS complexes. Fibrillation waves (F) can sometimes be seen. Note the irregularly irregular rhythm and the absence of P waves preceding the QRS complexes. The baseline may show an irregular fibrillating pattern. **(B)** Note the regular rhythm with a rate divisible into 300 (150 beats/min in this case). The P waves are seen in all three leads, but best in V1 at a rate of 300/min. Occasionally, the F (flutter) waves form a sawtooth-like pattern (not shown here). Note the F waves at 200-ms intervals (300/min), narrow QRS and regular RR intervals at 400 ms (150/min).

Continued

C Supraventricular re-entry tachycardia

lead V1

lead V2

lead V3

↑
X

Figure 8-4—cont'd **(C)** The rhythm is regular and fast (usually 140–240 beats/min). P waves can be seen; these can occur before or after the QRS. Point X shows reversion back to sinus rhythm – note that the following beat has a normal P wave preceding it.

Broad complex tachycardia can occur in atrial fibrillation or atrial flutter when there is also aberrant conduction across the AV node. However, any broad complex tachycardia should always be assumed to be ventricular in origin, because it is sometimes difficult to differentiate between the two.

The characteristic features of these tachyarrhythmias are listed in Fig. 8.5.

Adenosine administration

Adenosine is a purine nucleoside that acts to block the AV node. When administered intravenously it will achieve complete AV block. Its half-life is very short (only a few seconds), so this effect is very short lived.

Side effects of adenosine include bronchospasm, so avoid in asthmatics.

Echocardiography

This will reveal any valvular pathology. It also enables evaluation of left-ventricular function.

Fig. 8.5 Characteristic features of atrial fibrillation, atrial flutter and supraventricular re-entry tachycardia

	Atrial fibrillation	Atrial flutter	Supraventricular re-entry tachycardia
Rate	Any rate; pulse deficit if fast	Atrial flutter rate is 300/min; the ventricular response is therefore divisible into this (usually 100 or 150/min)	140–260 beats/min
Rhythm	Irregularly irregular	Regular	Regular
Response to adenosine or Valsalva manoeuvre	Slowing of ventricular rate reveals underlying lack of P waves	Slowing of ventricular rate reveals underlying flutter waves	Blocking the AV node might 'break' the re-entry circuit and terminate the tachycardia
AV node, atrioventricular node.			

Electrophysiological study

This is useful in investigating patients suspected of having tachyarrhythmias due to abnormal re-entry pathways. The technique enables localization of the re-entry circuit, which may then be ablated using a radiofrequency thermal electrode placed inside the heart.

Other investigations

Various other investigations may be required to identify a suspected cause of the palpitation. These depend upon the clinical evidence, for example:

- V/Q scan or CTPA, if a pulmonary embolus is likely.
- Coronary angiogram, if coronary artery disease is suspected.

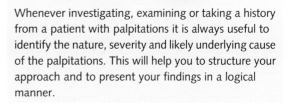

HINTS AND TIPS

Whenever investigating, examining or taking a history from a patient with palpitations it is always useful to identify the nature, severity and likely underlying cause of the palpitations. This will help you to structure your approach and to present your findings in a logical manner.

Peripheral oedema

By the end of this chapter you should:
- Be able to take a history and examine a patient who presents with peripheral oedema.
- Understand the causes of peripheral oedema.
- Understand the appropriate investigations for a patient who presents with peripheral oedema.

Peripheral oedema is caused by an increase in extracellular fluid. The fluid will follow gravity and, therefore, the ankles are the first part affected in the upright patient. Ankle swelling is indicative of oedema if there is not a local acute or chronic traumatic cause. Oedema may be a feature of generalized fluid retention or obstruction of fluid drainage from the lower limbs.

DIFFERENTIAL DIAGNOSIS OF OEDEMA

There are a number of causes of oedema that can be divided into five main groups (Fig. 9.1):
- Cardiac failure – this is due to increased sodium retention secondary to activation of the renin-angiotensin system.
- Hypoalbuminaemia – loss of oncotic pressure within the capillaries causes loss of fluid from the intravascular space.
- Renal impairment – reduction in sodium excretion results in water retention.
- Hepatic cirrhosis – there are a number of mechanisms involved: hypoalbuminaemia (occurs as the hepatic synthetic activity is reduced), peripheral vasodilatation and activation of the renin-angiotensin system with resulting sodium retention.
- Drugs (e.g. corticosteroids or calcium channel blockers).
- Venous disease, obesity and lymphoedema.

HISTORY TO FOCUS ON THE DIFFERENTIAL DIAGNOSIS OF PERIPHERAL OEDEMA

The first differentiation to be made is between cardiac and non-cardiac oedema. The cause of the oedema is usually revealed by a detailed systems review because there are often symptoms related to the underlying disorder. Associated breathlessness suggests:
- Pulmonary oedema – this can occur due to cardiac failure or renal failure.
- Chronic lung disease (e.g. chronic obstructive airways disease causes breathlessness).
- Primary and thromboembolic pulmonary hypertension – cause breathlessness and right heart failure.

Other important signs and symptoms include:
- Chest pain and palpitations – suggest underlying cardiac disease (ischaemia or arrhythmias, respectively).
- A history of alcohol or drug abuse or of previous liver disease – suggests a hepatic cause for the oedema.
- Diarrhoea – may be due to a protein-losing enteropathy.

Past medical history

A detailed history of all previous illnesses and operations will provide clues in a patient who has longstanding cardiac, hepatic or liver disease.

Drug history

Important points include the following:
- Some drugs may be renotoxic (e.g. NSAIDs, ACE inhibitors).
- Some drugs may be hepatotoxic (e.g. methotrexate).
- Dihydropyridine calcium channel blockers cause ankle oedema in approximately 8% of patients.

Social history

Important findings may include:
- Cigarette smoking – a risk factor for ischaemic heart disease.
- Intravenous drug abuse – a risk factor for hepatitis.
- Alcohol abuse – a risk factor for hepatic cirrhosis.

Fig. 9.1 Differential diagnosis of peripheral oedema

Pathology	Cause
Congestive cardiac failure	Myocardial infarction, recurrent tachyarrhythmias (particularly atrial fibrillation), hypertensive heart disease, myocarditis, cardiomyopathy due to drugs and toxins, mitral, aortic, or pulmonary valve disease
Right heart failure secondary to pulmonary hypertension (cor pulmonale)	Chronic lung disease, primary pulmonary hypertension
Hypoalbuminaemia	Excessive protein loss (due to nephrotic syndrome, extensive burns, protein-losing enteropathy), reduced protein production (due to liver failure) or inadequate protein intake (due to protein-energy malnutrition)
Renal disease	Any cause of renal impairment (e.g. hypertension, diabetes mellitus, autoimmune disease, infection)
Liver cirrhosis	Alcohol, hepatitis A, B, C, autoimmune chronic active hepatitis, biliary cirrhosis, Wilson disease, haemochromatosis, drugs
Idiopathic	Premenstrual oedema
Arteriolar dilatation (exposing the capillaries to high pressure, so increasing intravascular hydrostatic pressure)	Dihydropyridine calcium channel blockers (e.g. nifedipine, amlodipine)
Sodium retention	Cushing disease resulting in excessive mineralocorticoid activity, corticosteroids

HINTS AND TIPS

Causes of localized oedema in either the arms or legs include:
• Local venous thrombosis or compression.
• Local cellulitis.
• Local trauma.
• Lymphoedema secondary to obstruction of lymphatic drainage (e.g. secondary to malignancy).

EXAMINATION OF PATIENTS WHO HAVE OEDEMA

A thorough examination of all systems usually reveals the underlying disease.

Cardiovascular system

Check the pulse and blood pressure:
• The pulse is often fast in the patient who has cardiac failure.
• Blood pressure may be low.
• Patients who have chronic renal disease are often hypertensive.

Check the jugular venous pressure (JVP). A raised JVP indicates an increased right atrial pressure.

On examination of the praecordium:
• The apex may be dyskinetic and laterally displaced in the patient who has cardiac failure.
• There may be a left parasternal heave suggestive of right-ventricular strain.
• There may be added third and fourth heart sounds in cardiac failure (a 'gallop' rhythm).
• Audible murmurs may be present suggesting a valvular cause for cardiac failure.

Respiratory system

On inspection, consider the following:
• The patient may be tachypnoeic and cyanosed – this may be secondary to cardiac or respiratory disease.
• The lungs may be hyperinflated (due to emphysema) or show reduced expansion.

Expansion is reduced in all causes of lung disease, except perhaps primary pulmonary hypertension.

The lung bases may be stony dull (with absent breath sounds) indicating bilateral pleural effusions – these are a sign of generalized fluid retention.

Findings on auscultation of the lungs can include:
• Bilateral basal fine inspiratory crepitations suggesting left ventricular failure.

- Coarse crepitations or wheeze, which may be heard in bronchitis or emphysema.
- Mid-inspiratory crepitations, which may be heard in pulmonary fibrosis.

Gastrointestinal system

Inspect for:

- Signs of chronic liver disease, such as jaundice, spider naevi, gynaecomastia, loss of body hair and testicular atrophy.
- Signs of encephalopathy such as confusion and a liver flap.

Palpation of the abdomen may reveal ascites in patients who have liver, cardiac or renal disease. A *caput medusae* may be evident.

Renal system

On inspection:

- The patient may have earthy discolouration of the skin secondary to uraemia.
- Patients with renal failure may be anaemic (pale sclerae).
- There might be evidence of ongoing dialysis, either though the presence of fistulae (usually in the forearms) or tubing attached to the abdomen in ambulatory peritoneal dialysis.

On examination:

- Patients are occasionally hypertensive.
- The JVP may be raised as a result of fluid retention.
- Lung bases may be stony dull due to bilateral pleural effusions.
- Auscultation may reveal a pericardial rub.
- Bilateral basal inspiratory crepitations suggest pulmonary congestion.

Dip the urine – this is part of every examination of the cardiovascular system. Proteinuria is a feature of nephrotic syndrome and other causes of renal impairment. Haematuria is seen in some diseases causing renal impairment.

Examination of the oedema

Oedema of generalized fluid retention is pitting in nature. To demonstrate this, the area in question should be pressed firmly for at least 15 s – there will be an indent in the oedema after this. Be careful: ankle oedema may be tender. The severity of the ankle oedema can be roughly gauged by the extent to which the oedema can be felt up the leg. Lymphoedema and chronic venous oedema do not 'pit'. Fig. 9.2 summarizes the findings in patients who have ankle swelling.

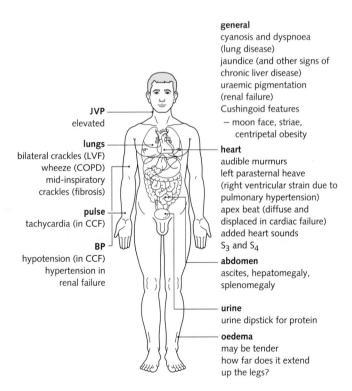

general
cyanosis and dyspnoea (lung disease)
jaundice (and other signs of chronic liver disease)
uraemic pigmentation (renal failure)
Cushingoid features
 — moon face, striae, centripetal obesity

JVP
elevated

lungs
bilateral crackles (LVF)
wheeze (COPD)
mid-inspiratory crackles (fibrosis)

heart
audible murmurs
left parasternal heave (right ventricular strain due to pulmonary hypertension)
apex beat (diffuse and displaced in cardiac failure)
added heart sounds S_3 and S_4

pulse
tachycardia (in CCF)

BP
hypotension (in CCF)
hypertension in renal failure

abdomen
ascites, hepatomegaly, splenomegaly

urine
urine dipstick for protein

oedema
may be tender
how far does it extend up the legs?

Fig. 9.2 Signs in patients who present with ankle swelling. BP, blood pressure; CCF, congestive cardiac failure; COPD, chronic obstructive pulmonary disease; JVP, jugular venous pressure; LVF, left ventricular failure.

When assessing a patient with peripheral oedema for the first time it is useful to ask about ankle swelling – as fluid follows gravity it is often first noticed in the lower limbs in the mobile patient, and may be most pronounced by the end of the day. In the supine patient this swelling may also be detectable around the sacrum.

INVESTIGATION OF PATIENTS WHO HAVE OEDEMA

An algorithm for the investigation of peripheral oedema is given in Fig. 9.3.

Blood tests

The following blood tests should be considered:

- Full blood count – anaemia is common in chronic renal disease and can precipitate cardiac failure.

- Renal function – this will be abnormal in primary renal disease, but also commonly in heart failure or liver disease.
- Liver function – this is abnormal in liver disease, but note that hepatic congestion due to cardiac failure also causes abnormal liver function tests.
- Plasma albumin concentration.
- Thyroid function – hyperthyroidism may precipitate cardiac failure, hypothyroidism can cause oedema.

Urine tests

With urine tests, note:

- A 24-h urine protein excretion test is mandatory if there is no evidence of cardiac disease and the plasma albumin is low.
- Nephrotic syndrome causes loss of at least 3 g protein in 24 h.
- The albumin:creatinine (A:Cr) ratio may also be used to estimate proteinuria, avoiding the need for 24-h collections.

Fig. 9.3 Algorithm for peripheral oedema. ACE, angiotensin-converting enzyme; CXR, chest X-ray; JVP, jugular venous pressure; LV, left ventricular.

Arterial blood gases

Looking for:

- Hypoxia, which may be caused by lung or cardiac disease.
- Carbon dioxide retention, which is a sign of chronic obstructive airways disease.
- Acidosis, which can occur with normal oxygen and carbon dioxide (metabolic acidosis) in both liver and renal failure.

Electrocardiography

This may show evidence of old myocardial infarction in a patient who has cardiac failure. Atrial fibrillation is common in patients with heart failure.

Chest radiography

Chest radiography may show:

- Cardiomegaly (increased cardiothoracic ratio).
- Signs of pulmonary oedema (Bat's wing shadowing, upper lobe blood diversion, Kerley B lines).
- Pleural effusions.
- Lung overexpansion.

Echocardiography

This may show impaired ventricular function, and a dilated ventricle. Valve lesions may also be seen.

Ultrasound

Regarding ultrasound:

- In a patient who has no evidence of cardiac, renal or liver disease and bilateral ankle oedema, a venous obstruction or external compression must be excluded.
- Doppler ultrasound to detect venous thrombosis and ultrasound of the pelvis to exclude a mass lesion causing compression are appropriate.

IMPORTANT ASPECTS

Salt and water retention

It is important to appreciate that oedema in heart failure is due to generalized salt and water retention, which results from the neurohumoral response to heart failure (see Ch. 19 and Fig. 9.4). The symptoms and signs do

Fig. 9.4   The vicious cycle of heart failure.

not, therefore, differ from those due to generalized salt and water retention in other conditions with similar neurohumoral response. A similar picture is obtained when the salt and water retention is primarily renal in origin.

Increase in extracellular water and intravascular blood volume

Salt and water retention cause an increase in extracellular water and intravascular blood volume. The increase in volume of blood in the heart and central vessels increases pressures, including right atrial pressure. This is appreciated clinically as raised JVP. It can be observed very simply that the appearance of oedema occurs first and that the increase in JVP follows as the central compartment subsequently fills up. When diuretics are administered, the JVP goes down first before the peripheral oedema disappears. Therefore, it is incorrect to diagnose right heart failure from a raised JVP in the presence of oedema, but only where the JVP is raised when oedema is absent or has been removed.

Hypertension treated with calcium antagonists

Oedema commonly appears in patients who have hypertension treated with the dihydropyridine calcium antagonists (e.g. nifedipine, amlodipine). This is due to disturbance of Starling's forces in the tissue, not to general fluid retention. This type of oedema should not be treated with diuretics, which cause electrolyte depletion.

Heart murmur 10

By the end of this chapter you should:
• Be able to take a history and examine a patient with a heart murmur.
• Understand the differential diagnosis for the causes of a heart murmur.
• Understand the appropriate investigations for a patient presenting with a heart murmur.

A heart murmur is the sound caused by turbulence of blood flow, which occurs when the velocity of blood is disproportionate to the size of the orifice it is moving through.

DIFFERENTIAL DIAGNOSIS OF A HEART MURMUR

Many conditions can give rise to a murmur:
• Valve lesions – either stenosis or regurgitation of any heart valve.
• Left-ventricular outflow obstruction – an example is hypertrophic cardiomyopathy (HCM).
• Ventricular septal defect.
• Vascular disorders – coarctation of the aorta, patent ductus arteriosus, arteriovenous malformations (pulmonary or intercostal) and venous hum (cervical or hepatic).
• Increased blood flow – normal anatomy, but increased blood flow as in high-output states. Examples of high-output states are anaemia, pregnancy, thyrotoxicosis or childhood.
• Increased flow across a normal pulmonary valve in atrial and ventricular septal defect.

HINTS AND TIPS

Cardiac sounds can be confused for murmurs. These include:
• Third and fourth heart sounds.
• Mid-systolic clicks, heard in mitral valve prolapse.
• Pericardial friction rub.

A differential diagnosis of heart murmur is shown in Fig. 10.1.

HISTORY TO FOCUS ON THE DIFFERENTIAL DIAGNOSIS OF A HEART MURMUR

HINTS AND TIPS

When taking a history from a patient who has a heart murmur, aim to answer the following questions:
• What is the possible aetiology of the murmur e.g. infective endocarditis, valve lesion secondary to rheumatic heart disease, high-output state, etc.?
• Are there any complications of valve disease e.g. cardiac failure, exacerbation of ischaemic heart disease, arrhythmias, syncope, etc.?

Presenting complaint

Common presenting complaints include:
• Shortness of breath – suggestive of cardiac failure; also ankle swelling, paroxysmal nocturnal dyspnoea and fatigue.
• Chest pain – due to ischaemic heart disease or atypical chest pain seen in patients who have mitral valve prolapse.
• Syncope – especially seen in patients who have left-ventricular outflow obstruction (e.g. aortic stenosis or HCM).
• Fever, rigors and malaise – common presenting complaints in patients who have infective endocarditis.
• Palpitations – for example, mitral valve disease is associated with atrial fibrillation.

Past medical history

Aim to elicit any history of cardiac disease with particular emphasis on possible causes of a murmur:
• History of rheumatic fever in childhood.

Fig. 10.1 Differential diagnosis of heart murmur

Phase of cardiac cycle	Nature of murmur	Valve lesion	Cause of valve lesion
Systolic	Ejection systolic	Aortic stenosis (AS)	Valvular stenosis, congenital valvular abnormality, rheumatic fever, supravalvular stenosis, subvalvular stenosis, senile valvular calcification
		Aortic sclerosis	Aortic valve roughening
		HCM	Left ventricular outflow tract (subaortic) stenosis, louder on standing or valsalva (increases gradient by emptying left ventricle)
		Increased flow across normal valve	High-output states (e.g. anaemia, fever, pregnancy, thyrotoxicosis)
	Pansystolic	Mitral regurgitation (MR)	Functional MR due to dilatation of mitral valve annulus Valvular MR: rheumatic fever, infective endocarditis, mitral valve prolapse, chordal rupture, papillary muscle infarct
		Tricuspid regurgitation (TR)	Functional TR Valvular TR: rheumatic fever, infective endocarditis
		VSD with left to right shunt	Congenital, septal infarct (acquired)
Diastolic	Early diastolic	Aortic regurgitation (AR)	Functional AR: dilatation of valve ring, aortic dissection, cystic medial necrosis (Marfan syndrome) Valvular AR: rheumatic fever, infective endocarditis, bicuspid aortic valve
		Pulmonary regurgitation (PR)	Functional PR: dilatation of valve ring, Marfan syndrome, pulmonary hypertension Valvular PR: rheumatic fever, carcinoid, tetralogy of Fallot
	Mid-diastolic	Mitral stenosis (MS)	Rheumatic fever, congenital
		Tricuspid stenosis (TS)	Rheumatic fever
		Left and right atrial myxomas	Tumour obstruction of valve orifice in diastole
Continuous		PDA	Congenital
		Arteriovenous fistula	
		Cervical venous hum	

HCM, hypertrophic cardiomyopathy; PDA, patent ductus arteriosus; VSD, ventricular septal defect.

- Previous cardiac surgery.
- Myocardial infarction in past – may cause ventricular dilatation and, therefore, functional mitral regurgitation or dysfunction of papillary muscle leading to mitral regurgitation.
- Family history of cardiac problems or sudden death – as may occur for patients who have HCM.
- Recent dental procedures or operations – may be a cause of infective endocarditis.

Social history

Ask in particular about:

- Smoking – an important risk factor for ischaemic heart disease.

- Alcohol intake – if excessive may result in dilated cardiomyopathy.
- History of intravenous drug abuse.

EXAMINATION OF PATIENTS WHO HAVE A HEART MURMUR

General observation

Look for signs of cardiac failure (i.e. dyspnoea, cyanosis or oedema). Look also for clues indicating the cause of the murmur:

- Anaemia – may cause a high-output state or be caused by infective endocarditis.

- Scars of previous cardiac surgery – median sternotomy, thoracotomy or valvuloplasty scars.

Examine the eyes for retinal haemorrhages (Roth spots) and conjunctival haemorrhages. These are signs of infective endocarditis.

Fig. 10.2 gives a summary of the findings on examination of a patient who has a heart murmur.

Hands

Look for peripheral stigmas of infective endocarditis:

- Splinter haemorrhages – more than five is pathological.
- Osler nodes (purplish raised papules on finger pulps).
- Janeway lesions (erythematous non-tender lesions on the thenar eminence).
- Finger clubbing.

Cardiovascular system

Pulse

Examine the pulse at both the radial site and the carotid artery. Examples of abnormal pulse due to valvular disease include:

- Slow rising or plateau pulse in aortic stenosis.
- Collapsing or waterhammer pulse in aortic regurgitation or patent ductus arteriosus.
- Bisferiens pulse in mixed aortic valve disease.
- A jerky pulse in HCM.

Blood pressure

This may also give important clues:

- A narrow pulse pressure associated with hypotension is a sign of severe aortic stenosis.
- A wide pulse pressure may be seen in aortic regurgitation or high-output states.

Jugular venous pressure

Remember the patient must be at 45° with the neck muscles relaxed. The jugular venous pressure is measured as the height of the visible pulsation vertically from the sternal angle. Possible findings include:

- An elevated jugular venous pressure in congestive cardiac failure.
- Large 'a' waves (see Fig. 2.4) in pulmonary stenosis and pulmonary hypertension.
- Large 'v' waves – a sign of tricuspid regurgitation.

Praecordium

Remember to look for scars of previous surgery. On palpation, the apex beat is the lowest and most lateral point at which the cardiac impulse can be felt. Possible abnormalities in a patient who has a murmur include:

- Displaced apex beat – due to mitral regurgitation and aortic regurgitation.
- Double apical impulse – due to HCM, also left ventricular aneurysm.
- Tapping apex beat – due to mitral stenosis.
- Heaving apex beat – due to aortic stenosis or LVH.
- Thrusting apex beat – due to aortic or mitral regurgitation or any high-output state.

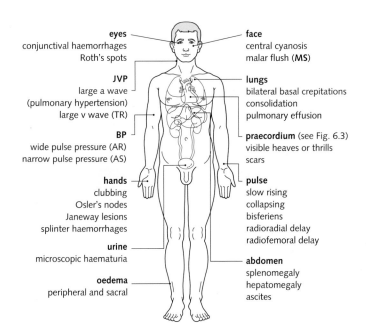

Fig. 10.2 Possible findings in a patient who has a heart murmur. AS, aortic stenosis; AR, aortic regurgitation; MS, mitral stenosis; TR, tricuspid regurgitation.

eyes
conjunctival haemorrhages
Roth's spots

face
central cyanosis
malar flush (**MS**)

JVP
large a wave
(pulmonary hypertension)
large v wave (TR)

lungs
bilateral basal crepitations
consolidation
pulmonary effusion

BP
wide pulse pressure (AR)
narrow pulse pressure (AS)

praecordium (see Fig. 6.3)
visible heaves or thrills
scars

hands
clubbing
Osler's nodes
Janeway lesions
splinter haemorrhages

pulse
slow rising
collapsing
bisferiens
radioradial delay
radiofemoral delay

urine
microscopic haematuria

abdomen
splenomegaly
hepatomegaly
ascites

oedema
peripheral and sacral

Right-ventricular heave is a sign of right-ventricular strain and may be felt in patients who have right-ventricular failure due to mitral valve disease.

Thrills (or palpable murmurs) may be felt in any of the cardiac areas where the corresponding murmurs are best heard. The positions of valve areas are shown in Fig. 10.3.

HINTS AND TIPS

Murmurs from valves on the left side of the heart (mitral and aortic) are heard best in expiration. Those from the right side of the heart (pulmonary and tricuspid) are heard best in inspiration.

Characteristics of common murmurs are listed in Fig. 10.4.

HINTS AND TIPS

Many students (and doctors!) find auscultation and interpretation of murmurs difficult. Don't worry – if you listen carefully to the cardiac cycle of every patient that you examine, to get a feel for the range of normal sounds, then you will start to pick up abnormal sounds more easily.

Peripheral vascular system

All peripheral pulses should be palpated. Radioradial delay and radiofemoral delay may be found with coarctation of the aorta. Also seen in this condition is discrepancy in the blood pressure taken in each arm. It is important to look for these signs as part of the cardiovascular examination.

HINTS AND TIPS

It is important to know these characteristics for each of the common murmurs:
• Location at which to listen for the murmur.
• Position of the patient for each murmur.
• Phase of respiration during which each murmur is best heard.
• Nature of the murmur and where it radiates.

Peripheral oedema

This may be elicited by applying firm pressure for at least 15 s, eliciting 'pitting oedema' can be painful for the patient – so be careful.

Respiratory system

The chest should be carefully examined. Possible findings include:

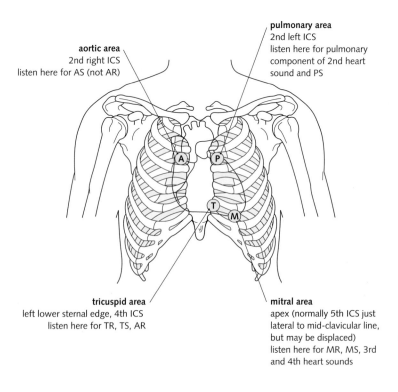

Fig. 10.3 Praecordium, illustrating the position of valve areas. AR, aortic regurgitation; AS, aortic stenosis; ICS, intercostal space; MR, mitral regurgitation; MS, mitral stenosis; PS, pulmonary stenosis; TR, tricuspid regurgitation; TS, tricuspid stenosis.

pulmonary area
2nd left ICS
listen here for pulmonary component of 2nd heart sound and PS

aortic area
2nd right ICS
listen here for AS (not AR)

tricuspid area
left lower sternal edge, 4th ICS
listen here for TR, TS, AR

mitral area
apex (normally 5th ICS just lateral to mid-clavicular line, but may be displaced)
listen here for MR, MS, 3rd and 4th heart sounds

Fig. 10.4 Important characteristics of common murmurs

Valve lesion	Murmur	Patient position	Phase of respiration	Radiation	Other features
MS	Mid-diastolic, low and rumbling, listen with bell of stethoscope, loud S_1, OS	Lying on left side	Expiration	None	Tapping non-displaced apex; often associated with atrial fibrillation; pulmonary hypertension may occur with loud P_2 and TR
MR	Pansystolic, listen with diaphragm of stethoscope, soft S_1	On back at 45°	Expiration	To axilla	Thrusting, displaced apex, may be associated with atrial fibrillation
AS	Ejection systolic murmur, listen with diaphragm, may get reversal of S_2 due to prolonged LV emptying	On back at 45°	Expiration	To carotid arteries	Heaving, non-displaced apex; slow-rising, low-volume pulse
AR	Soft, blowing early diastolic murmur, heard in tricuspid area, soft S_2, may hear Austin Flint murmur, listen with diaphragm	Sitting forward	Expiration	None	Thrusting, displaced apex; waterhammer (collapsing) pulse, wide pulse pressure, Duroziez sign, Quincke sign, pistol shot femorals, de Musset sign

The second heart sound (S_2) has two components: A_2 (aortic value closure) and P_2 (pulmonary valve closure). AS, aortic stenosis; AR, aortic regurgitation; LV, left ventricle; MR, mitral regurgitation; MS, mitral stenosis; OS, opening snap; S1, first heart sound; TR, tricuspid regurgitation.

- Bilateral basal fine end-inspiratory crepitations – suggests pulmonary oedema.
- Evidence of respiratory tract infection – sepsis may cause a high-output state.

Gastrointestinal system

Important findings include:

- Hepatomegaly or ascites, seen in right-sided heart failure or congestive cardiac failure.
- Splenomegaly, a feature of infective endocarditis.

Dipstick test of the urine should always be performed as part of the bedside examination. Microscopic haematuria is a common finding in patients who have infective endocarditis.

INVESTIGATION OF PATIENTS WHO HAVE A HEART MURMUR

An algorithm for the investigation of heart murmur is given in Fig. 10.5.

Blood tests

These include:

- Full blood count – anaemia may be seen as a sign of chronic disease in a patient who has infective endocarditis and is also a cause of hyperdynamic state; a leucocytosis is also a feature of infective endocarditis.
- Urea, creatinine and electrolytes – may be deranged in patients who have cardiac failure as a result of poor renal perfusion or diuretic therapy.
- Liver function tests – these may be abnormal in patients who have hepatic congestion secondary to cardiac failure.
- Blood cultures – at least three sets should be taken before commencement of antibiotic therapy in all patients in whom infective endocarditis is suspected.
- ESR and C-reactive protein (CRP) – these are markers of inflammation or infection and are useful in monitoring treatment of infective endocarditis.

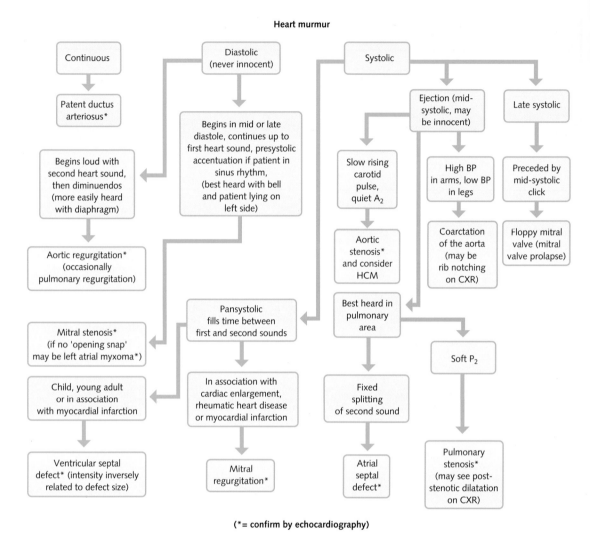

Fig. 10.5 Algorithm for heart murmur. BP, blood pressure; CXR, chest X-ray; HCM, hypertrophic cardiomyopathy.

Chest radiography

This may reveal an abnormal cardiac shadow (e.g. large left atrium and prominent pulmonary vessels in mitral stenosis, enlarged left ventricle in mitral or aortic regurgitation, or the abnormal aortic shadow in coarctation).

Abnormality in the lung fields may also be seen (e.g. pulmonary oedema, pulmonary effusion).

Electrocardiography

The 12-lead ECG may give useful information:

- Atrial fibrillation may be a sign of mitral valve disease.
- Left-ventricular strain pattern may be seen in aortic stenosis.
- P mitrale may be seen in the ECG if there is pulmonary hypertension secondary to valve disease (as occurs in severe mitral stenosis).

Echocardiography

Transthoracic echocardiography

Transthoracic echocardiography enables the valves to be visualized and pressure gradients across them to be assessed. Left-ventricular function and pulmonary artery pressure can be estimated. The presence of ventricular septal defect or patent ductus arteriosus may be more accurately assessed by cardiac catheterization, but they may be visualized using echocardiography.

Transoesophageal echocardiography

Transoesophageal echocardiography is very useful because it gives very detailed information on structures that are difficult to see using transthoracic echocardiography. Examples of its uses include:

- Assessment of prosthetic valves.
- Detailed evaluation of the mitral valve before mitral valve repair.

Cardiac catheterization

Before valve replacement this is performed to obtain information about the:

- Presence of coexisting coronary-artery disease.
- Degree of pulmonary hypertension in patients who have mitral valve disease.

This investigation can also be used to assess the severity of the left-to-right shunt in patients who have ventricular or atrial septal defects.

High blood pressure 11

By the end of this chapter you should:
• Understand the definition of hypertension.
• Be able to take a history and examine a patient with hypertension.
• Understand the complications associated with hypertension.
• Be able to list the causes of secondary hypertension.
• Understand the appropriate investigations for a patient with hypertension.

Hypertension is divided into 'stage 1', 'stage 2' and 'severe' categories. Note that stages 1 and 2 require both clinic and ambulatory blood pressure monitoring (ABPM) or home blood pressure monitoring (HBPM) readings greater than a certain value for a diagnosis. See Fig. 11.1 for details.

DIFFERENTIAL DIAGNOSIS

Systemic hypertension may be classified as:
• Primary hypertension, for which there is no identified cause. This accounts for 95% of cases.
• Secondary hypertension, for which there is a clear cause (Fig. 11.2).

HISTORY TO FOCUS ON THE DIFFERENTIAL DIAGNOSIS OF HIGH BLOOD PRESSURE

Presenting complaint

Hypertensive patients are often asymptomatic. Occasionally they complain of headaches, tinnitus, recurrent epistaxis or dizziness. In this situation a detailed systems review may reveal clues as to a possible cause of hypertension:
• Weight loss or gain, tremor, hair loss, heat intolerance or feeling cold may suggest the presence of thyroid disease.
• Paroxysmal palpitations, sweating, headaches or collapse may indicate the possibility of a phaeochromocytoma.

Ask the patient about symptoms that may indicate the presence of complications of hypertension such as:
• Dyspnoea, orthopnoea or ankle oedema suggesting cardiac failure.
• Chest pain indicating ischaemic heart disease.
• Unilateral weakness or visual disturbance (either persistent or transient) suggesting cerebrovascular disease.

Past medical history

To gain information about a condition that has so many varied causes it is crucial to ask about all previous illnesses and operations. Examples include:
• Recurrent urinary tract infections, especially in childhood, may lead to chronic pyelonephritis, a common cause of renal failure.
• A history of asthma may reveal chronic corticosteroid intake, leading to Cushing's syndrome.
• Thyroid surgery in the past.
• Evidence of peripheral vascular disease (e.g. leg claudication or previous vascular surgery may suggest the possibility of underlying renovascular disease).

Drug history

A careful history of all drugs being taken regularly is needed, including the use of proprietary analgesics (e.g. aspirin, non-steroidal anti-inflammatory drugs – a possible cause of renal disease, liquorice – can cause apparent mineralocorticoid excess).

Family history

Primary hypertension is a multifactorial disease requiring both genetic and environmental inputs. A family history of hypertension is, therefore, not an uncommon

Fig. 11.1 Categories of hypertension

Category	Clinic blood pressure	ABPM/HBPM
Stage 1	≥140/90 mmHg	≥135/85 mmHg
Stage 2	≥160/100 mmHg	≥150/95 mmHg
Severe	≥180 mmHg systolic or ≥110 mmHg diastolic	-

ABPM, ambulatory blood pressure monitoring; HBPM, home blood pressure monitoring.

Fig. 11.2 Causes of secondary hypertension

Mechanism	Pathology
Renal	Renal parenchymal disease (e.g. chronic atrophic pyelonephritis, chronic glomerulonephritis), renal artery stenosis, renin-producing tumours, primary sodium retention
Endocrine	Acromegaly, hypo- and hyperthyroidism, hypercalcaemia, adrenal cortex disorders (e.g. Cushing disease, Conn syndrome, congenital adrenal hyperplasia), adrenal medulla disorders (e.g. phaeochromocytoma)
Vascular disease	Coarctation of the aorta
Other	Hypertension of pregnancy, carcinoid syndrome
Increased intravascular volume	Polycythaemia (primary or secondary)
Drugs	Alcohol, oral contraceptives, monoamine oxidase inhibitors, glucocorticoids
Psychogenic	Stress

finding in these patients. Some secondary causes of hypertension have a genetic component:

- Adult polycystic kidney disease is an autosomal dominant condition associated with hypertension, renal failure and cerebral artery aneurysms.
- Phaeochromocytoma may occur as part of a multiple endocrine neoplasia syndrome (MEN 2, autosomal dominant) associated with medullary carcinoma of the thyroid and hyperparathyroidism.

Social history

Smoking, like hypertension, is a risk factor for ischaemic heart disease. Excessive alcohol intake can cause hypertension.

EXAMINATION OF PATIENTS WHO HAVE HIGH BLOOD PRESSURE

When performing the examination, look for:

- Signs of end-organ damage (i.e. cardiac failure, ischaemic heart disease, peripheral artery disease, cerebrovascular disease and renal impairment).
- Signs of an underlying cause of hypertension.

Blood pressure

Important points to note are that:

- The patient should be seated comfortably – preferably for 5 min before measurement of blood pressure in a quiet warm setting.
- The correct cuff size should be used – if it is too small a spuriously high reading will result.
- Whilst palpating the brachial artery, inflate the cuff. The point at which the pulse becomes impalpable is roughly equal to the systolic blood pressure.
- Deflate the cuff and now place your stethoscope over the brachial artery. Inflate the cuff to 20 mmHg above the systolic pressure you just measured.
- Systolic blood pressure is recorded as the point during bladder deflation where regular sounds can be heard (Korotkoff phase I).
- Diastolic blood pressure is recorded as the point at which the sounds disappear (Korotkoff phase V). In children and pregnant women muffling of the sounds is used as the diastolic blood pressure (Korotkoff phase IV).

HINTS AND TIPS

When performing the initial blood pressure measurements, measure blood pressure in both arms. A marked difference suggests coarctation of the aorta.

HINTS AND TIPS

The blood pressure in some patients goes up when they see a doctor - this is 'white coat hypertension'.

HINTS AND TIPS

Ambulatory blood pressure monitoring can help in the diagnosis of spurious 'white coat hypertension', and also establish efficacy of blood pressure control in patients on treatment.

Cardiovascular examination

Examine the pulses, considering the following:

- Rate – tachycardia or bradycardia may indicate underlying thyroid disease.
- Rhythm – atrial fibrillation may occur as a result of hypertensive heart disease.
- Symmetry – compare the pulses; radio-radial delay is a sign of coarctation as is the finding of abnormally weak foot pulses.

Bear in mind that:

- Weak or absent peripheral pulses along with cold extremities suggest peripheral vascular disease.
- Jugular venous pressure may be elevated in congestive cardiac failure; a complication of hypertension.
- A displaced apex is seen in left-ventricular failure due to dilatation of the left ventricle.
- Mitral regurgitation may occur secondary to dilatation of the valve ring that occurs during left-ventricular dilatation.
- In patients who have aortic coarctation, bruits may be heard over the scapulas and a systolic murmur may be heard below the left clavicle. There may also be a fourth heart sound (S4).

Respiratory system

Bilateral basal crepitations of pulmonary oedema may be heard on examination of the respiratory system.

Gastrointestinal system

Hepatomegaly and ascites may be seen in patients with congestive cardiac failure. Abdominal aortic aneurysm must be looked for because it is a manifestation of generalized atherosclerosis. Palpable kidneys may be evident in individuals who have polycystic kidney disease. A renal artery bruit may be heard in patients with renal artery stenosis.

Limbs

Peripheral oedema is a sign of congestive cardiac failure or underlying renal disease.

Eyes

A detailed examination of the fundi looking for hypertensive retinopathy is crucial in all patients who have hypertension because it provides valuable information about the severity of the hypertension (Fig. 11.3). Patients exhibiting grade III or IV hypertensive retinopathy have accelerated or malignant hypertension and need urgent treatment.

Fig. 11.3 Stages of hypertensive retinopathy. (A) Grade II, showing silver wiring (SW) and arteriovenous nipping (AVN) where an artery crossing above a vein causes apparent compression of the underlying vein. (B) Grade III, showing evidence of haemorrhages (H) and exudates (E). (C) Papilloedema – the optic disc (OD) is swollen and oedematous – a sign of malignant hypertension.

Fig. 11.4 highlights the features of the different grades of hypertensive retinopathy.

HINTS AND TIPS

When looking for features of hypertensive retinopathy in diabetic patients, be aware that they may also show separate features of diabetic retinopathy.

Fig. 11.4 Features of hypertensive retinopathy on ophthalmoscopy

Grade	Features
I	Narrowing of the arteriolar lumen occurs giving the classical 'silver wiring' effect
II	Sclerosis of the adventitia and thickening of the muscular wall of the arteries leads to compression of underlying veins and 'arteriovenous nipping'
III	Rupture of small vessels leading to haemorrhages and exudates
IV	Papilloedema (plus signs of grades I–IV)

Other findings on examination

When examining a patient who has a disorder that has many possible causes, a thorough examination of all systems is vital. Remember to look out for signs of thyroid disease, Cushing's syndrome, acromegaly, renal impairment, etc.

INVESTIGATION OF PATIENTS WHO HAVE HIGH BLOOD PRESSURE

Algorithms for the investigation of high blood pressure are given in Fig. 11.5. Look for evidence of end-organ damage and possible underlying causes.

Ambulatory blood pressure monitoring

24-h blood pressure monitoring is now used to confirm the diagnosis in most patients with suspected hypertension. The patient is fitted with a monitor and a cuff which takes readings as they carry out their normal day to day activities. Ambulatory blood pressure monitoring is also used to establish efficacy of blood pressure control in patients on treatment.

Home blood pressure monitoring

This is an alternative to ambulatory blood pressure monitoring. All readings must be taken with the patient seated, and are recorded twice daily, ideally for a period of seven days.

Blood tests

The following blood tests may help in the diagnosis:

- Electrolytes and renal function – many patients who have hypertension may be treated with diuretics and, therefore, may have hypokalaemia or hyponatraemia as a result. Renal impairment as a result of hypertension or its treatment must be excluded.
- Full blood count – polycythaemia may be present. Macrocytosis may be seen in hypothyroidism; anaemia may be a result of chronic renal failure.
- Blood glucose – elevated blood glucose may be seen in diabetes mellitus or in Cushing's syndrome.
- Thyroid function.
- Blood lipid profile – like hypertension, an important risk factor for ischaemic heart disease.

Fig. 11.5 Algorithm for investigating secondary causes of high blood pressure. BP, blood pressure; CT, computed tomography; MRI, magnetic resonance imaging; VMA, vanillylmandelic acid.

If treatment of hypertension with angiotensin-converting enzyme inhibitors causes a rise in serum creatinine, consider renal artery stenosis.

Urinalysis

Look for haematuria or proteinuria – a sign of underlying renal disease. If proteinuria is detected, record the level (e.g. trace or 3+). It can be quantified by completing a 24-h urine collection.

Electrocardiography

There may be evidence of left-ventricular hypertrophy. Features of left-ventricular hypertrophy, shown in Fig. 11.6, are:

- Tall R waves in lead V6 (>25 mm).
- R wave in V5 plus S wave in V2 >35 mm.
- Deep S wave in lead V2.
- Inverted T waves in lateral leads (i.e. I, AVL, V5 and V6).

There may be evidence of an old myocardial infarction or of rhythm disturbance (especially atrial fibrillation). In severe LVH there may be left axis deviation and ST changes (a 'strain pattern').

Chest radiography

Look for:

- An enlarged left ventricle – seen on the chest radiograph as an enlarged cardiac shadow. The normal ratio of cardiac width to thoracic width is 1:2.

- Evidence of coarctation of the aorta – this is seen as poststenotic dilatation of the aorta with an indentation above producing the reversed figure three, along with rib notching due to dilatation of the posterior intercostal arteries.

Echocardiography

This investigation can demonstrate:

- Left-ventricular hypertrophy (including left ventricular concentric hypertrophy, whereby the LV chamber size does not increase as the LV becomes more muscular, predisposing to diastolic dysfunction).
- Poor left-ventricular function.
- Enlarged left atrium (secondary to increased end-diastolic pressures on the ventricle).
- Show any ventricular-wall-motion abnormalities suggestive of old myocardial infarction (MI).

INVESTIGATIONS TO EXCLUDE SECONDARY HYPERTENSION

The above investigations may point to possible underlying causes of secondary hypertension, but they are not exhaustive. It would not, however, be cost-effective to investigate all hypertensive patients for these disorders, because over 95% of cases of hypertension are primary.

Careful selection of patients who are more likely to have secondary hypertension is, therefore, needed before embarking on more detailed and invasive

Fig. 11.6 Electrocardiographic features of left-ventricular hypertrophy (LVH). Note the three cardinal features indicating LVH: R wave in V5 plus S wave in V2 exceeds seven large squares; the R wave in V6 and S wave in V2 are greater than five large squares; T wave inversion in lateral leads V4–V6.

Fig. 11.7 Investigation of secondary hypertension

Underlying cause	Investigation	Notes/result
Renal parenchymal disease	24-h creatinine clearance 24-h protein excretion Renal ultrasound Renal biopsy	$\downarrow$ $\uparrow$ Bilateral small kidneys In some cases
Renal artery stenosis	Renal ultrasound Radionucleotide studies using DTPA Renal angiography or MRI angiography	Often asymmetrical kidneys Decreased uptake on affected side; this effect is highlighted by administration of an ACE inhibitor
Phaeochromocytoma	24-h urine catecholamines CT scan of abdomen MIBG scan	$\uparrow$, VMA measurements now rarely used Tumour is often large To identify extra-adrenal tumours (seen in 10% cases)
Primary hyperaldosteronism	Aldosterone:renin ratio	May be secondary to bilateral hyperplasia, or a single adenoma (Conn syndrome)
Cushing disease	24-h urinary free cortisol Dexamethasone suppression test 09:00 and 24:00 blood cortisol Adrenal CT scan Pituitary MRI scan Chest X-ray	$\uparrow$ Low-dose 48-h test initially, high-dose test to rule out ectopic source of ACTH Reveals loss of circadian rhythm in Cushing disease May show adrenal tumour May show enlarged pituitary May show oat cell carcinoma of bronchus (ectopic ACTH)

ACE, angiotensin-converting enzyme; ACTH, adrenocorticotrophic hormone; CT, computed tomography; DTPA, diethylenetriamine penta-acetate; MIBG, meta-iodobenzylguanidine; MRI, magnetic resonance Imaging; VMA, vanillylmandelic acid.

investigations. Secondary hypertension is more likely in patients who are under 40 years of age and also in patients who have:

- Symptoms of malignant hypertension (i.e. severe headaches, nausea and vomiting, blood pressure >180/110 mmHg or papilloedema).
- Evidence of end-organ damage (i.e. grade III or IV retinopathy, raised serum creatinine or cardiac failure).
- Signs of secondary causes (e.g. hypokalaemia in the absence of diuretics, signs of coarctation, abdominal bruit, symptoms of phaeochromocytoma, family history of renal disease or stroke at a young age).

- Poorly controlled blood pressure despite medical therapy.

Investigations for secondary hypertension are listed in Fig. 11.7.

HINTS AND TIPS

Failure of hypertension to respond to treatment might be because there is an underlying secondary cause or because of lack of compliance with therapy.

Fever associated with a cardiac symptom or sign

Objectives

By the end of this chapter you should:
- Be able to take a history and examine a patient that presents with fever, with specific relevance to symptoms and signs of cardiovascular disease.
- Understand the differential diagnosis of fever associated with cardiovascular disease.
- Understand the appropriate investigations to be used in the management of a patient with fever and cardiovascular symptoms.

DIFFERENTIAL DIAGNOSIS

The differential diagnosis includes:

- Infective endocarditis – bacterial or fungal infection within the heart (see Ch. 23).
- Myocarditis – involvement of the myocardium in an inflammatory process, which is usually infectious.
- Pericarditis – inflammation of the pericardium, which may be infective, post myocardial infarction or autoimmune.
- Other rare conditions, such as rheumatic fever, vasculitis, cardiac malignancy and cardiac myxoma.

The fever may be of non-cardiac origin.

HINTS AND TIPS

Some very serious and potentially fatal cardiac conditions are accompanied by fever. It is, therefore, important to have at hand a working list of differential diagnoses when presented with such a case.

Rare conditions

- Rheumatic fever – although common in developing countries, it is rare in the developed world. It is primarily a disease of childhood and is due to infection with Group A β-haemolytic streptococci. Most often this affects the mitral valve.
- Vasculitis – inflammation of the blood vessels. Kawasaki disease is an example of a vasculitis affecting children that can cause coronary arterial aneurysms.
- Cardiac malignancy.
- Cardiac myxomas – these are benign primary tumours of the heart, most often located in the atria. They may present with a wide variety of symptoms (e.g. dyspnoea, fever, weight loss and syncope)

and can cause complications, such as thromboembolic phenomena or sudden death. They are diagnosed by echocardiography and are treated with anticoagulation to prevent thromboembolic phenomena and resection (they may recur if incompletely resected).

HINTS AND TIPS

In the viva, a well-presented list of differential diagnoses implies that you can think laterally and adapt your knowledge of cardiac conditions to fit a clinical scenario.

HINTS AND TIPS

Whenever presenting a list of differential diagnoses, start with either the most dangerous or the most common disorder.

Leave the rare conditions to the end (even though these are invariably the ones that immediately spring to mind).

HISTORY TO FOCUS ON THE DIFFERENTIAL DIAGNOSIS OF FEVER

When presented with a set of symptoms that cover a potentially huge set of differential diagnoses, it is important to be systematic. Remember that sepsis is a common cause of atrial fibrillation and flutter. Patients who have sepsis may, therefore, present with fever and palpitations.

Presenting complaint

Common presenting complaints include:

- Fever– ask when it started and whether the patient can think of any precipitating factors (e.g. an operation or dental work).
- Chest pain – to differentiate between ischaemic and pericarditic pain, for example, establish the exact nature of the pain, where it radiates, duration and exacerbating factors (Fig. 12.1).
- Palpitations– ask about rate and rhythm to obtain information about the likely nature of the palpitations. Also ask about the possible complications of palpitations (e.g. dyspnoea, angina, dizziness).

Past medical history

It is crucial to obtain a detailed past medical history. In particular the following aspects of the past medical history are important in these patients:

- Recent dental work – this is a common source of bacteraemia and cause of infective endocarditis.
- Recent operations – these may also cause transient bacteraemia (e.g. gastrointestinal surgery, genitourinary surgery or even endoscopic investigations).
- History of rheumatic fever – although rare in the developed world now, this condition was common in the early twentieth century and is the cause of valve damage in many elderly patients. Such abnormal valves are vulnerable to colonization by bacteria.
- Previous myocardial infarction – a possible cause of pericarditis and Dressler syndrome (a nonspecific, possibly autoimmune, inflammatory response to cardiac necrosis in surgery).

- Recent viral infection (e.g. a sore throat or a cold) – myocarditis and pericarditis are commonly caused by viral infection.

Drug history

Ask about any recent antibiotics taken – obtain exact details of drugs and doses. Remember that some drugs may cause pericarditis, for example penicillin (associated with hypereosinophilia), hydralazine, procainamide and isoniazid.

Social history

Ask about:

- History of intravenous drug abuse, which is a risk factor for infective endocarditis.
- Risk factors for human immunodeficiency virus infection, which may be associated with infection due to unusual organisms.
- Smoking, which is a common cause for recurrent chest infection or myocardial infarction.

EXAMINATION OF PATIENTS WHO HAVE A FEVER ASSOCIATED WITH A CARDIAC SYMPTOM OR SIGN

Fig. 12.2 highlights the important features on examination of a patient who has fever and a cardiac sign or symptom.

Temperature

Examine the temperature chart to establish not only the severity of the fever, but also its trends (i.e. increasing, decreasing, cyclical variation, etc.).

Hands

Look for signs of infective endocarditis:

- Clubbing.
- Osler nodes (tender purplish nodules on the finger pulps).
- Janeway lesions (erythematous areas on palms).
- Splinter haemorrhages – up to four can be considered to be normal. The most common cause for a lesion that has the same appearance as a splinter haemorrhage is trauma, so they are common in keen gardeners.

All these are signs of vasculitis and may be found in other conditions causing vasculitis (e.g. autoimmune disease).

Condition	Pericarditis	Ischaemia
Location	Praecordium	Retrosternal ± radiation to left arm, throat or jaw
Quality	Sharp, pleuritic (may be dull)	Pressure pain (usually builds up)
Duration	Hours to days	Minutes, usually resolving (occasionally lasts hours)
Relationship to exercise	No	Yes, unless unstable angina or myocardial infarction
Relationship to posture	Worse when recumbent, relieved when sitting forward	Usually no effect

Fig. 12.1 Important features of ischaemic and pericarditic pain

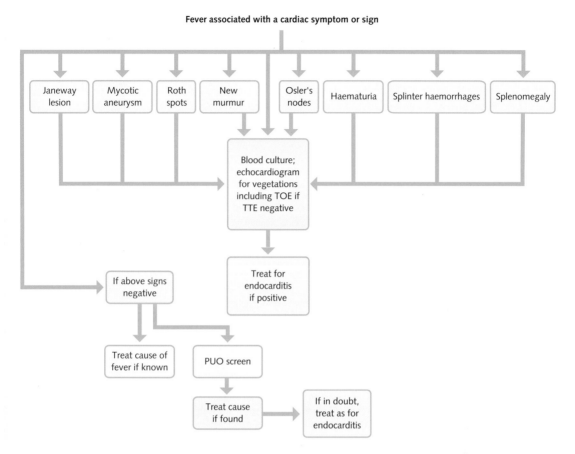

Fever associated with a cardiac symptom or sign

Fig. 12.2   Algorithm for fever. PUO, pyrexia of unknown origin; TOE, transoesophageal echocardiography; TTE, transthoracic echocardiography.

Facies

Look for:

- Conjunctival haemorrhages and Roth spots (retinal haemorrhages) – both signs of infective endocarditis.
- Central cyanosis – this may be a sign of a chest infection or cardiac failure.
- A vasculitic rash (e.g. the butterfly rash of systemic lupus erythematosus).

Cardiovascular system

Pulse

Check the:

- Rate and rhythm – may reveal underlying tachyarrhythmia (e.g. atrial fibrillation or, more commonly, sinus tachycardia – a common finding in a patient who has pyrexia).
- Quality of pulse – may reveal an underlying valve abnormality (e.g. waterhammer or collapsing pulse suggesting aortic regurgitation caused by endocarditis affecting the aortic valve).

Blood pressure

Hypotension may be found suggesting septic shock or cardiac failure.

A large pericardial effusion causing tamponade may result in pulsus paradoxus, which is an exaggeration of the normal variation of the blood pressure during respiration (i.e. the blood pressure falls during inspiration; a fall greater than 10 mmHg is abnormal).

Jugular venous pressure

Look for:

- Kussmaul sign – jugular venous pressure (JVP) increases with inspiration (normally, it falls), as seen in cases where pericardial effusion leads to cardiac tamponade.
- Friedreich sign – a rapid collapse of the JVP during diastole seen in aortic regurgitation. The JVP may be elevated due to cardiac failure.

Praecordium

Look for scars of previous valve replacement (prosthetic valves are more prone to infective endocarditis). The scar for these operations is the median sternotomy scar. Do not forget the mitral valvotomy scar under the left breast. Closed mitral valvotomy has been superseded by mitral valvuloplasty, which is undertaken via the femoral artery. However, there are still patients who have had closed mitral valvotomy to treat mitral stenosis in the past and these are also vulnerable to infective endocarditis. Listen for:

- Murmurs, especially those of valvular incompetence caused by infective endocarditis.
- Prosthetic valve sounds.
- Pericardial rub – this may be heard in patients who have pericarditis and has been described as the squeak of new leather. It is best heard with the diaphragm of the stethoscope and can be distinguished from a heart murmur because its timing with the heart cycle often varies from beat to beat and may appear and disappear from one day to the next.

Respiratory system

Examine carefully for signs of infection such as bronchial breathing, a pleural rub or pleural effusion.

Gastrointestinal system

Possible findings include:

- Splenomegaly, which is an important finding because it is a sign of infective endocarditis.
- Hepatomegaly, which may be found as a consequence of cardiac failure or of viral infection (e.g. infectious mononucleosis).

Skin

Infective endocarditis and many viral infections may be associated with a petechial rash.

INVESTIGATION OF PATIENTS WHO HAVE A FEVER ASSOCIATED WITH A CARDIAC SYMPTOM OR SIGN

An algorithm for the investigation of fever is given in Fig. 12.2.

Blood tests

Blood cultures

This is the most important diagnostic test in infective endocarditis.

At least three sets of blood cultures should be taken, if possible 1 h apart, from different sites before commencing antibiotics. This enables isolation of the causative organism in over 98% of cases of bacterial endocarditis. Therapy is often started immediately after this and can then be modified when the blood culture results are available.

Full blood count

A full blood count may reveal:

- Anaemia of chronic disease, which is commonly seen in patients who have infective endocarditis.
- A leucocytosis, which is an indicator of infection or inflammation.
- Thrombocytopenia, which may accompany disseminated intravascular coagulopathy in cases of severe sepsis.

Other blood tests

These include:

- Antistreptolysin O titres – may be useful in cases of rheumatic fever.
- Monospot test if Epstein-Barr virus infection is suspected as a possible cause of viral myocarditis.
- Clotting screen – clotting may be deranged in cases of sepsis associated with disseminated intravascular coagulation (DIC).
- Renal function tests – may be abnormal in infective endocarditis because the associated vasculitis may involve the kidneys causing glomerulonephritis. Autoimmune disease may also cause renal dysfunction and is a cause of pericarditis and myocarditis.
- Liver function tests – abnormal in many viral infections.
- Erythrocyte sedimentation rate and C-reactive protein measurements – these inflammatory markers are a sensitive indicator of the presence of infection or inflammation. They are also invaluable as markers of the response to treatment. Because C-reactive protein has a short half-life (approximately 8 h) it is often a more sensitive marker of disease activity than the erythrocyte sedimentation rate.
- Viral titres – taken in the acute and convalescent phase of the illness and may reveal the cause of pericarditis or myocarditis, e.g. coxsackie. If viral illness is suspected, throat swabs and faecal culture are also appropriate investigations to isolate the organism.

Urinalysis

No examination of a cardiovascular patient is complete without dipstick testing of the urine to look for microscopic haematuria. This is an extremely sensitive test for infective endocarditis and must not be forgotten. Urine microscopy almost always reveals red blood cells in infective endocarditis. Proteinuria may also be found.

Electrocardiography

In patients who have pericarditis the ECG may show characteristic ST segment elevation. This differs from that seen in myocardial infarction because it is:

- Concave.
- Present in all leads.
- Associated with upright T waves.

Eventually, with time, the ST segments may flatten or invert but, unlike infarction, there is no loss of R wave height.

Myocarditis may be associated with atrial arrhythmias or interventricular conduction defects. Rarely complete heart block may occur.

Chest radiography

This may reveal an underlying cause of cardiac disease:

- Pneumonia – a possible cause of atrial fibrillation.
- Lung tumour – may invade the pericardium causing pericardial effusion.
- Cardiac failure – an enlarged cardiac shadow and pulmonary oedema may be seen in patients who have valve disease or myocarditis.
- A globular heart shadow – characteristic of a pericardial effusion.
- Calcified heart valves – may be visible in a patient who has a history of rheumatic fever.

Transthoracic echocardiography

Transthoracic echocardiography is a very useful investigation in the patient who has fever and a cardiac symptom or sign:

- Left-ventricular function can be accurately assessed – in myocarditis this is found to be globally reduced (in patients who have left-ventricular failure due to ischaemic heart disease the left ventricle often shows regional dysfunction according to the site of the vascular lesion).

- Valve lesions may be identified and in cases of infective endocarditis the vegetations may be visualized on the valve leaflets. It is important to remember, however, that infective endocarditis cannot be excluded by the absence of vegetations on echocardiography. This investigation is by no means 100% sensitive and blood cultures remain the most important investigation for this condition.

Transoesophageal echocardiography

Transoesophageal echocardiography is more sensitive than transthoracic echocardiography because the resolution is much better. It allows a more detailed examination to be made and is especially useful in cases where transthoracic echocardiography does not provide adequate imaging, for example:

- Prosthetic heart valves – the acoustic shadows cast by these make imaging with transthoracic echocardiography very difficult.
- Localization of vegetations – transoesophageal echocardiography will visualize vegetations in many cases of infective endocarditis.

Pericardiocentesis

This may be appropriate if a pericardial effusion is found at echocardiography. The procedure is performed by an experienced operator and uses echocardiography as a guide for positioning of a catheter in the pericardial space. Pericardiocentesis can also be performed under fluoroscopic guidance. An ECG lead is often attached to the needle when attempting to enter the pericardium and will show an injury current (with ST elevation) if the myocardium is touched so enabling myocardial puncture to be avoided. Pericardiocentesis may be:

- Therapeutic – if it relieves cardiac tamponade.
- Diagnostic – if the pericardial fluid can be cultured to reveal an infective organism.

Angina pectoris 13

DEFINITION OF ANGINA PECTORIS

Angina pectoris is a crushing pain or discomfort felt in the anterior chest, commonly radiating to the left arm and jaw. The pain is caused by coronary arterial insufficiency leading to intermittent myocardial ischaemia. (Ischaemia refers to the effect of reduced delivery of oxygen and nutrients to an organ or cell.)

PATHOPHYSIOLOGY OF ANGINA PECTORIS

Myocardial ischaemia occurs when oxygen demand exceeds supply.

Supply may be reduced for a number of reasons:

- Stenotic atheromatous disease of epicardial coronary arteries – the most common cause of angina.
- Thrombosis within the arteries.
- Spasm of normal coronary arteries.
- Inflammation – arteritis.
- Small vessel disease – microvascular disease without the formation of large thrombi within the coronary system.

Demand may be increased for a number of reasons:

- In conditions requiring increased cardiac output – exercise, stress or thyrotoxicosis.
- In conditions necessitating greater cardiac work to maintain an adequate output – aortic stenosis.
- In conditions where peripheral vascular resistance is increased – hypertension.

The rest of this chapter discusses angina due to atherosclerotic narrowing of the coronary arteries because this is the most common cause of angina.

RISK FACTORS FOR CORONARY ARTERY DISEASE

Any modifiable risk factors should be sought and treated to reduce the risk of disease progression and eventual myocardial infarction (Fig. 13.1).

CLINICAL FEATURES OF ANGINA PECTORIS

Symptoms

These include:

- Chest pain – classically a tight, crushing, band-like pain across the centre of the chest. The pain may radiate to the left arm, throat or jaw. Precipitating factors include exercise, anxiety and cold air. As the coronary artery narrowing worsens, the amount of exertion required to produce angina reduces and the pain may occur even at rest or on minimal exertion. Relieving factors include rest and nitrates.
- Dyspnoea – often experienced. This occurs when the ischaemic myocardium becomes dysfunctional with an increase in left-ventricular filling pressure and, if severe, progression to pulmonary oedema.
- Fatigue – may be a manifestation of angina, which should be suspected if it occurs abnormally early into exercise and resolves rapidly at rest or to nitrates.

Signs

Most patients will have no obvious signs on examination. The patient may be breathless or sweaty and tachycardic, all due to overactivity of the sympathetic nervous

---

Fig. 13.1   Risk factors for coronary artery disease

Non-modifiable risk factors for coronary artery disease
Age: risk increases with age; older patients have a higher risk and therefore a potentially greater risk reduction if modifiable risk factors are treated
Sex: men > women (incidence in women increases rapidly after menopause)
Family history: this is a strong risk factor even when known genetic diseases (e.g. familial hypercholesterolaemia) are excluded

Modifiable risk factors for coronary artery disease
Hypertension
Diabetes mellitus
Smoking
Dyslipidaemia (includes hypercholesterolaemia and hypertriglyceridaemia): important studies include CARE (*N Engl J Med 335*), Helsinki Heart Study (*N Engl J Med 317*), LIPID (*N Engl J Med 339*), MRFIT (*JAMA 248*), SSSS (*Lancet 344*) and WOSCOPS (*N Engl J Med 333*)

CARE, Cholesterol and Recurrent Events Trial; LIPID, Long-tem Intervention with Pravastatin in Ischaemic Heart Disease; MRFIT, Multiple Risk Factor Intervention Trial; SSSS, Scandinavian Simvastatin Survival Study; WOSCOPS, West of Scotland Coronary Prevention Study.

---

system. There also might be evidence of an underlying cause:

- Hypertension.
- Corneal arcus (in those aged < 50) or xanthelasma–suggesting hypercholesterolaemia.

HINTS AND TIPS

Important points when diagnosing angina are:
• A sudden increase in exertional angina may be due to rupture of an atheromatous plaque in the coronary artery, which causes a steep decrease in its luminal diameter, and may even cause intermittent occlusion of the vessel. This condition may progress to myocardial infarction.
• Oesophageal pain is also relieved by nitrates.
• Any form of chest discomfort, even if atypical, could be angina, especially if it is related to effort.
There may be evidence of cardiac failure (third heart sound, raised jugular venous pressure, bilateral basal crepitations and possibly peripheral oedema due to fluid retention).

INVESTIGATION OF ANGINA PECTORIS

The investigation of patients presenting with chest pain is explained in detail in Ch. 5. A summary of investigations is given in Fig. 13.2. Coronary angiography is described in further detail below.

Coronary angiography

This is the most specific and sensitive test of coronary artery anatomical lesions and, as such, is the 'gold standard' in terms of diagnosis. Coronary angiography is used in patients who have positive stress tests and in patients who have negative stress tests in whom the diagnosis of angina is still suspected as stress tests may give false-negative results. Angiography is also considered a first-line investigation for patients who are deemed high risk.

An arterial puncture is made under local anaesthetic in the femoral or radial artery and a guide-wire is passed under X-ray control to the aortic root. A series of pre-shaped catheters is used to locate the right and left coronary ostia and radio-opaque contrast is injected into each in turn. Images are taken from several angles to obtain a full view of all branches of the two coronary arteries.

Information on left-ventricular function is obtained by measurement of the left-ventricular end-diastolic pressure (this is elevated in patients with poor left-ventricular function). Injection of contrast into the left-ventricle allows the pattern of left-ventricular contraction can be seen and gives an assessment of function.

It is important to remember that coronary angiography is invasive and there is a small risk of morbidity and mortality associated with the procedure.

Fig. 13.2   Investigations for angina pectoris

Investigation	Finding in angina pectoris
ECG	T wave flattening/ inversion ST segment depression Partial or complete left bundle branch block
Exercise ECG	Horizontal ST depression of >1mm when walking on a treadmill
Myocardial perfusion imaging (used with exercise or pharmacological stress agents such as dobutamine)	Poor perfusion of radionucleotide in ischaemic myocardium during exercise
Stress echocardiography (used with exercise or dobutamine)	Wall-motion abnormalities, decreased ejection fraction
Multi-slice CT/CT angiography	Coronary atheroma/ thrombus

MANAGEMENT OF ANGINA PECTORIS

Management of angina involves two areas that are addressed simultaneously:

1. Management of any modifiable risk factors.
2. Management of the angina itself.

Management of the risk factors

- Stop smoking. Patients who smoke should – at all stages of management – be actively discouraged. All health professionals should be involved, and positive encouragement, advice on the complications of smoking and information about self-help groups should all be made available to smokers. Smoking-cessation clinics (which often work on a self-referral basis) are now commonplace.
- Hypertension should be diagnosed. Lifestyle modifications are important (weight loss, reduced dietary sodium intake and increased physical activity). Medications (often multiple) may be needed to bring the blood pressure into the desired range (<140/ <90 mmHg). Regular monitoring is required to ensure that targets are met and maintained.
- Diabetes mellitus – blood glucose levels should be tightly controlled, by careful dietary control, oral medications and/or injected insulin.
- Hypercholesterolaemia should also be treated. The National Institute for Health and Clinical Excellence (NICE) recommend that patients who have coronary artery disease should have total cholesterol maintained under 4 mmol/L with low-density lipoprotein (LDL) maintained below 2 mmol/L. Lipid-lowering therapy should be offered to all patients irrespective of their cholesterol as part of a secondary prevention strategy. Drugs used to lower cholesterol include HMG-CoA reducatase inhibitors (statins, the first line therapy), fibrates, and ezetimibe. The trials mentioned in Fig. 13.1 should be read because they have dramatically altered the way hypercholesterolaemia is treated.

Treatment of the angina

Drug therapy

The main drugs used in the treatment of angina are aspirin, β-blockers (β-adrenoceptor antagonists), calcium channel antagonists, nitrates and potassium channel openers.

Aspirin

Aspirin acts to reduce platelet aggregation, which is a risk factor for the development and progression of atherosclerotic plaques.

β-Blockers

These agents are negatively inotropic and chronotropic and, therefore, reduce myocardial oxygen demand; swinging the balance of demand and supply. They are also effective antihypertensive agents and in some patients can perform a dual role reducing the need for multiple drug therapy. Remember that β-blockers are contraindicated in:

- Unstable cardiac failure.
- Asthma (COPD without bronchospasm may not be a contraindication).
- Peripheral vascular disease – a relative contraindication as the more β_1-selective agents may be used (e.g. bisoprolol).

Other side effects include:

- Nightmares – use a non-fat-soluble agent (e.g. atenolol).
- Loss of sympathetic response to hypoglycaemia – use a more cardioselective agent.
- Male impotence.
- Postural hypotension – especially in elderly patients who should start on a small dose initially.

Calcium channel antagonists

The slowing of calcium influx to the myocardial cells results in a negative inotropic response. The blockade of calcium channels in peripheral arteries results in relaxation and, therefore, vasodilatation. This improves blood flow. The blockade of calcium channels in the atrioventricular node increases the refractory period and, therefore, slows the heart rate. Agents in this group have actions on one or more of these areas and this affects the way they should be used:

- Nifedipine – dilates both coronary and peripheral vessels and can be used as an antihypertensive and anti-anginal drug. Main side effects are flushing, reflex tachycardia and ankle oedema.
- Diltiazem – dilates coronary arteries and has some negative inotropic and chronotropic effects. It is, therefore, a good anti-anginal drug. It has less effect on peripheral vessels. It causes less flushing and oedema and no reflex tachycardia.
- Verapamil – has almost no peripheral effects; its main effects are on the atrioventricular node and myocardium. It can, therefore, be used as an anti-anginal agent, but is used mainly as an antiarrhythmic.
- Amlodipine – a long-acting agent with actions similar to those of nifedipine. It is an effective anti-anginal and antihypertensive agent.

Nitrates

These act by conversion to nitric oxide, which is a potent vasodilator (so mimicking the endothelial release of nitric oxide). The vasodilatation affects:

- Veins – shifting blood from the central compartment (heart, pulmonary vessels) to peripheral veins.
- Arteries – reducing arterial pressure.
- Coronary arteries – improving myocardial perfusion.

There are a variety of preparations:

- Sublingual – glyceryl trinitrate or isosorbide dinitrate can both be taken sublingually from where they are absorbed and rapidly enter the blood. There is no risk of tolerance. Glyceryl trinitrate tablets should be changed every 6 months because they have a short shelf-life. Sublingual sprays do not have this problem.
- Transdermal – these take the form of patches or cream that allows the drug to be absorbed through the skin. Care should be taken to vary the location of the application each day.
- Oral nitrates – these may be once, twice or three times a day dosages. A drug free period is built into the dosing schedule to prevent tolerance.

Potassium channel openers

There are many families of potassium channels found in cardiac and vascular smooth muscle, and these are still incompletely understood. Nicorandil is a potassium channel opener that has been increasingly used to treat angina. The action of potassium channel openers results in venous and arterial dilatation (coronary and systemic). Potassium channel openers also act to precondition the myocardium against ischaemia, so limiting the area of myocardium vulnerable to ischaemia.

Side effects of potassium channel openers are generally similar to those of nitrates (i.e. headache and flushing). Tolerance does not occur. Recently, there have been reports of oral and peri-anal ulceration with nicorandil and this is now a recognised side effect.

New anti-anginals

Several new anti-anginal drugs have been introduced in the last few years.

- Ivabradine – acts on the sinoatrial node to lower heart rate and therefore decrease myocardial demand.
- Ranolazine – mechanism of action not fully understood but affects late sodium currents in myocardial cells, independently of heart rate. Therefore can be safely used in combination with drugs that lower heart rate.

Management plan for angina pectoris

A possible plan of action is, therefore, the following:

- Prescribe all patients aspirin.
- Prescribe all patients a GTN spray and advise them to use it for the relief of angina or prior to any activity which is known to bring angina on.
- Prescribe a β-blocker if not contraindicated.

- If β-blockade fails to control the symptoms or is contraindicated, there is a choice to start either a calcium antagonist, and be prepared to add a long-acting nitrate, or nicorandil, if the effect is still insufficient, or to prescribe nicorandil, which has effects similar to those produced by a combination of calcium antagonist and nitrate. Exercise caution when using rate-limiting calcium antagonists in combination with β-blockers as there is a risk of precipitating bradycardia.

Revascularization

There are two main ways of mechanically improving myocardial blood supply. Coronary angiography is used to help decide which revascularization technique to use:

1. Percutaneous intervention (PCI), which consists of both percutaneous transluminal coronary angioplasty (PTCA), which forces the lumen open by means of an inflated intraluminal balloon, and intracoronary stent implantation.
2. Coronary artery bypass grafting (CABG).

Percutaneous intervention

PCI achieves revascularization by the inflation of a small balloon placed across a stenotic lesion; following balloon dilatation of the stenosis a balloon mounted intracoronary stent is implanted. The procedure is carried out in the catheter laboratory under local anaesthetic and light sedation. A guide-wire is passed into the aorta via the femoral or radial artery and the balloon catheter is passed over it. Once the balloon catheter has been positioned across the stenotic plaque to be treated the balloon is inflated.

Advantages of PCI

The advantages of this technique over CABG are as follows:

- The patient avoids major surgery, general anaesthesia and cardiopulmonary bypass.
- There is a shortened hospital stay compared with CABG.

- Patients who have clotting disorders or who have recently had thrombolysis can be treated in an emergency.
- If PTCA is unsuccessful, CABG can still be performed (whereas a second CABG operation carries a much higher risk).

Disadvantages of PCI

- Not all patients will have coronary artery disease that is amenable to PCI. Patients with complex coronary disease, such as stenosis of the left main stem, multi-vessel disease and chronically occluded vessels may be better served by CABG.
- Approximately 10% of patients who have had PCI will develop 'in-stent restenosis' (ISR). This rate is higher in diabetic patients, and those that have long segments of stent and smaller calibre stents. ISR can be treated by further PCI. The rate of ISR has been reduced by the introduction of stents coated with drugs that inhibit the endothelial response to stent implantation; these are known as drug eluting stents (DES). DES are significantly more expensive than their bare metal counterparts and, thus, in the UK their use is rationed to patients who are deemed at the highest risk of ISR.
- Thrombosis at the site of stenting may occur and is partly prevented by the rigorous use of intravenous heparin at the time of PCI, and long-term oral anti-platelet aggregation agents (Fig. 13.3).
- Although it may provide symptomatic relief, PCI does not confer any prognostic benefit over medical therapy in stable angina (COURAGE trial – see further reading below).

Complications of PCI

These include major adverse effects such as:

- Myocardial infarction – secondary to thrombosis, spasm of the coronary artery, or dissection of the coronary artery by the balloon.
- Coronary artery perforation.
- Stroke.
- Less severe, but more common adverse effects such as:
  - arrhythmias
  - dye reactions (allergy and nephrotoxicity)
  - haemorrhage or infection at the puncture site.

Coronary artery bypass grafting

CABG aims to achieve revascularization by bypassing a stenotic lesion using grafts.

The patient undergoes a full general anaesthetic and the heart is exposed via a median sternotomy.

Cardiopulmonary bypass is achieved by inserting a cannula into the right atrium and another into the proximal aorta. The two cannulae are connected to the bypass machine, which oxygenates the venous blood from the right atrium and feeds it back to the aorta.

The heart is stopped using cooling and cardioplegic solutions.

Vein grafts harvested from the great saphenous vein or arterial grafts are used to bypass the occlusive coronary lesions.

Arterial grafts are preferred given that they have much better long-term patency than vein grafts. The arteries commonly used for grafting include the left and right internal mammary arteries, and to a lesser extent the radial arteries.

Fig. 13.3 Antiplatelet agents used to prevent thrombosis following PTCA ± stenting

Class of drug and examples	Action	Side effects
NSAIDs (e.g. aspirin)	Irreversible inactivation of cyclooxygenase – within platelets this enzyme is needed for the production of thromboxane (a stimulator of platelet aggregation)	Gastritis (possibly with ulcer formation and bleeding), renal impairment, bronchospasm, rashes
Platelet ADP receptor antagonists (e.g. clopidogrel)	When activated the adenylcyclase-coupled ADP receptor causes binding of fibrinogen to the platelet and initiation of thrombus formation – this is irreversibly inhibited by these agents	Haemorrhage, diarrhoea, nausea, neutropenia, hepatic dysfunction
Platelet membrane glycoprotein IIb/ IIIa receptor inhibitors (abciximab is a monoclonal antibody that binds to and blocks this receptor)	The GP IIb/IIIa platelet receptor binds fibrinogen, von Willebrand factor and other adhesive molecules – blockade therefore inhibits platelet aggregation and thrombus formation	Haemorrhage

ADP, adenosine diphosphate; NSAIDs, non-steroidal anti-inflammatory drugs.

Complications of coronary artery bypass grafting

These are:

- Death – mortality rates are approximately 1%.
- Myocardial infarction, stroke and peripheral thromboembolism.
- Wound infection.
- Complications related to cardiopulmonary bypass – these are related to the haemodilution involved and the exposure of the blood to synthetic materials in the oxygenating process; they include clotting and pulmonary abnormalities, and impaired cognitive function.

Minimally invasive coronary artery bypass grafting

Minimally invasive CABG (MICABG) is a new technique that involves a smaller incision, usually a left anterior minithoracotomy. The left or right internal mammary artery is used to graft the occluded vessel (usually the left anterior descending coronary artery because this is situated within easy reach). Cardiopulmonary bypass is not used – instead the heart is slowed using β-blockers and a specifically designed instrument is used to immobilize the small area around the anastomosis.

UNSTABLE ANGINA

This condition is one of the acute coronary syndromes. The pathophysiology underlying unstable angina involves rupture of an atherosclerotic plaque within the coronary artery and the subsequent formation of a thrombus over this. The result is a rapid reduction in the size of the lumen of the vessel.

Clinically, unstable angina is defined as:

- New onset (<6 weeks) angina at exertion or at rest.
- Angina at rest in previously exercise-induced angina.
- Exertional angina that is not responding to increasing anti-anginal medications.

Plasma troponin levels (troponin T or troponin I) are now being determined routinely. A raised troponin level suggests myocardial necrosis and the patient is then said to have sustained a myocardial infarction rather than unstable angina.

Management

The following management plan should be followed (but be aware that most hospitals have their own specific protocols which should be adhered to):

- Admit the patient to the coronary care unit for observation and strict bed rest – remember that if the thrombus extends and completely occludes the vessel lumen a myocardial infarction will occur.
- Provide analgesia with intravenous morphine (2.5–5 mg intravenously) if required to calm the patient and relieve pain – remember to give metoclopramide too.
- Give aspirin – it has been shown to reduce the incidence of myocardial infarction and death in patients who have unstable angina (300 mg soluble aspirin).
- Give clopidogrel (300 mg loading dose followed by 75 mg OD) – it has been shown to reduce mortality in acute coronary syndrome.
- Give nitrates – 2 puffs of GTN spray. Patients with ongoing pain may require an intravenous infusion of nitrates (e.g. glyceryltrinitrate 0.5–10 mg/h) to dilate the coronary arteries and reduce the load on the heart by peripheral vasodilatation and venodilatation. The blood pressure will drop so it should be carefully monitored.
- Give antithrombin (fondaparinux– a factor Xa inhibitor), low-molecular weight heparin (LMWH) or unfractionated heparin (if renal failure present) to prevent further thrombus formation.
- Consider the newer drugs used in the treatment of unstable angina such as glycoprotein IIb/IIIa antagonists (tirofiban, eptifbatide and abciximab) and bivalirudin – a direct thrombin inhibitor. Both are used in patients undergoing coronary angiography.
- Once the patient is more stable start oral anti-anginal therapy and arrange early angiography if appropriate.

Further reading

The Clopidogrel in Unstable Angina to Prevent Recurrent Events Trial Investigators, August 2001. Effects of clopidogrel in addition to aspirin in patients with acute coronary syndromes without ST-segment elevation. N. Engl. J. Med. 345, 494–502.

COURAGE Trial Research Group, 2007. Optimal Medical Therapy with or without PCI for Stable Coronary Disease. N. Engl. J. Med 356, 1503–1516.

National Institute for Health and Clinical Excellence (NICE), 2010. Guideline Number 67. Lipid Modification: cardiovascular risk assessment and the modification of blood lipids for the primary and secondary prevention of cardiovascular disease. http://www.nice.org.uk/CG67.

National Institute for Health and Clinical Excellence (NICE), 2010. Guideline Number 94. Unstable angina and NSTEMI the early management of unstable angina and non-ST-segment elevation myocardial infarction. http://www.nice.org.uk/CG94.

Scottish Intercollegiate Guideline Network (SIGN), 2010. Guideline Number 96. Management of stable angina. http://sign.ac.uk/pdf/sign96.pdf.

Acute myocardial infarction

Objectives

By the end of this chapter you should:
- Be able to describe the temporal changes of the various cardiac biomarkers after myocardial infarction.
- Be able to recognize the common cardiac complications that occur in the first 48 h following acute myocardial infarction and understand their management.
- Understand the common cardiac complications that occur in the first 7 days following acute myocardial infarction.
- Understand the emergency management for patients presenting with acute myocardial infarction.
- Understand the different revascularization strategies available to treat acute myocardial infarction.

DEFINITION OF ACUTE MYOCARDIAL INFARCTION

Acute myocardial infarction (MI) is the term used for cell death secondary to ischaemia. The most common cause of MI is atherosclerotic narrowing of the coronary arteries. The immediate precursor to MI is rupture of an atherosclerotic plaque and the formation of thrombus over the plaque resulting in rapid occlusion of the vessel.

Traditionally acute MI has been defined according to the 1971 World Health Organization criteria based on the presence of at least two of clinical syndrome, ECG changes and elevations in relatively non-specific markers of myocardial damage such as creatine kinase. This definition has recently been updated to include cardiac troponins as a more sensitive and specific biomarker for myocardial necrosis (Fig. 14.1).

Depending on the rate of vessel occlusion (if an atherosclerotic plaque grows slowly, over months, collateral vessels develop and protect the myocardium) and the degree of occlusion of the vessel by thrombus, a number of clinical conditions can result from plaque rupture. These conditions are termed the acute coronary syndromes. Acute MI is the most serious of this spectrum of acute illnesses (Fig. 14.2).

For simplicity, and to make the management algorithm work (see below), these are divided into two categories:

1. ST elevation.
2. No ST elevation.

All these syndromes present as severe central chest pain of typical cardiac type (see Ch. 5) and patients usually present at the accident and emergency department with one of the following:

- Severe angina – there is a history of angina and the pain usually subsides spontaneously with rest and nitrates without permanent change to the ECG or evidence of activation of coagulation or myocardial damage.
- A sudden increase in exertional angina – there is rupture of an atheromatous plaque in the coronary artery, which causes a step decrease in its luminal diameter; the pain usually subsides spontaneously with rest and nitrates, without permanent change to the ECG or evidence of activation of coagulation or myocardial damage. The condition may progress to full infarction.
- Widespread subendocardial ischaemia – ST depression may be present in all ECG leads except AVR. This is a manifestation of critical stenoses in all three coronary arteries.

There is no evidence of activation of coagulation or myocardial damage, but the prognosis is very poor without emergency treatment.

- Unstable angina due to coronary arterial thrombosis – there is no ST elevation, but microinfarcts may be occurring due to embolization of thrombi from the site of plaque rupture downstream.
- Non-ST-elevation myocardial infarction (NSTEMI) – this is necrosis caused by thrombotic coronary artery occlusion in which the myocardial cell death is confined to the endocardial layers and is not full thickness. It occurs because the occluded artery is a relatively small branch, because there is good collateral flow around the occluded vessel or because intervention for ST elevation has been early and effective.
- ST-elevation myocardial infarction (STEMI) – this represents a developing full-thickness MI, which

Fig. 14.1 Joint European Society of Cardiology/American College of Cardiology criteria

Criteria for acute, evolving, or recent myocardial infarction (MI) – one of the following:

1. Typical rise and fall of biochemical markers of myocardial necrosis with at least one of the following:
   a. ischaemic symptoms
   b. Q waves
   c. ischaemic ECG changes
   d. coronary artery intervention
2. Pathological findings of an acute MI

Criteria for established MI – any of the following:

1. Development of new pathological Q waves on serial ECGs
2. Pathological findings of a healed or healing MI

Fig. 14.2 Acute coronary syndromes in order of severity (↑)

ST-elevation myocardial infarction
Non-ST-elevation myocardial infarction
Unstable angina due to coronary arterial thrombosis
Widespread subendocardial ischaemia
Sudden increase in severity of exertional angina
Severe angina episode in a patient who has exertional angina

can lead to arrhythmia, death or leave the patient with severe heart failure. This is a common ECG to see in Finals as making the diagnosis and rapidly instigating management is absolutely crucial. Delayed intervention leaves dead muscle, which shows as permanent Q waves on the ECG (Fig. 14.3). Remember that new LBBB with chest pain should also be treated as acute MI.

CLINICAL FEATURES OF ACUTE MYOCARDIAL INFARCTION

History

The history is very important because it provides clues about the severity of the infarction and the time of onset (important when deciding on therapy). The following are classic features of the history of acute MI.

Presenting complaint

The main presenting complaint is of chest pain. The following characteristics are common:

- Usually severe in nature.
- Normally lasts at least 30 min.
- Usually tight, crushing and band-like in nature.
- Retrosternal in location.
- May radiate to the left arm, throat or jaw.
- Associated features include sweating, breathlessness and nausea.

Elderly patients may have relatively little pain, but present with features of left ventricular failure (profound breathlessness) or syncope.

Past medical history

Important features include a history of angina or intermittent chest pain that often increases in severity or frequency in the few weeks preceding this event.

Risk factors for ischaemic heart disease are smoking, hypertension, diabetes mellitus, hypercholesterolaemia and positive family history. (Although some of these do not belong in this section of the clerking, it is important not to forget these and, therefore, easier to ask about them all together at the same time.)

The patient may have a history of previous MI or of cardiac intervention, such as angiography, percutaneous coronary intervention (PCI) or CABG.

Also ask about any bleeding risks at this stage.

Examination

On inspection, the patient is often extremely anxious and distressed and will often be restless; he or she may be in severe pain. Breathlessness suggests the presence of pulmonary oedema, as does the presence of pink frothy sputum. The patient may be pale, clammy and sweaty, suggesting cardiogenic shock. Look for scars of previous surgery.

Cardiovascular system

The pulse may be tachycardic secondary to anxiety or left ventricular failure, or it may be bradycardic in the case of an inferior MI as there is a large increase in vagal tone, which suppresses the AV node (the Bezhold-Jarisch reflex).

Although the blood pressure may be normal, in some patients it is raised due to anxiety. If there is cardiogenic shock the blood pressure may be low.

The jugular venous pressure may be elevated in cases of congestive cardiac failure or in pure right-ventricular infarction.

Examination of the praecordium may reveal the following:

- A displaced diffuse apex in cases of left ventricular failure.

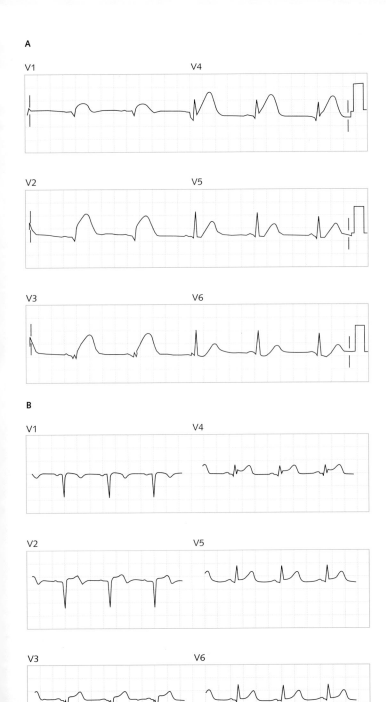

Fig. 14.3 (A) ECG showing acute anterior myocardial infarction (MI). (B) ECG 24 h after anterior MI. Note the resolution of the ST elevation and the development of Q waves. The loss of the R wave in this ECG suggests that a significant left-ventricle muscle mass has undergone necrosis.

- In anterior infarction a paradoxical systolic outward movement of the ventricular wall may be felt parasternally.
- Audible murmurs.
- The murmur of mitral regurgitation – may occur as a new murmur due to rupture of the papillary muscle.
- A pericardial rub – may be audible in some patients because it is not uncommon for an MI to be complicated by pericarditis.
- A fourth heart sound (Fig. 14.4) – common in MI due to reduction of left-ventricular compliance.
- A third heart sound – occurs in the presence of left ventricular failure.
- Further evidence of cardiac failure (e.g. bilateral basal crepitations, peripheral oedema and poor peripheral perfusion).

INVESTIGATION OF ACUTE MYOCARDIAL INFARCTION

Blood tests

Indicators of myocardial damage

Troponin T and troponin I

Troponin T and troponin I are proteins that form part of the myocardial cell structure. Release of these proteins into the bloodstream indicates that there has been myocardial cell damage. The levels rise within 6–14 h of the onset of MI and remain elevated for up to 14 days. This test is now widely available and is used in both diagnosis and risk stratification, as the increase in cardiac troponin is related to the risk of cardiac complications. Recently, high-sensitivity troponin measurement has been introduced to many hospitals. A high-sensitivity troponin that rises between serial measurements, after an episode of chest pain is strongly indicative of ACS. However, the test is so sensitive that it may be positive in a variety of pathological (i.e. PE, pericarditis, tachyarrhythmias, sepsis) and non-pathological situations (i.e. after running a marathon). Renal failure reduces the excretion of troponin and will raise plasma levels,

however a raised troponin in patients with end-stage renal failure is still an indicator of coronary risk and should not be ignored.

Creatine kinase

The MB isoenzyme of creatine kinase (CK) increases and falls within 72 h. The source of CK-MB isoenzyme is cardiac muscle, whereas CK-MM is found in skeletal muscle and CK-BB is in brain and kidney. Many laboratories provide only total CK measurements for routine use and this is not specific. The CK-MB isoenzyme does not begin to increase until at least 4 h after infarction and is, therefore, no longer used to make the initial diagnosis in most cases.

Renal function and electrolytes

These are important in all patients who have MI. Renal function may be deranged or may worsen due to poor renal perfusion in cardiogenic shock. Hypokalaemia may predispose to arrhythmias and must be corrected because acute MI is in itself a proarrhythmogenic condition.

Blood glucose

Diabetes mellitus must be controlled aggressively after MI and all patients who have diabetes mellitus benefit from insulin therapy either using an intravenous sliding scale or, if stable, four times daily subcutaneous insulin.

Full blood count

Anaemia may precipitate an acute MI in a patient who has angina. There is often a leucocytosis after acute MI.

Serum cholesterol

This should be measured within 24 h of an MI; hypercholesterolaemia is a risk factor for MI and needs to be treated. Cholesterol level falls to an artificially low level 24 h after MI, so after this time a true reading can only be obtained 2 months after MI.

Fig. 14.4 Notes on third and fourth heart sounds

Heart sound	Mechanism	When heard	Causes
Fourth	Represents atrial contribution to ventricular filling	Heard in any condition that causes a stiff left ventricular wall	Hypertension, aortic stenosis, acute MI
Third	Rapid filling of the ventricle as soon as the mitral valve opens	Normal finding in the young and heard in conditions where there is rapid ventricular filling	Mitral regurgitation, ventricular septal defect, left ventricular failure, MI

MI, myocardial infarction.

Electrocardiography

The ECG is the main diagnostic test in acute MI (Fig. 14.5) and it is, therefore, important to have a thorough knowledge of the ECG appearances of different types of MI. Delay in the diagnosis wastes precious time because treatment should be given as soon as possible for maximum benefit - "time is muscle"!.

Classic ECG changes of a full-thickness MI are as follows:

- ST segment elevation – this is due to full-thickness myocardial injury and may appear within minutes of the onset of infarction; it is almost always present by 24 h. The criteria for acute thrombolysis are a good history and ST segment elevation greater than 1 mm in two or more consecutive leads. Reciprocal ST segment depression may be present at the same time and represents the mirror image of the ST elevation as seen from the opposite side of the heart.
- Over 24 h the ST elevation resolves and the T waves begin to invert.
- Q waves develop within 24–72 h of MI.

Fig. 14.5B ST elevation in leads

Location of MI	ECG changes
Anterior (LAD)	ST elevation in leads V1–4
Inferior (RCA or circumflex coronary artery)	ST elevation in leads II, III, AVF
Lateral (circumflex coronary artery)	ST elevation in leads V4–6
Posterior (RCA or circumflex coronary artery)	Prominent R wave in V1 and V2 with ST depression (mirror image of anterior MI)
Anterolateral (proximal LAD) above diagonal branch	ST elevation V1–6
Right ventricular infarction (suspect in inferior or posterior MI)	Perform right-sided ECG using lead V1 (as normal), leads V3–6 placed on the right side, limb leads as normal

HINTS AND TIPS

Persistent elevation of ST segments after 1 week indicates either reinfarction or a left-ventricular aneurysm.

HINTS AND TIPS

Posterior MI can be missed. Flip the ECG upside down, looking through the back of the paper – the anterior ST depression of posterior MI looks like an anterior STEMI when looked at from behind.

ECG changes in non-ST-elevation myocardial infarction

These are variable and the absence of Q waves does not necessarily indicate that full-thickness infarction has not occurred. The conventional view used to be that this represented subendocardial damage only.

The ECG changes tend to be in the form of persistent T wave inversion accompanied by an increase in cardiac enzymes.

Chest radiography

This should be performed on all patients who have acute MI. Points to note are:

- Widening of the mediastinum – suggests a likelihood of aortic dissection, which is an absolute contraindication for thrombolysis.
- Signs of pulmonary oedema – signify the need for antifailure therapy (intravenous diuretics, oxygen and possibly a nitrate infusion).
- An enlarged heart – suggests cardiac failure.

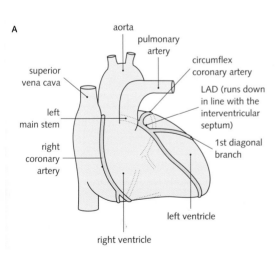

A

aorta
pulmonary artery
circumflex coronary artery
LAD (runs down in line with the interventricular septum)
1st diagonal branch
superior vena cava
left main stem
right coronary artery
left ventricle
right ventricle

Fig. 14.5 (A) Location of coronary arteries. Note the left anterior descending coronary artery branch (LAD) supplies the anterior aspect of the heart (the left ventricle and the septum), the right coronary artery (RCA) usually supplies the inferoposterior aspect and the circumflex supplies the lateral part of the left ventricle. (B) ST elevation in leads.

Echocardiography

This is not a first-line investigation, but is very useful early on to assess left-ventricular function or investigate valve lesions (mitral regurgitation may occur after MI as a result of papillary muscle infarction).

MANAGEMENT OF ACUTE MYOCARDIAL INFARCTION

Acute MI is a medical emergency and, therefore, you must know its acute management thoroughly (Fig. 14.6). It is one of the few occasions in an examination when you will be expected to know the doses of drugs given.

In the context of cardiac chest pain, ST segment elevation on the 12-lead ECG usually signifies complete occlusion of a proximal epicardial coronary artery. If untreated myocardial necrosis commences within 30 min, affecting full myocardial thickness within 6 h. Forty per cent of patients die before reaching hospital.

Treatment

Urgent restoration of coronary blood flow (reperfusion) prevents further left-ventricular damage and improves prognosis. The amount of myocardium that can be salvaged falls exponentially with time, the greatest benefit being within 3 h of symptom onset, and little benefit after 12 h.

Options for reperfusion include the following:

- Primary percutaneous coronary intervention (primary PCI) – this is the preferred reperfusion strategy and is superseding thrombolysis throughout the UK. Patients may be transferred as an emergency to larger centres for this treatment.
- Thrombolysis – where timely primary PCI is not realistically achievable, thrombolysis may be

---

Fig. 14.6 Acute management of acute myocardial infarction

Administer oxygen via a facial mask
Give the patient aspirin 300 mg and clopidogrel 600 mg or prasugrel 60 mg
Establish IV access and connect patient to cardiac monitor
If patient is distressed or in pain give morphine 5–10 mg IV with 10 mg metoclopramide
Urgent cardiology review for primary angioplasty where available
Otherwise, if patient satisfies the criteria for thrombolysis and has no contraindications, administer thrombolysis with rt-PA

IV, intravenous; rt-PA, recombinant tissue plasminogen activator.

---

attempted in the absence of contraindications. Transfer to a larger centre remains an option if chest pain persists or recurs ('failed thrombolysis').

Indications for primary PCI

Patients for primary PCI will be assessed by a specialist but they should be alerted about patients with the following:

- History of chest pain lasting less than 24 h.
- One of the following – ST elevation >1 mm in standard leads or in two adjacent chest leads, new bundle branch block on ECG.

Contraindications

Patients will be assessed on a case-by-case basis, and there are few absolute contraindications to primary PCI, but the following should be sought and documented:

- History of haemorrhagic cerebrovascular event – ever.
- History of any type of cerebrovascular event – in the past 6 months.
- Recent gastrointestinal bleed.
- Bleeding diathesis.
- Recent surgery – a relative contraindication.
- Pregnancy.
- Any other invasive procedure in the past month (e.g. organ biopsy, dental extraction) – consult a senior before proceeding.

Other agents used for acute myocardial infarction

Aspirin

300 mg of aspirin should be chewed and absorbed under the tongue. The antiplatelet aggregation action of aspirin makes it effective in all acute coronary syndromes where the primary event is clot formation. This drug has relatively few side effects and should be administered promptly to all patients as soon as the ECG is found to be positive. Aspirin was found to reduce the mortality rate in the ISIS 2 study.

Other antiplatelet agents

Clopidogrel acts on the ADP receptor, and so has an additive antiplatelet effect compared to aspirin alone. Some patients are genetically resistant to clopidogrel and so a newer drug, prasugrel, may be given to patients in high-risk groups (e.g. STEMI, NSTEMI with diabetes) or with those with particularly high-risk lesions (e.g. left main stem disease).

Diamorphine

A powerful anxiolytic and analgesic, this drug is extremely effective in patients with cardiac pain. It has venodilating properties and is, therefore, also an effective antifailure agent. If unavailable, morphine can be used as an alternative.

β-Blockers (β-adrenoceptor antagonists)

These drugs were shown to reduce mortality rate acutely after MI in the ISIS 1 study. The following are contraindications to the administration of β-blockers:

- Unstable or acute cardiac failure.
- Bradycardia (heart rate <60 beats/min).
- Hypotension (systolic blood pressure <90 mmHg).
- Asthma.

Oxygen

Oxygen should be administered to all patients who have hypoxaemia (i.e. arterial oxygen saturation 90%). There is no good evidence that patients who are normoxic benefit from extra oxygen and there is some evidence of harm.

Non-acute management

The first 3 days after MI are spent in hospital because this is when most complications (Fig. 14.7) will arise. Before primary PCI patients generally spent 5–7 days in hospital.

Fig. 14.7 Complications of an acute myocardial infarction
Early (0–48 h)
Arrhythmias – VT, VF, SVT, heart block Cardiogenic shock due to left or right ventricular failure
Medium term (2–7 days)
Arrhythmias – VT, VF, SVT, heart block Pulmonary embolus (4–7 days) Rupture of papillary muscle (3–5 days) Rupture of interventricular septum (3–5 days) Free wall rupture (3–5 days) Note: Rupture of the above structures usually presents with acute cardiac failure and progresses rapidly to death; some patients may survive after surgery
Late (7 days)
Arrhythmias – VT, VF, SVT, heart block Cardiac failure Dressler syndrome (3–8 weeks) Left ventricular aneurysm (after several weeks) Mural thrombosis and systemic embolization
SVT, supraventricular tachycardia; VF, ventricular fibrillation: VT, ventricular tachycardia.

The following points of management must be observed. The patient must be seen and examined every day by a cardiologist. Particular points to look for on examination and questioning are:

- Chest pain – further pain indicates the possibility of another MI and should be investigated early with urgent coronary angiography.
- Breathlessness or signs of cardiac failure – diuretics should be commenced and urgent echocardiography performed to exclude septal defect or mitral regurgitation secondary to papillary muscle rupture.
- New murmurs – a ruptured papillary muscle causes mitral regurgitation; a ruptured septum causes ventricular septal defect.
- Pericardial rub – pericarditis.
- Hypotension – drug induced or secondary to cardiogenic shock. Cardiac rupture is thankfully uncommon but leads rapidly to shock and death.
- Bradycardia – heart block after an inferior MI (or very large anterior MI with septal necrosis).

Patients should have daily ECGs to look for arrhythmias including heart block.

A continuous cardiac monitor should be used for the first 5 days because fatal arrhythmias are common after MI (usually ventricular tachycardia or fibrillation).

Early mobilization (after 48 h) is instituted to prevent venous stasis.

If a patient has had a large MI, or if there is clinical evidence of cardiac failure (and provided there is no renal failure or hypotension), an angiotensin-converting enzyme inhibitor should be introduced at day 3 after MI. This improves outcome (as seen in the ISIS 4 and GISSI 3 studies).

All patients should be given a high-potency statin, regardless of measured blood cholesterol, as statins give benefit after MI separate to their lipid-lowering effects. NICE guidelines recommend that aspirin and clopidogrel should be continued for at least four weeks, with aspirin alone after this period. If the patient has received coronary stenting, clopidogrel (or prasugrel) may be continued for longer periods (typically one year). Omega 3 fatty acids may also be given. Patients with reduced ejection fraction after an MI should be considered for an aldosterone antagonist (either spironolactone or eplerenone). DVLA guidelines state that the patient cannot drive for at least one week if they have been treated with angioplasty, or four weeks if not (as long as ejection fraction is greater than 40%).

Follow-up care should include:

- An exercise test at about 6 weeks after MI to assess the risk of further ischaemia – if positive coronary angiography should be performed.
- Access to the rehabilitation programme.

Fig. 14.8 Drugs on discharge after myocardial infarction

Aspirin plus clopidogrel/prasugrel
β-Blocker
ACE inhibitor
A statin lipid-lowering drug

ACE, angiotensin-converting enzyme.

Cardiac rehabilitation

All good cardiac units have an integrated rehabilitation programme available to all cardiac patients that consists of:

- Progressively increasing exercise level to a maintenance level of as much regular rapid walking as possible every day.
- Dietary advice, particularly emphasizing the value of fish and olive oil, and fresh fruit and vegetables. Carbohydrate restriction for non-insulin-dependent diabetes mellitus and insulin resistance. Calorie restriction for patients who have diabetes mellitus or who are obese.
- Advice on medications (Fig. 14.8), their role in improving prognosis, and the importance of compliance.
- Advice from a clinical psychologist on how to cope with the illness.
- Group gymnasium sessions may help some patients by encouraging exercise and giving psychological support to each other.
- A subsequent support group may be continued as long as each individual patient finds it helpful; a doctor's input is important from time to time.

SUMMARY OF MANAGEMENT OF ISCHAEMIC CHEST PAIN

An algorithm summarizing the management of ischaemic chest pain is given in Fig. 14.9.

HEART BLOCK AFTER MYOCARDIAL INFARCTION

Ischaemic injury can occur at any point in the conducting system – the sinoatrial node, the atrioventricular node or anywhere from the bundle of His downwards. It is, therefore, not surprising that heart block after MI may be:

- First- or second-degree atrioventricular block.
- Complete heart block with atrioventricular dissociation.
- Interventricular block (complete or partial right or left bundle branch block).

Atrioventricular block is most associated with inferior MI. This is commonly thought to be due to ischaemia of the AV node, but in fact is caused by the Bezhold–Jarisch reflex; abnormally high vagal tone causes bradycardia and AV block, and is associated with reperfusion.

Anterior MI may cause heart block if there is marked septal necrosis (indicating a large anterior MI).

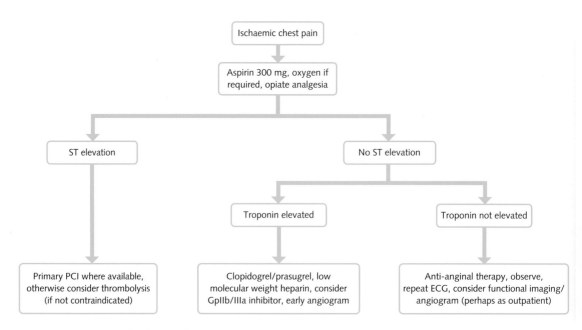

Fig. 14.9 Management of ischaemic chest pain. IV, intravenous.

Management of postmyocardial infarction heart block

Patients who have Mobitz type II or complete heart block and are hypotensive or clinically compromised should have temporary pacing wires inserted as soon as possible. Patients with a high degree of AV block who remain clinically stable should be carefully monitored.

The need for a permanent pacemaker depends upon the site of the MI.

Patients who have anterior MI and septal necrosis often need permanent pacing because the atrioventricular node rarely recovers.

Patients who have an inferior MI may not need permanent pacing because many recover normal function of the atrioventricular node. Current practice is to wait 10–14 days to allow intrinsic conduction to recover prior to a final decision regarding permanent pacemaker implantation.

CARDIOGENIC SHOCK AFTER MYOCARDIAL INFARCTION

Patients with cardiogenic shock due to a reversible cause like MI may be treated with an intra-aortic balloon pump (IABP). This balloon sits in the descending aorta and, using the ECG for timing, inflates during diastole. This forces blood back to the coronary arteries and forward to the renal arteries, increasing perfusion of the heart and kidneys.

Supraventricular tachyarrhythmias ⑮

By the end of this chapter you should:
- Know the definition of supraventricular tachyarrhythmias.
- Understand how different supraventricular tachyarrhythmias are generated.
- Be able to identify the different types of arrhythmia from the ECG.
- Know the difference between rate control and rhythm control strategies for the treatment of AF.
- Be able to outline the use of anticoagulation in patients with AF.
- Know which drugs to use for the treatment of supraventricular tachyarrhythmias and when to avoid certain drugs.
- Be able to list the major side effects.

Supraventricular tachyarrhythmias (SVTs) are fast rhythms characterized by narrow QRS complexes (unless aberrant conduction is present).

A tachycardia is defined as a rate of 100 beats/min or greater. In order of increasing atrial electrical dysfunction, these are:

- Sinus tachycardia.
- Atrial ectopics.
- Nodal ectopics.
- Atrial tachycardia.
- Junctional tachycardia and supraventricular re-entry tachycardia.
- Atrial flutter.
- Atrial fibrillation.

SINUS TACHYCARDIA

Points of importance are:

- The sinus node fires at over 100 beats/min.
- Every complex is preceded by a normal P wave.
- The PR interval is within normal limits and remains stable (Fig. 15.1).

Causes

Causes of sinus tachycardia include:
- Fever.
- Thyrotoxicosis.
- Hypotension.
- Hypoxia.
- Any form of stress (e.g. pain, anxiety and exertion).

These are all physiological responses. Occasionally, an inappropriate resting sinus tachycardia occurs. This is due to an abnormality of sinus node discharge or another atrial focus of activity located near the sinus node.

PREMATURE ATRIAL COMPLEXES

These are seen on the ECG as a premature P wave (which may be normal or abnormal in appearance) followed by a PR interval, which may be prolonged or short, depending upon where in the atrium the impulse arises (Fig. 15.2). This is followed by a pause because the atrioventricular (AV) node is refractory and cannot conduct. In contrast to ventricular premature complexes this pause is not fully compensatory (i.e. the next sinus beat occurs earlier than it otherwise would have done; after premature ventricular complexes the sinus beats continue on as normal).

Premature atrial complexes can be precipitated by many conditions including:

- Stress.
- Caffeine.
- Alcohol.
- Myocardial ischaemia.
- Myocardial inflammation.

Treatment is not indicated unless the patient is very symptomatic, in which case β-blockers (β-adrenoceptor antagonists) may be of benefit.

Fig. 15.1 Sinus tachycardia.

Fig. 15.2 ECG illustrating an ectopic atrial beat. Note that the premature atrial beat fires an abnormally shaped P wave and a normal QRS complex. A compensatory pause follows.

atrial ectopic

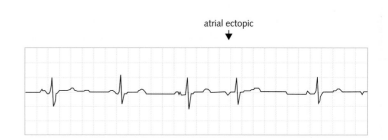

NODAL AND JUNCTIONAL ECTOPICS

The AV node is a compact structure and lying close to it is the AV junctional area. It is from this area and from the node itself that these ectopic beats originate. These structures have the ability to fire autonomously, but they have a slower rate of firing than the sinoatrial (SA) node; therefore, they are usually suppressed.

In some conditions, impulses arise ectopically from the AV node and junctional region. The impulse is conducted to the atrium where a retrograde P wave is produced and also to the ventricle where a narrow complex QRS is produced (Fig. 15.3). Depending on the speed of conduction, the P wave may occur just before, after or simultaneously with the QRS.

Again, treatment is not usually indicated.

ATRIAL TACHYCARDIA

Atrial tachycardia is a tachyarrhythmia generated in the atrial tissue. The atrial rate is 150–200 beats/min.

Because the origin of the tachycardia is not the SA node, the P-wave morphology is different from normal (Fig. 15.4). The P wave axis may also be abnormal, for example when the atrial focus is in the left atrium the P wave in lead V1 is positive.

Causes

The following may lead to atrial tachycardia:

- Structural heart abnormality.
- Coronary artery disease.
- Digitalis toxicity.

Investigation and diagnosis

On examination the pulse is rapid and of variable intensity:

- Jugular venous pressure may reveal many a waves to each v wave if there is a degree of atrioventricular (AV) block.
- ECG may show 1:1 conduction or variable degrees of AV block.
- It may be difficult to differentiate atrial tachycardia from atrial flutter.

retrograde P

nodal ectopic

Fig. 15.3 A nodal ectopic. The ectopic complex is similar to the normal QRS, suggesting that it originates from the atrioventricular or junctional region. The P wave is retrograde and is seen just after the ectopic QRS superimposed on the T wave. The ectopic beat is followed by a compensatory pause.

Fig. 15.4   Atrial tachycardia.

Abnormal P wave superimposed on T wave

Diagnosis may be aided by enhancing AV block and, therefore, making it easier to visualize the P wave morphology and rate. There are two effective methods of doing this:

1. Carotid sinus massage – increases vagal stimulation of the SA and AV node.
2. Intravenous adenosine – results in transient complete AV block.

HINTS AND TIPS

Remember that atrial flutter usually has an atrial rate of 300/min with a degree of AV block. Atrial tachycardia has a slightly slower atrial rate with abnormal P waves.

Management

The patient will present with palpitations. Any underlying cause should be treated (e.g. check digoxin levels and stop the drug).

Drugs used to treat atrial tachycardia include:

- Atrioventricular blocking drugs, such as digoxin, β-blockers (β-adrenoceptor antagonists, e.g. metoprolol) and calcium channel blockers (e.g. verapamil) – these slow the ventricular response rate, but do not affect the atrial tachycardia itself.
- Class IA (e.g. disopyramide), IC (e.g. flecainide) or III (e.g. amiodarone) drugs, which can be used to try to terminate the atrial tachycardia.

Electrical cardioversion is often successful.

ATRIOVENTRICULAR JUNCTIONAL TACHYCARDIA

Tachycardias arising from the junctional area occur when there is a focus of activity with a discharge rate that is faster than that of the SA node. This is an abnormal situation and is usually due to ischaemic heart disease or digitalis toxicity.

Clinical features

The following features are seen:

- Rate is usually up to 130 beats/min.
- Gradual onset.
- Terminates gradually.
- ECG shows a narrow complex tachycardia occasionally with retrogradely conducted P waves. It is difficult to distinguish this from an AV nodal re-entry tachycardia and you will not be expected to do so. The main point is to realize that the junctional tissue may be a site of ectopic electrical activity.

Management

Treatment is aimed at the underlying cause:

- Antiarrhythmic agents such as digoxin, β-blockers and calcium channel antagonists may be tried.
- Electrical cardioversion may be successful.

ATRIOVENTRICULAR NODAL RE-ENTRY TACHYCARDIA

These tachycardias involve a re-entry circuit that lies in or close to the AV node and allows impulses to travel round and round triggering the ventricles and the atria (in a retrograde manner) as they go.

Clinical features

These tachycardias display the following features:

- Rate is 150–260 beats/min.
- Usually sudden onset and offset.
- QRS complexes are narrow unless there is aberrant conduction and the P waves may occur just before, just after, or within the QRS (it is not always easy to see these) (Fig. 15.5).

Causes of re-entry tachycardia are caffeine, alcohol and anxiety.

Fig. 15.5 Atrioventricular nodal re-entry tachycardia.

P wave occur after QRS complex

Diagnosis

Differentiation from atrial flutter and atrial fibrillation (AF) can be made by either:

- performing carotid sinus massage or Valsalva manoeuvre

or

- giving intravenous adenosine.

These procedures block the AV node and, therefore, the P waves of atrial flutter can be seen or the baseline fibrillation of AF can be seen. Blockade of the AV node in re-entrant tachycardia breaks the re-entry circuit and terminates the tachycardia in most cases. Re-entry tachycardia will also be terminated by a ventricular ectopic beat.

Management

These tachycardias often terminate spontaneously with relaxation.

Vagal manoeuvres, such as carotid sinus massage and the Valsalva manoeuvre, are often effective in terminating the tachycardia and patients can be taught to do these themselves.

In hospital the following treatments can be effective:

- Vagal manoeuvres.
- Intravenous adenosine.
- Atrioventricular node blocking agents (e.g. β-blockers, digoxin and calcium channel blockers).
- Direct current (DC) cardioversion if less invasive methods have been unsuccessful.

In a patient who has recurrent troublesome AV nodal re-entry tachycardia, electrophysiological testing can locate the site of the abnormal circuit and this can then be ablated. This is a curative procedure. The main risk is AV node ablation resulting in complete heart block and requiring a permanent pacemaker.

WOLFF–PARKINSON–WHITE SYNDROME

In this condition there is an abnormal connection between the atrium and the ventricle along which the impulse can travel. This is known as an accessory pathway. In Wolff–Parkinson–White syndrome the accessory pathway is known as the bundle of Kent.

Characteristics of the bundle of Kent

The bundle of Kent is capable of:

- Anterograde conduction – that is it can conduct from the atrium to the ventricle; it is also capable of retrograde conduction.
- Conducting impulses faster than the normal His conductive tissue. Therefore, the ventricle is activated sooner than normal.

If, however, the impulse does not travel down the bundle of Kent, the P wave and QRS complex are normal. Therefore, it can be seen that the impulse can travel via two different routes from the atrium to the ventricle.

The impulse often travels both routes simultaneously; this results in a short PR interval and a slurred upstroke to the R wave (known as a delta wave; Fig. 15.6).

Tachycardias associated with Wolff–Parkinson–White syndrome

A number of tachycardias may occur:

- Atrioventricular re-entry tachycardia – the impulse is conducted from the atrium to the ventricle via the AV node then back to the atrium via the accessory pathway; this results in a narrow complex tachycardia.
- A similar tachycardia with conduction in the opposite direction (i.e. from the atrium to the ventricle via the accessory pathway) results in a broad complex tachycardia because the ventricle is depolarized from a point away from the bundle of His.
- Atrial fibrillation and atrial flutter may occur and may present a potential risk because the atrial impulses can be conducted rapidly via the accessory pathway giving ventricular rates of 300 beats/min or greater (avoiding the AV node which usually regulates conduction). This rapid ventricular rate predisposes to ventricular fibrillation.

delta wave

V1 V4

V2 V5

V3 V6

Fig. 15.6 Wolff–Parkinson–White syndrome. Note the short PR interval (0.08 s) and the slurred upstroke of the QRS complex (the δ wave). This is caused by part of the impulse travelling down the accessory pathway and causing pre-excitation (early excitation) of the ventricle (represented by the δ wave). The rest of the impulse travels via the atrioventricular node and is represented by the main QRS complex.

Clinical features

Wolff–Parkinson–White syndrome is a congenital condition. Patients present with recurrent palpitations or syncope. Sudden death is a risk due to ventricular tachyarrhythmias. The accessory pathway may cease to conduct as patients grow older, but other patients continue to have problems.

Management

Treatment of Wolff–Parkinson–White syndrome is indicated only in patients who have tachyarrhythmias; some patients have ECG evidence of the accessory pathway (short PR and delta waves), but no tachyarrhythmia, and these do not require treatment. There are a number of treatment options; the main ones to consider are drug therapy and ablation therapy.

Drug therapy

The aim of drug therapy is to slow conduction in the accessory pathway as well as to slow AV conduction. Drugs that do both are Vaughan Williams classification IA, IC, and III drugs.

Drugs such as digoxin and verapamil block the AV node, but do not affect the accessory pathway, so increasing the risk of rapid conduction of AF and flutter via the accessory pathway.

So remember that digoxin and verapamil should not be used as single agents in the treatment of tachycardias in Wolff–Parkinson–White syndrome.

Ablation therapy

This is the preferred method of treatment and is used to abolish accessory pathways. It may be surgical or electrical:

- Electrical ablation (or radiofrequency catheter ablation) is performed after the accessory pathway has been located by electrophysiological testing. This procedure is usually performed under light sedation using local anaesthetic, with access being via the femoral vein.
- Surgical ablation is rarely performed, but may be useful if electrical ablation is not successful.

ATRIAL FLUTTER

Atrial flutter has the following characteristics:

- Atrial contraction rate is regular and is 250–350 beats/min (usually 300 beats/min).

- Ventricular response is rarely 1:1 (300 beats/min), but more commonly 2:1 (150 beats/min), 3:1 (100 beats/min), etc.
- Severity of the symptoms – this depends on the ventricular response rate (i.e. a rapid ventricular response is likely to cause palpitations, angina and cardiac failure).

Causes include:

- Structural heart disease (e.g. valve disease, cardiomyopathy).
- Pulmonary disease (e.g. pulmonary embolus, pneumothorax, infection).
- Toxins (e.g. alcohol, caffeine).

Investigations and diagnosis

The ECG findings (Fig. 15.7) are:

- Regular sawtooth atrial flutter waves (P waves).
- Narrow QRS complexes (unless there is coexistent bundle branch block).

Diagnosis is confirmed by performing AV nodal blocking manoeuvres (e.g. adenosine or carotid sinus massage). This slows the ventricular response so that the sawtooth P waves are revealed on the ECG.

Management

Cardioversion back to sinus rhythm is the best treatment, but if this is not possible then slowing of the ventricular rate will provide symptomatic relief and protect against cardiac failure. Direct current cardioversion using a synchronized shock will rapidly and safely restore sinus rhythm in some cases. Class IA, IC or III drugs may be useful:

- Where DC cardioversion is unsuccessful to cardiovert to sinus rhythm chemically.

- To maintain sinus rhythm after successful electrical cardioversion.

Where cardioversion is not possible or not sustained AV blocking agents are used to slow the ventricular response rate (class II, class IV or digoxin). Note that some drugs (e.g. flecainide may slow the flutter rate, leading to 1:1 conduction of flutter beats and a corresponding *increase* in ventricular rate).

There is an increased risk of thrombus formation in atrial flutter so anticoagulation is recommended before DC cardioversion, as with atrial fibrillation.

ATRIAL FIBRILLATION

Atrial fibrillation has the following features:

- It is a common arrhythmia found in over 5% of the population over 70 years of age.
- There is disorganized random electrical activity in the atria resulting in a lack of effective atrial contraction.
- Stasis of blood in the atria predisposes to thrombus formation and embolic episodes.

The rhythm disturbance may be paroxysmal (transient), persistent (lasting longer than 1 week) or permanent (chronic).

Causes

Common causes are as follows:

- Ischaemic heart disease.
- Valvular heart disease, especially mitral valve disease.

Fig. 15.7 Atrial flutter. Note the sawtooth F waves at a rate of just over 300 beats/min and the ventricular response of 4:1. Leads II and V1 often show P waves best (but not in this case).

- Hypertensive heart disease.
- Pulmonary disease (e.g. embolus, infection, pneumothorax).
- Any form of sepsis.
- Thyrotoxicosis.
- Alcohol excess.

Investigations and diagnosis

The ECG shows no P waves and an irregular baseline with a variable ventricular response rate (hence the irregularly irregular pulse; Fig. 15.8). Ventricular response ranges from 90 to 170 beats/min, but can be faster or slower. The actual AF rate may be from 300 to 600 beats/min. Because of the absence of atrial contraction there are no a waves in the jugular venous pressure waveform and there cannot be a fourth heart sound.

Management

The decision needs to be made between a rhythm control strategy (aiming to restore and maintain sinus rhythm) or for rate control (controlling the ventricular response) alone (Fig. 15.9). The likelihood of successful cardioversion depends upon:

- Persistence of the underlying cause (e.g. a patient who has untreated mitral stenosis is unlikely to cardiovert successfully whereas a patient who has angina treated with medication or angioplasty is).
- Duration of the AF (i.e. the longer the duration the smaller the chance of cardioversion).

Treatment options (Fig. 15.10) are similar to those of atrial flutter:

- Rate control alone (usually with either β-blocker or a rate-slowing calcium channel antagonist, e.g. verapamil).
- DC cardioversion (often requiring higher energy than for atrial flutter) may cardiovert the patient into sinus rhythm.
- Pharmacological agents from group IC (e.g. flecainide, propafenone) if no structural heart disease or group III (e.g. amiodarone, sotalol) can be used to cardiovert or to maintain sinus rhythm after electrical cardioversion.

- Patients who have resistant AF may be treated with an AV node blocking agent to slow the electrical response (group II or IV drugs or digoxin).

Anticoagulation and atrial fibrillation

Atrial fibrillation carries an increased risk of thromboembolism because of cerebrovascular and peripheral embolization in particular. Benefits of anticoagulation must be balanced against risk of haemorrhage before the decision to anticoagulate is made. The following points must be recognized (in order to stratify the risk to the patient):

- Patients who have structural heart disease (e.g. valve lesion, dilated left ventricle) and AF have a higher risk of thromboembolic complications than those who have lone AF (i.e. AF with no obvious underlying cause).
- Patients who have other risk factors for thromboembolism (e.g. hypertension, diabetes mellitus and previous cerebral embolus) have a higher risk of thromboembolism.
- Older patients who have AF are at a greater risk.
- Warfarin reduces the risk of cerebral embolus by approximately 60–80%.
- Aspirin reduces the risk of cerebral embolus by approximately 40%.

Clinicians use the CHADS2 criteria (see Further reading) to help in the anticoagulation decision-making process. A CHADS2 score of 2 or more is considered high risk and all these patients are started on warfarin unless there are contraindications. A score of 1 is considered moderate risk; these patients can be treated with either warfarin or aspirin. A score of 0 is considered low risk and these patients are treated with aspirin only or no anticoagulation at all. Anticoagulation should be carefully monitored especially in the elderly. As mentioned above this group of patients have a higher risk of haemorrhage with anticoagulation. The international normalized ratio (INR) should be maintained at between 2 and 3. More recently, an extended scoring system, the CHA2DS2-VASc score, has also been employed by clinicians (see Further reading).

Fig. 15.8 Atrial fibrillation. Note the irregular baseline and the lack of P waves. The rhythm is irregularly irregular.

Fig. 15.9 Factors to consider when deciding to treat AF with rate or rhythm control

Rate control	Older patients Pre-existing coronary disease Contraindications to cardioversion
Rhythm control	Younger patients First episode of AF AF secondary to a treatable cause

Anticoagulation and cardioversion of AF

There is an increased risk of thromboembolism after cardioversion of AF to sinus rhythm. This is thought to be due to the formation of atrial thrombus before cardioversion and the persistence of inefficient contraction in certain parts of the atrium (e.g. left atrial appendage) for a few weeks after apparently successful cardioversion. Therefore, there is a risk of intracardiac clot forming for a few weeks, even after successful cardioversion. Points to note are as follows:

- If the AF is of recent onset (within 48 h) it is reasonable to anticoagulate the patient with intravenous heparin and cardiovert straightaway.
- If the patient has a longer history full anticoagulation should be given (warfarin with an INR 2–3)

for at least 4 weeks before cardioversion and continued for at least 6 months after cardioversion.

- In patients where emergency cardioversion is required (i.e. patients who have severe heart failure secondary to AF) cardioversion should be performed with heparin cover immediately.
- Transoesophageal echocardiography is a reliable way of excluding intracardiac clot and can be used to see whether it is safe to proceed to cardioversion immediately in an unanticoagulated patient.

HINTS AND TIPS

Heart rhythm disturbances are a cause of great concern to patients who worry about the possibility of sudden death. In general, supraventricular tachyarrhythmias are not life threatening; the main risk is of stroke, and this is reduced effectively with the treatment strategies discussed. The only life-threatening supraventricular tachyarrhythmia is pre-excited AF in patients with an accessory pathway, as this may degenerate into ventricular fibrillation. Therefore, symptomatic patients are usually treated on an inpatient basis with radiofrequency ablation.

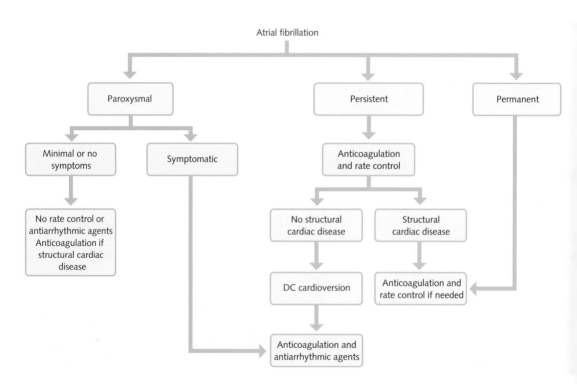

Fig. 15.10 Algorithm for the treatment of atrial fibrillation. Patients with troubling symptoms refractory to the depicted treatment should be considered for radiofrequency ablation therapy.

INVESTIGATION OF PATIENTS WHO HAVE SUPRAVENTRICULAR TACHYARRHYTHMIAS

The following investigations are appropriate for all patients who have a supraventricular tacharrhythmia (SVT).

Blood tests

These include:

- Electrolytes – hypokalaemia may predispose to tachyarrhythmias and also to digoxin toxicity.
- Thyroid function tests.
- Full blood count – anaemia may precipitate ischaemia.
- Liver function tests, particularly γ-glutamyltransferase, which is abnormal in patients who have excess alcohol intake.

Electrocardiography

Features that may be evident include:

- The arrhythmia.
- Ischaemic changes – these are usually accentuated during a tachycardia due to increased cardiac oxygen demand.
- Hypertensive changes.
- Pre-excitation.

24- or 48-h electrocardiography

This may be useful in identifying paroxysmal tachyarrhythmias.

Chest radiography

Notable features may include:

- Cardiomegaly or pulmonary oedema.
- Valve calcification.

Echocardiography

This may be useful because:

- Valve lesions and dilated cardiac chambers may be identified.
- Transoesophageal echocardiography will exclude intracardiac clot.

Electrophysiological studies

These are useful for arrhythmias when it is difficult to identify the mechanism and any possible focus or accessory pathway suitable for ablation.

Atrioventricular nodal blocking manoeuvres

These are used diagnostically and therapeutically:

- Diagnostically – they slow the ventricular response and enable P wave morphology to be seen.
- Therapeutically – they are used to terminate arrhythmias with re-entry circuits involving the AV node.

The following manoeuvres are appropriate:

- Carotid sinus massage.
- Valsalva manoeuvre – straining against a closed glottis.
- Adenosine administration (rapid intravenous injection).

Carotid sinus massage

This increases vagal tone and so prolongs AV node conduction time. The patient should be lying comfortably with the neck extended. Carotid bruits must be excluded (carotid artery occlusion may cause a stroke if the opposite side is heavily diseased).

The patient should preferably be connected to a 12-lead ECG running all 12 leads simultaneously. The P waves might not be seen if only a few leads are running.

Initial gentle and then firm pressure is applied to the carotid pulse just below the angle of the jaw. Remember – never do this on both sides simultaneously.

Pressure is applied for a maximum of 5–10 s.

Adenosine administration

Again the patient should be supine and connected to a 12-lead ECG continuous trace. Warn the patient that he or she may experience chest pain, flushing and dyspnoea for a few seconds after administration.

Establish intravenous access in a good-sized vein (antecubital fossa is ideal). Start with 6 mg rapid intravenous injection; follow with a rapid normal saline flush of 20 mL. If there is no response this may be followed by a 12 mg bolus, followed by another 12 mg bolus if necessary.

Actions of adenosine

Adenosine activates potassium channels and hyperpolarizes the cell membrane. It acts to slow AV conduction time.

The half-life of adenosine is very short (6 s) and it can be safely used to differentiate ventricular tachycardia from SVT with aberrant conduction. After adenosine the P waves will be revealed in SVT or the SVT may be terminated.

If verapamil is used for this purpose there is a risk of fatal myocardial depression in patients who have ventricular tachycardia.

HINTS AND TIPS

Adenosine can precipitate bronchospasm and should be avoided in asthmatic patients.

DRUGS USED TO TREAT TACHYARRHYTHMIAS

The older Vaughan Williams classification is still sometimes used:

- Class I – inhibitors of sodium current (like a local anaesthetic).
- Class II – β-adrenergic receptor antagonists.
- Class III – inhibitors of repolarization, which prolong the action potential and refractory period.
- Class IV – inhibitors of calcium current.
- Digitalis glycosides.

A summary of the electrophysiological actions of antiarrhythmic drugs is given in Fig. 15.11. It can be seen that class IA, IC and III drugs affect conduction in the atria and ventricular tissue – they are, therefore, useful for cardioverting many rhythms to sinus by breaking re-entry circuits or reducing the excitability of ectopic foci. Class III drugs have the added advantage of slowing AV conduction and, therefore, slowing ventricular response as well.

Class II and IV drugs and digoxin act as AV node blockers. This is useful in slowing the ventricular response and will cardiovert rhythms that are caused by re-entry circuits involving the AV node (e.g. AV nodal re-entry tachycardias and AV re-entry tachycardias).

A summary of the pharmacokinetics and side effects of antiarrhythmic agents is shown in Fig. 15.12.

HINTS AND TIPS

Antiarrhythmic agents can cause bradyarrhythmias as well as being arrhythmogenic and extreme caution should be exercised when using them and especially in combination.

Fig. 15.11 Electrophysiological actions of antiarrhythmic drugs

Vaughan Williams class of drug	Examples	Site of action	Sinus node rate	Atrial conduction rate	AV node refractory period	Ventricular conduction rate
IA	Quinidine, procainamide, disopyramide	Block fast sodium channels	No effect	Decreased	Increased	Decreased
IB	Lidocaine (lignocaine) mexiletine, tocainide	Block fast sodium channels	No effect	No effect	Not much effect (may slightly increase or decrease)	Decreased
IC	Flecainide, propafenone	Block fast sodium channels	Reduced	Decreased	Increased	Decreased
II	Atenolol, metoprolol, sotalol, propranolol	Block β-adrenergic receptors	Reduced	No effect	Increased	No effect
III	Amiodarone, sotalol, bretylium	Block potassium channels; mechanism not entirely understood	Reduced	Decreased	Increased	Decreased
IV	Verapamil, diltiazem	Block slow calcium channels	Small reduction	Slightly reduced	Increased	No effect
Digoxin		Blocks Na/K ATPase	No effect	Increased	Increased	Slows AV conduction

ATPase, adenosine triphosphatase.

Fig. 15.12   Pharmacokinetics and adverse effects of antiarrhythmic drugs

Drug	Route of administration	Half-life	Mode of excretion	Interactions	Adverse effects
Procainamide	Oral, IV or IM	3–5 h	Renal	Amiodarone reduces clearance	Skin rashes, Raynaud syndrome, hallucinations; toxicity – cardiac failure, long QT, ventricular tachyarrhythmias
Lidocaine (lignocaine)	IV (extensive first-pass metabolism in liver)	1–2 h	Hepatic	Cimetidine reduces clearance	Myocardial depression, cardiac failure, long QT; toxicity – dizziness, confusion, paraesthesia
Flecainide	Oral, IV	20 h	Renal (partly hepatic)	Cimetidine reduces clearance	Myocardial depression, ventricular arrhythmias (a major problem, especially in patients who have ischaemic heart disease)
Atenolol	Oral, IV		Renal	May precipitate asthma or peripheral ischaemia	Myocardial depression, bronchospasm, peripheral vasoconstriction
Sotalol	Oral, IV	10–15 h	Renal	May precipitate asthma or peripheral ischaemia	Myocardial depression, long QT, ventricular tachyarrhythmias
Amiodarone	Oral, IV	3–6 weeks	Hepatic	Reduces digoxin excretion, reduces warfarin excretion (need to watch INR closely)	Pulmonary fibrosis, liver damage, peripheral neuropathy, hyper- or hypothyroidism, corneal microdeposits, photosensitivity, myocardial depression (but safe in cardiac failure), long QT
Verapamil	Oral, IV	3–7 h	Renal	Reduces digoxin excretion	Myocardial depression, constipation
Digoxin	Oral, IV	36–48 h	Renal	Amiodarone, verapamil and propafenone decrease renal clearance; erythromycin increases absorption; captopril decreases renal clearance	Toxicity – heart block, atrial tachycardia, ventricular arrhythmia, xanthopsia

Note that a common complication of all antiarrhythmic agents is bradycardia, which can be severe. Care must always be used when increasing dosage or combining more than one agent.
IM, intramuscular; INR, international normalized ratio; IV, intravenous.

Further reading

Delacretaz, E., 2006. Supraventricular tachycardia. N. Engl. J. Med. 354, 1039.

National Institute of Clinical Excellence (NICE), 2006. Clinical Guideline 36. Atrial Fibrillation. http://guidance.nice.org.uk/CG36.

The Taskforce for the Management of Atrial Fibrillation of the European Society of Cardiology (ESC), 2010. Guidelines for the management of atrial fibrillation. Eur. Heart. J. 31, 2369–2429.

Ventricular arrhythmias 16

● **Objectives**

By the end of this chapter you should:
- Understand the clinical significance of ventricular ectopic beats.
- Know the key points for the ECG diagnosis of ventricular tachycardia.
- Know the management steps of broad complex tachycardia.
- Understand the role of different pharmacological and non-pharmacological management of ventricular arrhythmias.
- Understand the causes and clinical importance of a prolonged QT interval.

VENTRICULAR ECTOPIC BEATS

Also known as ventricular premature complexes, these beats have certain ECG characteristics (Fig. 16.1) such as:

- They occur before the next normal beat would be due.
- They are not preceded by a P wave.
- The QRS complex is abnormal in shape and has a duration of greater than 120 ms.
- They are followed by a compensatory pause so that the RR interval between the normal beats immediately preceding and immediately following the ectopic beat is exactly twice the normal RR interval (in atrial premature complexes the RR interval is less than this).

Clinical features

It is thought that ventricular ectopics occur in over half the normal population. This prevalence increases with age. These extra beats do not in themselves imply underlying heart disease.

Most people are entirely asymptomatic; others may complain of missed or extra beats. Alternatively, others may experience thumping or heavy beats because the beat immediately following the ectopic does so after a compensatory pause during which there is a prolonged filling time resulting in an increased stroke volume plus postextrasystolic potentiation of contractility.

A number of precipitating causes of ventricular premature beats are recognized, including:

- Low serum potassium.
- Excess caffeine consumption.
- Febrile illness.
- Underlying cardiac abnormality (e.g. myocardial ischaemia, cardiomyopathy, mitral or aortic valve disease).

Management

The clinical significance of ventricular ectopic beats is unclear and the general rule is that, in a patient who has no underlying cardiac abnormality, no treatment is needed unless symptoms are severe (in this situation a small dose of β-blocker should suppress ectopic activity).

In the post-myocardial infarction (MI) situation there is controversy about whether ventricular ectopics are significant or need treatment. Treatment with anti-arrhythmics may in fact increase the mortality rate: in the CAST trial, encainide/flecainide increased the risk of death 3.6-fold. In any case, all post-MI patients must have their serum electrolytes (especially potassium and magnesium) checked and should be given a β-blocker unless contraindicated.

DEFINITION OF VENTRICULAR TACHYARRHYTHMIAS

A ventricular tachyarrhythmia is an abnormal rapid rhythm that originates in the ventricular myocardium or the His-Purkinje system.

Ventricular tachyarrhythmias are broad complex – the QRS complex is greater than 120 ms in duration or three small squares on a standard ECG trace.

There are three basic types of ventricular tachyarrhythmia:

1. Monomorphic ventricular tachycardia.
2. Polymorphic ventricular tachycardia including 'Torsades de pointes'.
3. Ventricular fibrillation.

117

Fig. 16.1 Ventricular ectopic beats, which are indicated by arrows.

ventricular ectopic beats

VENTRICULAR TACHYCARDIA

Ventricular tachycardia (VT) is defined as three or more consecutive ventricular beats occurring at a rate greater than 120 beats/min (Fig. 16.2). Again the complexes are abnormally wide - their duration is longer than 120 ms.

Clinical features

Patients may tolerate this rhythm well and experience only palpitations or rarely nothing at all. However, the reduction in cardiac output caused by this arrhythmia often causes dizziness or syncope. Common precipitants include acute MI, cardiomyopathy or inherited conduction disorders.

Diagnosis

VT may be monomorphic (complexes on the surface ECG have the same shape) or polymorphic (beat-to-beat variations in morphology). The main differential diagnosis for VT is supraventricular tachycardia with aberrant conduction (or bundle branch block, usually RBBB) (Fig. 16.3). This causes much confusion and concern amongst junior doctors and final-year students alike. It helps if you remember the following points:

- Both arrhythmias are potentially fatal so treat each with respect.
- The use of carotid sinus massage or adenosine may briefly block the atrioventricular node and, therefore, slow the ventricular response in supraventricular tachycardia (it will have no effect on VT).

Fig. 16.2 ECG illustrating ventricular tachycardia. Note the concordance shown in the chest leads. No fusion or capture beats are visible.

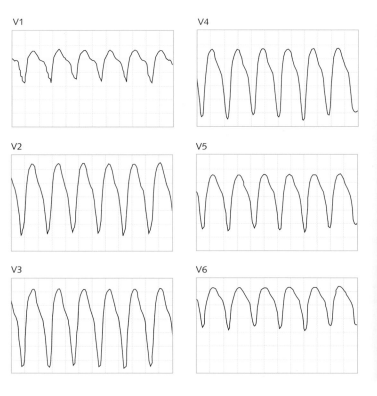

V1

V4

V2

V5

V3

V6

Fig. 16.3 Differences between ventricular tachycardia (VT) and supraventricular tachycardia (SVT) with bundle branch block (BBB)

Arrhythmia	VT	SVT with BBB
AV association	AV dissociation (no relationship between P waves and QRS)	P waves, if seen, are associated with the QRS
Variety of complexes	Capture beats (where a P wave is followed by a normal QRS); fusion beats (where a normal sinus beat occurs simultaneously with a ventricular beat, the resulting complex having an intermediate appearance that is a combination of the two component beats)	No capture or fusion beats
ECG pattern	May be RBBB or LBBB	Usually RBBB
Concordance	Present (the QRS complexes retain the same axis throughout the chest leads)	Absent (some QRS complexes will be positive, others will be negative)
QRS waveform	May vary from beat to beat	Constant

AV, atrioventricular; LBBB, left bundle branch block; RBBB, right bundle branch block.

- Never use verapamil or lidocaine (lignocaine) to slow the ventricular response in this situation: the negative inotropic effect of this drug could have disastrous effects if the rhythm is, in fact, VT, causing rapid development of cardiac failure.

Management

VT is very dangerous and if allowed to continue will result in cardiac failure or even death. Treatment must, therefore, be prompt and the nature of the treatment depends upon the clinical scenario:

- Patient conscious with VT and no haemodynamic compromise – treatment should be with drugs (these are discussed on p. 121).
- Patient conscious with VT, but haemodynamic compromise – triggered (synchronized) direct current (DC) cardioversion under general anaesthetic (fast bleep the anaesthetist).
- Patient unconscious with ongoing VT and no cardiac output ('pulseless VT') – praecordial thump followed by triggered (synchronized) DC cardioversion as per cardiac arrest protocol (see Resuscitation Council guidelines (Ch. 17)).

HINTS AND TIPS

It is vital to correct hypokalaemia promptly for all patients who have ventricular arrhythmias – potassium can be given orally or in a very dilute form via a peripheral vein. In the emergency situation larger doses of potassium can be given via a central line with careful monitoring of cardiac rhythm and serum potassium levels. Warning: intravenous potassium can cause ventricular fibrillation.

Electrophysiological studies

These studies involve inserting multiple electrodes into the heart via the great veins and positioning them at various intracardiac sites. Electrical activity can then be recorded from the atria, ventricles, bundle of His and so on to provide information on the type of conduction defect or rhythm disturbance. These studies are used mostly:

- To elucidate the mechanism of tachyarrhythmias.
- Therapeutically to terminate a tachyarrhythmia by overdrive pacing or shock.
- Therapeutically to ablate an area of myocardium thought to be propagating a recurrent tachyarrhythmia.
- Diagnostically to evaluate the risk of sudden cardiac death in patients who have possible ventricular tachyarrhythmias.
- Diagnostically to determine conduction defects in patients who have recurrent syncope.

Increasingly nowadays, patients who have survived a cardiac arrest will be treated with an implantable cardioverter defibrillator (ICD) without an electrophysiological study beforehand.

TORSADES DE POINTES

This rhythm is usually self-terminating, but can occasionally lead to VF and death. It is an irregular rapid rhythm with a characteristic twisting axis seen on the ECG (Fig. 16.4). In between episodes the ECG usually shows a long QT interval.

Fig. 16.4 Torsades de pointes. Note the irregular rhythm and twisting axis.

The QT interval corresponds to the time from depolarization to repolarization (beginning of the Q wave to end of T wave, i.e. action potential duration; see *Crash course: Cardiovascular system)* and varies according to the heart rate. Therefore, a long QT interval is approximated by a corrected QT interval (QTc) of greater than 0.44 s. QTc = QT/square root of RR interval.

Clinical features

The patient usually feels faint or loses consciousness as the result of a drop in cardiac output. Attacks may occur during periods of adrenergic stimulation (e.g. fear) or in some cases in the context of bradycardia or during a compensatory pause following an ectopic beat. There are many possible causes, all of which act through a prolonged QT interval (Fig. 16.5).

Fig. 16.5 Causes of a long QT interval

Cause	Examples
Congenital	Jervell and Lange–Nielsen syndrome (autosomal recessive and sensorineural deafness) Romano–Ward syndrome (autosomal dominant, no deafness)
Drugs	Class IA (e.g. quinidine, procainamide) Class III (e.g. amiodarone, sotalol) Tricyclic antidepressants (e.g. amitriptyline) Phenothiazines (e.g. chlorpromazine) Terfenadine
Electrolyte abnormalities	Hypokalaemia Hypomagnesaemia Hypocalcaemia
Others	Acute myocardial infarction Central nervous system disease Mitral valve prolapse Organophosphate insecticides

Management

Treatment of torsades de pointes differs from that of the other ventricular arrhythmias and is as follows:

- Identify and treat any precipitating factors (stop offending drugs, correct electrolyte imbalance).
- Atrial or ventricular pacing to maintain a heart rate of no less than 90 beats/min to prevent lengthening of the QT interval – intravenous isoprenaline may also be used to reduce the QT interval.
- In congenital long QT syndromes high-dose β-blockers (β-adrenoceptor antagonists) or left stellectomy may be used and there is increasing use of permanent pacemakers and cardioverter defibrillators.

Do not use antiarrhythmic drugs.

VENTRICULAR FIBRILLATION

Ventricular fibrillation (VF) is irregular rapid ventricular depolarization (Fig. 16.6). There is no organized contraction of the ventricle; therefore the patient has no pulse. This arrhythmia rapidly causes loss of consciousness and cardiorespiratory arrest.

Clinical features

The most common cause of VF is acute MI. However, it is also seen at the end-stage of many disease processes and signifies the presence of severe myocardial damage (this is sometimes referred to as secondary VF and usually results in death despite resuscitation attempts). It may be precipitated by:

- A ventricular ectopic beat or blow to the chest (commotio cordis) - rare.
- Ventricular tachycardia.
- Torsades de pointes.

Management

VF must be treated promptly with simple (non-synchronized) DC cardioversion (the resuscitation protocol is discussed in Ch. 17). A single praecordial thump may be given in a witnessed arrest but it is vital to start effective chest compressions as soon as possible while the defibrillator is charging.

Coarse VF

Fine VF

Fig. 16.6 Ventricular fibrillation (VF) can have a coarse or a fine pattern.

For secondary prevention an ICD is indicated (see p. 122).

DRUGS USED TO TREAT VENTRICULAR TACHYCARDIA AND FIBRILLATION

In the acute situation, if the patient is unconscious or has no cardiac output, give prompt DC cardioversion. Effective chest compressions should be given while the defibrillator is charging. 200 J is the normal starting voltage for a biphasic defibrillator, but each hospital will have a published protocol which you should follow. If the arrhythmia persists further resuscitation is carried out according to the set protocol. This is discussed in Ch. 17.

The drugs used to treat ventricular tachyarrhythmias other than torsades de pointes fall into two main classes:

1. Class I.
2. Class III.

In the acutely ill patient who has VT or VF, antiarrhythmic agents may be given after sinus rhythm has been established by DC cardioversion (Fig. 16.7) in an effort to stabilize the myocardium. Amiodarone or β-blockers are commonly used, but alternative agents include flecainide and lidocaine (lignocaine). Amiodarone is a good choice for the patient who has cardiac failure, because it has little negative inotropic effect. If given intravenously, amiodarone after the initial bolus dose should be given centrally, because it is damaging to peripheral veins:

- Amiodarone has a very long half-life (25 days) and oral loading takes at least 1 month. Intravenous loading is faster.

- In a patient who has no contraindication for β-blockers, sotalol is a good long-term agent because it has none of the long-term side effects of amiodarone. It must be used in high doses to gain the class III effect, but should be uptitrated gradually, measuring the QT interval before each dose increase.
- Flecainide is an effective agent but is avoided in patients who have suspected ischaemic heart disease because this may increase its proarrhythmic effects. For secondary prevention an ICD should be considered.

The Vaughan Williams classification of antiarrhythmic drugs allows agents to be grouped according to their mode of action on the myocardium and also makes selection of appropriate agents for the treatment of any given arrhythmia more straightforward.

Drug treatment alone for the secondary prevention of ventricular arrhythmia has been shown to be ineffective, although β-blockers should be used where possible in patients post MI or with heart failure, and drugs are a useful adjunct to reduce the frequency of arrhythmic events in conjunction with ICD therapy.

NON-PHARMACOLOGICAL TREATMENTS OF VENTRICULAR TACHYARRHYTHMIAS

Non-pharmacological treatments are used in patients who have recurrent VT or VF because:

- If successful, complete cure is achieved without the need for drugs.
- Localization of the arrhythmogenic focus is becoming possible in more cases due to increased understanding of the mechanisms of these arrhythmias.

Fig. 16.7 Main features of common antiarrhythmic drugs classed using Vaughan Williams classification

Class of agent	Class I	Class II	Class III	Class IV	Digoxin
Examples	IA – quinidine, procainamide, disopyramide; IB – lidocaine (lignocaine) mexiletine, tocainide; IC – flecainide, propafenone	β-blockers (e.g. atenolol, bisoprolol, metoprolol); sotalol also has some class III activity	Amiodarone, sotalol, bretylium	Calcium channel blockers (e.g. diltiazem, verapamil)	Not classified by the Vaughan Williams system
Mode of action	Variable action on the His-Purkinje system	Increase AV node refractory period	Increase both AV node and His-Purkinje refractory period	Increase AV node refractory period	Slows AV conduction; increases AV node refractory period; positively inotropic
Adverse effects	Quinidine – nausea, diarrhoea; procainamide – development of antinuclear antibodies and SLE; flecainide – higher incidence of proarrhythmic effects than other class I drugs; all may lengthen QT and cause torsades; all are negatively inotropic	Negatively inotropic, may induce bronchospasm, exacerbation of peripheral vascular disease	Amiodarone – pulmonary fibrosis, hypo-/hyperthyroidism, hepatic toxicity, cutaneous photosensitivity; corneal microdeposits (reversible), peripheral neuropathy; sotalol – as for other β-blockers; both may lengthen QT and cause torsades	Verapamil and diltiazem – complete AV block, negatively inotropic	Nausea, vomiting if blood levels too high, visual disturbances (xanthopsia), complete heart block positively inotropic

AV, atrioventricular; SLE, systemic lupus erythematosus.

The two methods commonly used are:

1. Radiofrequency ablation.
2. Implantable cardioverter defibrillator (ICD).

Radiofrequency ablation

This involves localization of the proarrhythmic focus using intracardiac electrodes introduced via a central vein followed by the use of radiofrequency energy to cauterize the myocardium in that area. The successful result is the ablation of the focus, therefore rendering the patient cured and no longer needing antiarrhythmic agents. This technique is commonly used in patients who have Wolff–Parkinson–White syndrome (a supraventricular arrhythmia) who are young and have a discrete accessory pathway that can be localized easily. Ventricular arrhythmias can also sometimes be prevented by ablation, though this does not in itself reduce the incidence of sudden death.

Implantable cardioverter defibrillators

ICDs are now being increasingly used in the treatment of sustained or life-threatening ventricular arrhythmias, because they have been shown in some studies to prolong survival in such patients. These devices are slightly larger than a permanent pacemaker and are implanted in the same way (i.e. the box is situated superficial to the pectoralis major muscle on the patient's non-dominant side and the leads are positioned in the atrium and ventricle via the cephalic or subclavian vein). The device can sense VT and VF and can attempt to cardiovert the arrhythmia by pacing the ventricle or by delivering a DC shock.

The implantation and subsequent programming and monitoring of these devices should be performed in specialist centres. The indications are complicated and you certainly don't need to memorise them. An ICD may be indicated for primary prevention (prophylaxis) as well as secondary prevention (previously documented episode). Current NICE guidelines recommend the use of an ICD in survivors of VT/VF arrest, patients who have collapsed or had a documented significant blood pressure drop due to VT, in patients with severe heart failure (ejection fraction <35%) where sustained VT has been recorded, as long as their functional state is reasonable (NYHA class I-III), and in those who have suffered an acute MI in whom ejection fraction is < 30% 3 months post-MI (and where the QRS interval is >120 ms).

COMMUNICATION

Patients need counselling and advice before implantation of an ICD (in order to give fully informed consent) because the sensation when the ICD discharges a shock can be extremely unpleasant and comes without warning. This may result in marked psychological problems in some patients.

Further reading

Bardy, G.H., Lee, K.L., Mark, D.B., et al., 2005. Amiodarone or an implantable cardioverter-defibrillator for congestive heart failure. N. Engl. J. Med. 352, 225–237.

DiMarco, J.P., 2003. Implantable cardioverter-defibrillators. N. Engl. J. Med. 349, 1836–1847.

Edhouse, J., Morris, F., March 2002. ABC of clinical electrocardiography: Broad complex tachycardia. Part I, BMJ 324, 719–722, Part II, BMJ 324, 776–779.

Moss, A.J., Zareba, W., Hall, W.J., et al., 2002. Prophylactic implantation of a defibrillator in patients with myocardial infarction and reduced ejection fraction. N. Engl. J. Med. 346, 877–883.

National Institute for Health and Clinical Excellence (NICE), 2000. Guidance on the use of implantable cardioverter defibrillators for arrhythmias. National Institute for Health and Clinical Excellence, London.

Objectives

By the end of this chapter you should:
- Know the main steps of basic life support.
- Understand management of upper airway obstruction by foreign material.
- Know the placement of defibrillator pads.
- Be able to outline the ALS algorithm.
- Be able to list the potentially reversible causes of cardiac arrest.

Cardiopulmonary arrest results in a rapid decline in oxygen delivery to the brain. Permanent disability or death results if the period of cerebral hypoxia lasts longer than 3 min.

Cardiopulmonary resuscitation (CPR) is the term used to describe the maintenance of adequate breathing and circulation in a patient who cannot do so for him-or herself. The aim of CPR is to restore respiration and adequate cardiac output as soon as possible to prevent death or permanent disability. Cardiopulmonary resuscitation involves two types of protocol:

1. Basic life support (BLS) – no special equipment required.
2. Advanced life support (ALS) – requires specialist skill and equipment.

In any type of resuscitation protocol the following three areas must be assessed and supported in order of priority:

- Airway.
- Breathing.
- Circulation.

BASIC LIFE SUPPORT

BLS refers to the maintenance and support of airway, breathing and circulation without the aid of any specialized equipment (Fig. 17.1). The aim of BLS is to maintain adequate ventilation and cardiac output until the underlying problem can be reversed. There are a number of points to note relating to Fig. 17.1:

- If trauma to the cervical spine is a possibility, the airway should be maintained without tilting the head.
- If there are two operators, one should go for help as soon as possible. If there is only one the operator should shout for help and if necessary *very* quickly

(i.e. taking seconds) go to obtain help after establishing that the victim is not breathing. If, however, the victim is a child, then 1 min of CPR should be given before the operator goes for help – in these situations the collapse is likely to be due to respiratory arrest and rescue breaths, if given early, will improve prognosis.

- Check and, if necessary, open the airway.
- Assessment of the carotid pulse should take no more than 10 s.
- If there is no pulse, chest compressions are performed by placing the heel of the hand over the lower half of the sternum. Enough pressure should be applied to depress the sternum 5–6 cm and no more.
- The operator should be vertically above the victim's chest and the arms should be kept straight. The rate of compressions should be 100–120/min. After each compression the pressure should be released and the chest wall allowed to rise back up. The sequence is 30 compressions followed by 2 rescue breaths.
- Each rescue breath is given by mouth-to-mouth inflation with the nose occluded and should deliver approximately 700 mL expired air into the lungs of the victim. The operator should watch the chest wall of the victim to ensure that it rises and falls with each breath. Each breath will take approximately 1–1.5 s. It is important to allow the chest wall to fall back completely before taking the next breath.

Principle of chest compressions

The current theory suggests that chest compression increases intrathoracic pressure and it is this that propels blood out of the thorax. The veins collapse, but the arteries remain patent and flow is, therefore, in a forward direction.

Fig. 17.1 Algorithm for adult basic life support. (With permission from The Resuscitation Council (UK).)

 2010 Resuscitation Guidelines

 Resuscitation Council (UK)

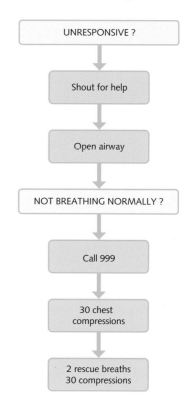

Adult Basic Life Support

UNRESPONSIVE ?

Shout for help

Open airway

NOT BREATHING NORMALLY ?

Call 999

30 chest compressions

2 rescue breaths 30 compressions

Recovery position

The function and features of the recovery position are shown in Fig. 17.2. This should be adopted if an unresponsive patient is both breathing and has a pulse whilst the rescuer goes for help. It has several important functions, including keeping the patient's airway straight, allowing the tongue to fall forward and not obstruct the airway, and minimising risk of aspiration of gastric contents.

HINTS AND TIPS

The final examinations are likely to test BLS techniques, so practise these until you are competent. Inability to perform BLS satisfactorily in finals almost always results in a fail.

Management of upper airway obstruction by foreign material

The management of choking in a conscious victim, although not strictly BLS, is extremely important because it is a common occurrence both in the community and in the hospital where aspiration of stomach contents or blood may occur (Fig. 17.3).

Points to note in the management of choking:

- If the patient becomes cyanosed then immediate positive action is needed with administration of oxygen and back blows followed by the Heimlich manoeuvre.
- Back blows are performed during expiration with the patient either standing or sitting, and with the head bent down below the level of the chest.

hand under cheek keeps head tilted back

Airway straight with no obstruction from tongue – minimises risk of aspiration

lower arm not under body

upper leg, hip and knee are at right angles

Manoeuvres

1. Remove victim's spectacles

2. Ensure airway is open by lifting chin

3. Kneel beside victim

4. Tuck one hand under the victim's buttock (arm should be straight with palm facing up)

5. Bring other forearm across victim's chest and hold back of hand against the victim's nearest cheek

6. With your other hand bring far leg into a bent position with foot still on the ground and, keeping the hand pressed against the cheek, pull on the leg to roll the victim towards you onto his or her side

Fig. 17.2 The recovery position.

2010 Resuscitation Guidelines

Resuscitation Council (UK)

Fig. 17.3 Algorithm for the management of choking. (With permission from The Resuscitation Council (UK).)

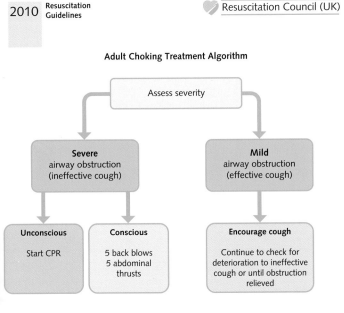

Adult Choking Treatment Algorithm

Assess severity

Severe
airway obstruction
(ineffective cough)

Mild
airway obstruction
(effective cough)

Unconscious

Start CPR

Conscious

5 back blows
5 abdominal
thrusts

Encourage cough

Continue to check for deterioration to ineffective cough or until obstruction relieved

- Heimlich manoeuvre – this may be performed with the patient standing, sitting or lying down. Sharp upward pressure is applied in the midline just beneath the diaphragm with the operator behind the patient. This procedure can result in damage to abdominal viscera and should not be attempted in small children or pregnant women.

ADVANCED LIFE SUPPORT

The ALS method of resuscitation requires specialist training and equipment, and has recently been reviewed and modified. The 2010 Resuscitation Council (UK) guidelines use a universal algorithm that is dependent upon the presence or absence of a shockable or non-shockable rhythm (Fig. 17.4).

2010 Resuscitation Guidelines

Resuscitation Council (UK)

Adult Advanced Life Support

Unresponsive?
Not breathing or
only occasional gasps

Call
resuscitation team

CPR 30:2
Attach defibrillator / monitor
Minimise interruptions

Assess
rhythm

Shockable
(VF / Pulseless VT)

Non-Shockable
(PEA / Asystole)

1 Shock

Return of
spontaneous
circulation

Immediately resume
CPR for 2 min
Minimise interruptions

Immediate post cardiac arrest treatment
• Use ABCDE approach
• Controlled oxygenation and ventilation
• 12-lead ECG
• Treat precipitating cause
• Temperature control / therapeutic hypothermia

Immediately resume
CPR for 2 min
Minimise interruptions

During CPR
• Ensure high-quality CPR: rate, depth, recoil
• Plan actions before interrupting CPR
• Give oxygen
• Consider advanced airway and capnography
• Continuous chest compressions when advanced airway in place
• Vascular access (intravenous, intraosseous)
• Give adrenaline every 3-5 min
• Correct reversible causes

Reversible Causes
• Hypoxia
• Hypovolaemia
• Hypo-/hyperkalaemia/metabolic
• Hypothermia

• Thrombosis - coronary or pulmonary
• Tamponade - cardiac
• Toxins
• Tension pneumothorax

Fig. 17.4 Algorithm for advanced adult life support. VF, ventricular fibrillation; VT, ventricular tachycardia. (With permission from The Resuscitation Council (UK).)

Make sure you have seen all of the pieces of equipment used for ALS.

Points to note about advanced life support

Protocol

The protocol for ALS (see Further reading) consists of 2-min cycles of CPR (30 compression:2 breaths) irrespective of the initial rhythm. However, if the rhythm shows ventricular fibrillation (VF) or ventricular tachycardia (VT) (i.e. a 'shockable' rhythm) then the CPR is preceded by 1 shock. Following the shock, it is no longer advised to stop and check the rhythm. This is done at the end of the cycle of CPR. Adrenaline (10 mL of 1:10 000 IV) is given every 4 min (i.e. every two cycles).

Airway ventilation and protection

During these cycles of CPR:

Adequate ventilation must be established.
The airway must be protected by an operator (preferably an anaesthetist) who remains at the patient's head.

The optimal method of protecting the airway is by insertion of a cuffed endotracheal tube. This device minimizes the risk of aspiration of the gastric contents and allows effective ventilation to be carried out. Endotracheal intubation can be a hazardous procedure and a laryngeal mask airway is an alternative.

Intravenous access must also be established either via a large peripheral vein or preferably via a central vein.

Placing the defibrillator pads

Placement of the defibrillator pads is important because only a small proportion of the energy reaches the myocardium during transthoracic defibrillation and every effort should be made to maximize this:

- The right pad should be placed below the clavicle in the mid-clavicular line.
- The left pad should be placed on the lower rib cage on the anterior axillary line.

Regardless of the setting, it is crucial that basic life support is commenced immediately and, once a cardiac monitor is available, that defibrillation of VT/VF is administered immediately. It is these two factors that affect the eventual outcome of resuscitation.

The ventricular tachycardia/fibrillation arm of the advanced life support algorithm

In the event of VF or VT (so-called 'shockable' rhythms), one DC shock should be administered. The energy should be 360 J for a monophasic defibrillator, or 150–200 J for a biphasic defibrillator. Following this shock, CPR should be restarted immediately. Pulse and rhythm are then assessed after one cycle of 2-min CPR. The algorithm then restarts with one further shock if indicated, or continuation of CPR for a further 2 min. Adrenaline is given every 4 min. If the arrhythmia persists, antiarrhythmics such as amiodarone may be used.

The non-VT/VF arm of the ALS algorithm

This arm includes asystole, pulseless electrical activity (previously termed electromechanical dissociation) and profound bradyarrhythmias. Prognosis for patients in this arm is much poorer than in the VF/VT arm. Defibrillation is not required unless VT/VF supervenes and 2-min cycles of CPR are given. During this period, possible underlying causes must be excluded or treated:

- Asystole is treated initially with IV adrenaline 1 mg. During subsequent cycles of CPR adrenaline may be repeated.

Pulseless electrical activity (PEA) occurs when there is a regular rhythm on the monitor (that is not VT), but no cardiac output arising from it. Underlying causes must be sought because these may be easily treated. The following are possible underlying causes of PEA:

- Hypovolaemia – rapid administration of IV fluids is required.
- Electrolyte imbalance (e.g. hypokalaemia, hypocalcaemia) – check ABG.
- Tension pneumothorax – suspect in trauma cases or after insertion of central line; also seen spontaneously in fit young men. Look for absence of chest movements and breath sounds on one side. Treat with cannula into the pleural space at the second intercostal space in mid-clavicular line followed by insertion of chest drain.
- Cardiac tamponade – suspect in trauma cases and post-thoracotomy patients. Need rapid insertion of pericardial drain.
- Pulmonary embolism – if strongly suspected thrombolysis should be administered.

It is helpful in the event of a cardiac arrest for an experienced member of the team to discuss the course of events early on with the patient's relatives or next of kin if possible. Discussing the situation at an early stage can facilitate breaking bad news if the resuscitation attempt is unsuccessful.

In-hospital cardiac arrest

When a cardiac arrest occurs in hospital, a call is put out to the arrest team. Most hospitals in the UK have a standard number (2222), which is a direct line to the switchboard operator. The caller should state in a clear voice, 'Cardiac arrest, ward X'. The switchboard operator will then repeat the information back to the caller before calling the arrest team. Generally the arrest team comprises an anaesthetist, a medical registrar, a senior house officer and an FY1, as well as a porter who can take urgent blood samples to the laboratory. The anaesthetist or registrar are usually in charge of the resuscitation effort, and will direct the other members of the team.

Many hospitals now use audit forms to analyse the response to each cardiac arrest call. These forms collect information on the condition of the patient on arrival (were they breathing and did they have a pulse?), events during the arrest (what was their heart rhythm and did they require defibrillation?), and whether it was successful or not. The results of audit sheets are used to direct further training of the arrest team.

Further reading

Resuscitation Council (UK), 2010. Adult Advanced Life Support Resuscitation Guidelines. http://www.resus.org.uk/pages/mediMain.htm.

By the end of this chapter you should:

- Know the pathological causes of sinus bradycardia.
- Understand the difference between Mobitz I and Mobitz II heart block and how they are managed.
- Be able to describe the management of complete heart block.
- Be able to recognize the ECG appearance of left and right bundle branch block.
- Be aware of different types of pacemakers.

DEFINITION OF BRADYARRHYTHMIAS

The bradyarrhythmias (Fig. 18.1) are slow rhythms.

SINUS BRADYCARDIA

Sinus bradycardia occurs when the resting heart rate is less than 60 beats/min; this can be physiological (e.g. during sleep) and is also seen in young athletes. Pathological causes include:

- Sinus node disease (especially in the elderly).
- Raised intracranial pressure.
- Severe hypoxia.
- Hypothyroidism (myxoedema).
- Hypothermia.
- Tumours (cervical, mediastinal).
- Sepsis.
- Drugs (β-blockers, calcium channel blockers and other antiarrhythmic agents).
- Ischaemic heart disease affecting the SA node (in 60% of patients the SA node is supplied by the right coronary artery).

Patients are usually asymptomatic and no treatment is required. Occasionally, however, syncope, hypotension or dyspnoea may occur. In these circumstances, treatment with IV atropine or isoprenaline, or insertion of a temporary pacing wire might be required to speed up the heart rate until the underlying condition is treated.

Sinus node disease

The sinoatrial (SA) node is the natural cardiac pacemaker. It is a crescent-shaped structure approximately 1 mm × 3 mm in size. The SA node is located just below the epicardial surface at the junction of the right atrium and the superior vena cava.

The rate at which the SA node generates impulses is determined by both vagal and sympathetic tone. The impulses are conducted via the atrial myocardium to the atrioventricular (AV) node.

Disease of the SA node may be due to:

- Age-related degeneration and fibrosis.
- Ischaemia and infarction.
- Excessive vagal stimulation.
- Myocarditis.
- Rarely, conduction disease including sinus node disease may be genetic.

This can result in pauses between consecutive P waves (>2 s). There are degrees of SA node conduction abnormality:

- Sinoatrial exit block – an expected P wave is absent, but the following one occurs at the expected time (i.e. the pauses are exact multiples of the basic PP interval).
- Sinus pause or sinus arrest (Fig. 18.2) – the interval between the P waves is longer than 2 s and is not a multiple of the basic PP interval.

Tachy-brady syndrome (sick sinus syndrome)

This is a combination of sinus node disease and abnormal tachyarrhythmias. It is most commonly caused by degenerative fibrosis of the SA node in the elderly.

Management

Patients who have symptomatic sinus pauses or evidence of recurrent sinus pauses require permanent pacing with a dual-chamber pacemaker (assuming rate-slowing drugs have been discontinued). Single chamber (ventricular) pacemakers are usually reserved only for patients who have atrial fibrillation. It is worth

Fig. 18.1 Bradyarrhythmias listed in ascending order of electrical dysfunction

Bradyarrhythmia	Features
Sinus bradycardia	Heart rate <60 beats/min during the day
Sinoatrial node disease and sick sinus syndrome	Prolonged PP interval, may be associated with tachyarrhythmias and, intermittently, with tachy-brady syndrome
First-degree heart block Second-degree heart block – Mobitz type I	PR interval >0.20 s Wenckebach phenomenon – progressive prolongation of PR interval with eventual dropped beat
Second-degree heart block – Mobitz type II	Dropped beats, no prolongation of PR interval
Second-degree heart block –2:1 heart block/ 3:1 heart block	Every second or third beat conducted, the rest are not
Complete heart block, third-degree heart block	Complete AV dissociation
Asystole	No beats conducted, no ventricular activity
Ventricular standstill P wave aystole	Visible P waves but no QRS complex

AV, atrioventricular.

noting that many patients with SA node disease have more distal conduction disease, hence why dual- (rather than single-) chamber pacemakers are usually used.

Antiarrhythmic drugs may also be needed if the patient has sick sinus syndrome. Pacemaker insertion should be considered before commencing these because they will make the SA node conduction defect worse. Paroxysmal AF often coexists with sinus node disease, so such patients will often also need anticoagulation.

ATRIOVENTRICULAR BLOCK

The AV node is a complex structure that lies in the right atrial wall on the septal surface between the ostium of the coronary sinus and the septal leaflet of the tricuspid valve. In 90% of patients the AV node is supplied by the right coronary artery. The rest are supplied via the circumflex coronary artery.

The AV node acts as a physiological gearbox conducting impulses from the atria to the ventricular conductive tissue.

First-degree atrioventricular block

In this conduction disturbance (Fig. 18.3), conduction time through the AV node is prolonged, but all impulses are conducted. The PR interval is longer than 0.20 s.

This condition does not require treatment in a healthy patient, but should be watched because it can herald greater degrees of block (this occurs in approximately 40% of cases). This is particularly important in patients who have evidence of other conducting tissue disease, e.g. bundle branch block.

Second-degree atrioventricular block

In this type of block some impulses are not conducted from the atria to the ventricles.

Mobitz type I heart block – Wenckebach phenomenon

Wenckebach phenomenon is characterized by progressive prolongation of the PR interval; eventually resulting in a non-conducted P wave (dropped QRS complex). The cycle is then repeated. This is a common phenomenon and can occur in any cardiac tissue, including the SA node.

HINTS AND TIPS

In a patient who has infective endocarditis serial ECGs are performed to observe the PR interval. Prolongation of this can occur secondary to the formation of a paravalvular abscess (the conducting tissue is in close proximity to the valve ring) and this usually heralds rapid development of complete heart block and valve dehiscence. In these patients progressive prolongation of the PR interval therefore requires an urgent ECG and temporary pacing wire.

Fig. 18.2 Sinus pause or arrest. Note the interval of more than 2s between P waves.

P   P

Fig. 18.3 ECGs of bradyarrhythmias. (A) First-degree heart block. Note the long PR interval. (B) Mobitz type I (Wenckebach) partial heart block caused by inferior myocardial infarction (raised ST segments in leads II, III and AVF). (C) 2:1 heart block; arrows point to dropped P waves. There are two P waves (A) from the atrium for every QRS (V) from the ventricles.

Wenckebach phenomenon can occur in athletes and children, and is due to high vagal tone. It is usually benign and is not usually an indication for pacing.

When it occurs after an inferior myocardial infarction (MI), pacing is not usually required unless the patient is symptomatic. In anterior MI any newly developed heart block suggests massive septal necrosis and temporary pacing is required.

Mobitz type II heart block

The PR interval remains constant and P waves are dropped intermittently. This type of heart block carries a risk of progressing to complete heart block and requires insertion of a pacemaker.

2:1 or 3:1 heart block

This represents a more advanced degree of block and requires pacing because there is a high risk of complete heart block.

Third-degree or complete heart block

Complete heart block (CHB) (Fig. 18.4) results in dissociation of the atria from the ventricles.

The ECG shows that the P waves and the QRS complexes are independent from one another. The P and QRS complexes are regular, but bear no temporal relationship to one another. There is a ventricular 'escape' rhythm, which usually gives rise to wide QRS complexes. Note that if the AV block is proximal ('high') the complexes may be narrow.

On examination there might be some classic features:

- The first heart sound has a variable intensity.
- There are intermittent cannon waves in the jugular venous pulse. These correspond to a large a wave caused by the right atrial contraction against a closed tricuspid valve.

Management depends upon the underlying cause:

- After an inferior MI a temporary pacemaker should only be inserted in the event of haemodynamic compromise. Usually, the AV block is high (at the level of

the AV node itself), temporary and the escape rate is reasonable. Most of these cases revert back to normal conduction within a few weeks and a permanent pacemaker is rarely needed. If the heart block is due to drugs (e.g. β-blockers) it may resolve once these are withdrawn.
- After an anterior MI a permanent pacemaker (PPM) will be required and should be inserted promptly (unless the patient is unstable in which case a temporary wire is inserted first, followed by a permanent system some days later). The AV block is lower, generally permanent, and the escape rate unsustainably low.
- In the absence of MI, symptomatic CHB requires a permanent pacemaker. A PPM will also be required in asymptomatic CHB with documented asystole ('pauses') >3 s, or an escape rate <40 beats/min. Note that congenital CHB often has a high AV block, is asymptomatic and does not require a PPM.

> **HINTS AND TIPS**
>
> Bradyarrhythmias do not usually compromise cardiac output if the rate is over 50/min and the ventricles have normal function.

BUNDLE BRANCH BLOCK

Bundle branch block is an interventricular conduction disturbance. The bundle of His arises from the AV node and at the level of the top of the muscular interventricular septum it divides into the left and right bundle branches (Fig. 18.5), which supply the left and right ventricles, respectively. The left bundle divides again into anterior and posterior divisions.

Damage to one or more of these bundles due to ischaemia or infarction (or any other condition disturbing electrical conduction; see SA node disease, above) results in a characteristic ECG picture as the pattern of depolarization of the ventricles is altered. In either complete left or complete right bundle branch block the QRS complex is widened to greater than 0.12 s.

Fig. 18.4 Complete heart block. Atrial P waves (A) and ventricular QRS (V) complexes are completely dissociated.

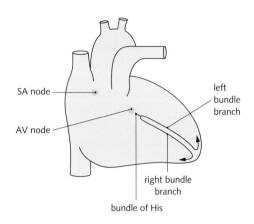

Fig. 18.5 Location of conductive tissue in the heart. AV node, atrioventricular node; SA node, sinoatrial node.

Left bundle branch block

In the normal situation the septum is depolarized from left to right. If the left bundle is blocked the septum is depolarized from right to left and the right ventricle depolarized before the left. This results in the classic M-shaped complex in lead V6 (Fig. 18.6).

Remember that V6 is on the left side of the chest and that a positive deflection occurs when current flows towards the lead. The initial upstroke is due to septal depolarization from right to left and, therefore, towards lead V6. Depolarization of the right ventricle occurs next, which is in a centre to right direction and,

therefore, causes a negative deflection. Finally, the left ventricle is depolarized, which is from right to left, causing the final upstroke.

It is possible to see isolated block of the left anterior or left posterior fascicles of the left bundle branch on the ECG. Left anterior hemiblock causes a left axis deviation on the ECG and left posterior hemiblock causes right axis deviation.

Right bundle branch block

This results in the classic RSR pattern in leads V1 and V2 (Fig. 18.7), which lie to the right of the left ventricle. The septum is depolarized from left to right as normal (resulting in an upstroke in V1), but as there is no conduction down the right bundle the left ventricle depolarizes first, which causes a current to the left resulting in a negative stroke in V1. Finally, the delayed right ventricular depolarization of the right ventricle occurs, causing another upstroke in V1.

HINTS AND TIPS

An easy way of determining if an ECG is showing left or right bundle branch block is to look at the QRS complexes in V1 and V6. Remember the phrase WILLIAM MARROW. If there is a W in V1 and an M in V6 it is LBBB. If there is an M in V1 and a W in V6 it is RBBB.

Fig. 18.6 Complete left bundle branch block. This is characterized by widening of the QRS complex. The R wave is positive in I (to the left) and negative in V1 (posterior) (i.e. the delayed depolarization is to the left ventricle). Note the widened complexes and the M-shaped complexes in V6.

Fig. 18.7 Right bundle branch block. Note the wide QRS. The late part of the QRS in time is negative in I (i.e. to the right) and positive in V1 (i.e. anterior). The delayed depolarization is to the right ventricle. Note the widened QRS complexes and the RSR pattern in V1 and V2.

Bundle branch block may progress to complete heart block; intermittent heart block should be suspected in patients who present with syncope and bundle branch block.

INVESTIGATION OF BRADYARRHYTHMIAS

Electrocardiography

This may show evidence of heart block. However, if the heart block is intermittent the ECG may be normal.

In a patient who has unexplained syncope it is important to exclude intermittent conduction disturbances using continuous ambulatory ECG monitoring. These devices can be used to record the ECG over at least 24 h continuously.

Blood tests

Liver function and thyroid function tests may reveal causes of sinus bradycardia.

Chest radiography

This may reveal cardiomegaly in patients who have ischaemic cardiomyopathy or myocarditis. Pulmonary oedema may be a result of the bradycardia.

Echocardiography

This may reveal regional wall hypokinesia due to areas of ischaemia or infarction. This is especially relevant if it involves the septum.

PACEMAKERS

Indications for a permanent pacemaker

A pacemaker is used to deliver electrical stimuli via leads in contact with the heart. The leads not only deliver energy, but are also able to sense spontaneous electrical activity from the heart. The aim of inserting a pacemaker is to mimic as closely as possible the normal electrical activity of the heart in a patient who has a potentially life-threatening conduction disturbance. The indications for a permanent pacemaker are listed in Fig. 18.8.

Indications for temporary pacing

The following indications for temporary pacing are appropriate:

- All of the above (see Fig. 18.8) if there is no facility for permanent pacing immediately available.
- Drug-induced symptomatic bradyarrhythmias – a temporary wire is used until the effect of the drug has worn off, for example after a trial or overdose of a β-blocker (β-adrenoceptor antagonist).
- Heart block after inferior MI if there is haemodynamic compromise.

Fig. 18.8 Indications for a permanent pacemaker

Complete AV block – should be permanently paced whether symptomatic or not unless following inferior MI (may recover)
Mobitz type II block and 2:1 and 3:1 block with symptoms
Symptomatic bifascicular BBB (i.e. RBBB and left anterior or posterior hemiblock)
Trifascicular block, if symptomatic (i.e. first-degree heart block, RBBB and left anterior or posterior hemiblock)
Sinus node pauses ± tachycardia
Symptomatic sinus bradycardia with no treatable cause
After inferior MI with persistent complete heart block or persistent Mobitz type II block after trial with temporary pacing wire
After anterior MI with persistent complete heart block or persistent Mobitz type II block: trial with temporary pacing is unnecessary as conduction very rarely recovers
Symptomatic bradyarrhythmia following drug treatment of a serious tachyarrhythmia: continue the antiarrhythmic drug and combine with a permanent pacemaker

MI, myocardial infarction; RBBB, right bundle branch block.

Pacemaker insertion

Both temporary and permanent pacemakers are inserted via a venous route by introducing first a sheath and then a pacing wire into one of the great veins.

Permanent pacemakers are most often inserted into the cephalic or subclavian veins. In an emergency situation a temporary wire may be inserted into the internal jugular, subclavian or femoral vein (using the Seldinger technique).

In the case of the temporary pacemaker, the pacemaker box sits externally. In the case of the permanent pacemaker it is buried under the fat and subcutaneous tissue overlying one of the pectoralis major muscles (usually on the patient's non-dominant side).

Complications of pacemaker insertion

The following are recognized complications of pacemaker insertion:

- Complications of wire insertion such as pneumothorax, haemorrhage, brachial plexus injury (during subclavian vein puncture), arrhythmias as the wire is manipulated inside the heart and infection (may progress to infective endocarditis).
- Complications of permanent pacemaker box positioning (e.g. haematoma formation, infection and erosion of the box through the skin).
- Difficulties with the wire, such as wire displacement and loss of ability to pace or sense (need to reposition wire), fracture of the wire insulation (usually due to tight sutures or friction against the clavicle – need to replace wire) and perforation of the myocardium (uncommon unless after MI when the myocardium is friable – need to reposition wire).

Types of pacemaker

Pacemakers are generally of three main types:

- Fixed rate – work irrespective of the heart's underlying activity.
- On demand – work only in certain circumstances e.g. below a rate of 50 beats/min.
- Rate responsive – which adapt to exertional needs of the patient by decreasing or increasing rate as appropriate.

Pacemakers are either single chamber (with a wire into either the ventricles (more common) or the atria (less common)), or dual chamber (with one wire into the atria and one wire into the ventricles).

Ventricular pacemakers stimulate ventricular contraction only and patients who have these, have no atrial contribution to the cardiac output. The atrial contribution can, however, be very important (up to 25% of total cardiac output). It is generally accepted now that a dual-chamber pacemaker should be fitted in patients in whom the atrium can be paced and sensed.

Patients who have chronic atrial fibrillation cannot have an atrial wire because the constant random electrical activity cannot be appropriately sensed.

Pacemakers are classified according to a three-letter code. The first letter refers to the chamber paced, the second, to the chamber sensed, and the third, to the pacing response of the pacemaker. The response is referred to either as T (triggered) or I (inhibited). Triggered means that when an event is sensed, the pacemaker will trigger an output. Inhibited means that any sensed event will inhibit an output from the pacemaker. Dual chamber pacemakers can have both a triggered and an inhibitory pacing response – an atrial impulse will inhibit the atrial wire and trigger the ventricular wire. Common types of pacemaker are listed in Fig. 18.9.

HINTS AND TIPS

Biventricular pacemakers have leads going into both left and right ventricles and are useful in the treatment of patients with heart failure (cardiac resynchronisation therapy – CRT) and ventricular conduction abnormalities such as bundle branch block.

HINTS AND TIPS

Evidence has shown that pacemaker leads implanted in the right ventricular apex worsens left ventricular function and increases the risk of heart failure. Therefore leads are now placed away from this area.

Fig. 18.9 Common types of pacemakers.

Code	Chamber paced	Chamber sensed	Pacing response	Indication
AAI	Atrial	Atrial	Inhibited	SA node dysfunction
DDD	Dual (A&V)	Dual (A&V)	Dual (triggered and inhibited)	Poor AV synchrony

Pacemaker syndrome

Permanent single-chamber right ventricular pacing in a patient who has intact atrial function can lead to atrial activation by retrograde conduction from the ventricle – so-called pacemaker syndrome. There is a cannon wave with every beat, pulmonary arterial pressure rises and cardiac output is impaired. This is managed by replacing the pacemaker with a dual-chamber device.

COMMUNICATION

Patients must be informed of the need to notify the DVLA following pacemaker insertion. Car drivers may drive after one week but HGV drivers must wait 6 weeks before driving. Patients must also promise to attend follow-up pacemaker checks.

Further reading

ACC/AHA/NASPE Committee Members, and Task Force Members, October 2002. ACC/AHA/NASPE 2002 Guideline update for implantation of cardiac pacemakers and antiarrhythmia devices. Circulation 106, 2145–2161.

Chan, J.Y.S., Fang, F., Zhang, Q., et al., 2011. Biventricular pacing is superior to right ventricular pacing in bradycardia patients with preserved systolic function: 2 year results of the PACE trial. Eur. Heart J. 32, 2533–2540.

Da Costa, D., Brady, W.J., Edhouse, J., 2002. ABC of clinical electrocardiography: bradycardias and atrioventricular conduction block. BMJ 324, 535–538.

Mangrum, J.M., DiMarco, J.P., 2000. The evaluation and management of bradycardia. N. Engl. J. Med. 342, 703–709.

Heart failure 19

● Objectives

By the end of this chapter you should:
- Be able to list the main causes of heart failure and understand the mechanisms by which it develops.
- Be able to recognize the main clinical signs of left-ventricular and right-ventricular failure.
- Know the management steps of acute pulmonary oedema.
- Be able to list the drugs used in the treatment of chronic heart failure.

DEFINITION OF HEART FAILURE

Heart failure is the inability of the heart to perfuse metabolizing tissues adequately. The most common cause of this is myocardial systolic failure, which can be caused by a wide variety of disease states.

Myocardial failure can affect the left and right ventricles individually or both together. If left untreated, left-ventricular failure (LVF) will lead to right-ventricular failure (RVF) due to high right-ventricular pressure load. Occasionally there is no abnormality of myocardial function, but cardiac failure occurs. This is due to a sudden excessive high demand on the heart (Fig. 19.1) or acute pressure load.

The remainder of this chapter discusses myocardial failure.

COMMUNICATION

Patients may find the term heart failure frightening. You might find it helps to say something like: 'That doesn't mean it's going to stop, it just means it's not pumping as well as it should'.

PATHOPHYSIOLOGY OF HEART FAILURE

Normal myocardial response to work

During exercise and other stresses there is an increased adrenergic stimulation of the myocardium and cardiac pacemaker tissue. This results in tachycardia and increased myocardial contractility.

Venoconstriction shifts blood to the central compartment resulting in an increased end-diastolic volume of the left ventricle, resulting in stretching of the myocytes. This stretch causes an increase in myocardial performance – as predicted by the Frank-Starling law (Fig. 19.2).

HINTS AND TIPS

The terms 'preload' and 'afterload' are commonly used. Load is a force – in this case the force in the wall of the cardiac chambers. Preload = diastolic force. Afterload = systolic force. Preload and afterload always change together because of the LaPlace relationship (e.g. increasing venous return increases volume and, therefore, systolic wall force). Vasodilatation shifts blood from the heart and decreases diastolic and systolic wall force.

At the same time, vasodilatation in the exercising muscles reduces peripheral vascular resistance resulting in a marked increase in cardiac output with relatively little increase in systemic blood pressure.

The failing heart's response to work

The adrenergic system is already at an increased level of activity in cardiac failure in an attempt to boost cardiac output. During stress this stimulation increases, but cardiac reserve does not permit a significant increase in contractility. The result is tachycardia with its increased energy consumption and a small increase in cardiac output (Fig. 19.3).

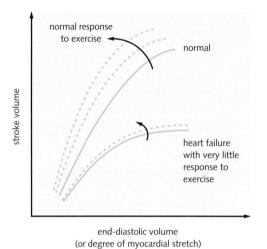

Fig. 19.2   Relationship between end-diastolic volume and stroke volume in normal and failing myocardium (Frank-Starling relationship).

Similarly, the response to increased myocardial stretch is impaired in the failing heart. During stress the impairment results in inadequate contractile response and a large increase in pulmonary capillary pressure (back pressure). This predisposes to the development of pulmonary oedema.

The elevated catecholamine activity may result in peripheral vasoconstriction. Cardiac output is redistributed towards vital organs (e.g. the brain and heart) with vasoconstriction in the skin and skeletal muscle; therefore, the blood flow to less crucial organs is reduced, and this underperfusion leads to formation of lactic acid and weakness and fatigue – classic symptoms in all patients who have cardiac failure.

The result is:

- An inadequate myocardial response to stress.
- Increased and wasteful myocardial energy consumption.
- Possible pulmonary oedema.

Salt and water retention in heart failure

Salt and water retention causes the characteristic raised jugular venous pressure (JVP) and oedema of congestive cardiac failure (CCF).

The renin-angiotensin system is activated in heart failure for two reasons:

1. Stimulation of the β_1-adrenergic receptors on the juxtaglomerular apparatus.
2. Reduced renal perfusion leads to activation of the baroreceptors in the renal arterioles so stimulating renin production.

Renin acts to convert angiotensinogen to angiotensin I. The subsequent action of angiotensin-converting enzyme (predominantly in the lung) converts angiotensin I to angiotensin II. Angiotensin II has a variety of actions:

- It is a potent vasoconstrictor.
- It may increase noradrenaline release (which in turn causes vasoconstriction and myocardial stimulation).
- It is the major stimulus for aldosterone release from the adrenal cortex. Aldosterone causes sodium retention in the distal convoluted tubule. Water is retained with the sodium resulting in increased intravascular volume, which leads to increased cardiac load, so exacerbating heart failure.

Other neurohumoral factors

Heart failure is still relatively poorly understood and, as our understanding improves, it has become apparent that many different hormones and chemical messengers have a role to play. These are often referred to as 'neurohumoral factors' – this term is fine so long as you appreciate that the identities of these factors are not known and that we do not even know exactly how many there are. Natriuretic peptides, cytokines and endothelin are all thought to have a role in cardiac failure.

Natriuretic peptides

There are three such peptides known currently:

1. Atrial natriuretic peptide (ANP).
2. Brain natriuretic peptide (BNP).
3. C-natriuretic peptide (C-NP).

Both ANP and BNP cause sodium excretion (natriuresis), resulting in water excretion; they also cause peripheral vasodilatation; therefore, reducing cardiac load. The exact role of C-NP is unclear.

Levels of all three peptides are increased in patients who are in heart failure. It is generally accepted that these peptides play a protective role in cardiac failure by attempting to break the vicious cycle, as illustrated in Fig. 19.3.

Cytokines

Cytokines (such as tumour necrosis factor α) are thought to be involved in causing cardiac dysfunction. Levels are increased in patients who have heart failure.

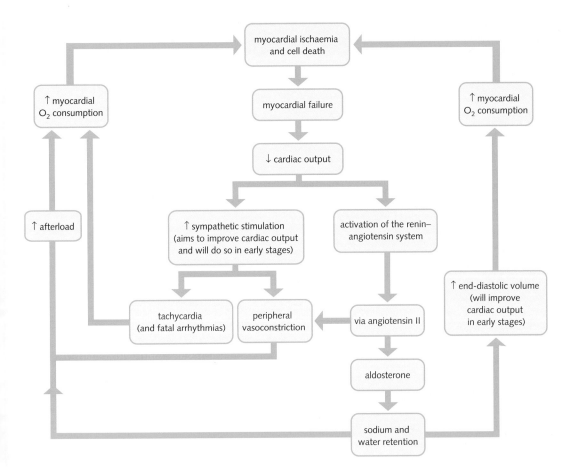

Fig. 19.3 Pathophysiology of heart failure.

Endothelin

This peptide is a powerful vasoconstrictor. It is produced by endothelial cells and there are a number of different subtypes. Endothelin levels are raised in patients who have heart failure. The resulting increase in load may cause increased myocardial strain in heart failure.

Galectin-3

One of the lectin family that is expressed in multiple cellular compartments and with a role in cell adhesion and activation, as well as cell growth and apoptosis. It has recently been proposed to be involved in fibrosis, inflammation and adverse remodelling in the failing heart.

CAUSES OF CARDIAC FAILURE

Any cardiac disease can lead to heart failure, but a few common causes are:

- Ischaemic heart disease – remember that a right-ventricular infarction will give isolated RVF, which requires different acute management to LVF.
- Valve disease – aortic valve disease will lead to CCF, as will mitral regurgitation. Remember that mitral stenosis causes RVF, but leaves the left ventricle unharmed.
- Hypertensive heart disease.
- Cardiomyopathy – hereditary, e.g. dilated or hypertrophic cardiomyopathy, or acquired, e.g. secondary to viral myocarditis, drugs, inflammatory disorders, thyotoxicosis, etc. (see Ch. 20).

Heart failure may occur without impairment of systolic myocardial function. Heart failure with preserved systolic function (also known as diastolic heart failure) is thought to occur due to impaired relaxation of the ventricle in diastole, or increased passive stiffness of the myocardium. It usually occurs in elderly people with hypertension, and is more common in women.

Precipitants

In most cases, an acute exacerbation of heart failure is related to a precipitating event other than the underlying cause. Common precipitants are:

- Reduction of or non-compliance with therapy, or fluid retention due to drugs, such as NSAIDs.
- Recent infection – especially pulmonary infection (which patients with cardiac failure are prone to). Infection increases metabolic rate and causes tachycardia, and both increase demand on the heart.
- Myocardial ischaemia – a new ischaemic event or myocardial infarction (MI) may trigger heart failure.
- Tachy- or bradyarrhythmias – these are common in such patients because the underlying diseases are often associated with arrhythmias. Atrial fibrillation results in a loss of the atrial component to cardiac output by reducing the efficiency of ventricular filling. Bradycardia requires an increase in stroke volume to maintain cardiac output with a lower heart rate and this may not be possible in the failing heart.

CLINICAL FEATURES OF HEART FAILURE

The symptoms and signs of cardiac failure vary depending upon a number of factors:

- Severity of heart failure.
- Which ventricle is involved (isolated right heart failure is less common and a pulmonary cause should be excluded).
- Age of the patient.

Regardless of the cause of heart failure, it is possible to predict the effects if the mechanics of pump failure are considered. The effects can be divided into forward and backward effects.

Forward effects

Forward effects refer to the failure of the pump to provide an adequate output. This applies to the left ventricle resulting in:

- Poor renal perfusion predisposing to prerenal failure.
- Poor perfusion of extremities resulting in cold extremities.
- Secondary changes in skeletal muscle structure leading to weakness and fatigue.
- Hypotension.

Forward failure of the right ventricle results in reduced pulmonary flow leading to dyspnoea and underfilling of the left ventricle resulting in hypotension, and so on (as above).

Backward effects

Failure of the left and right ventricles results in congestion of the systemic and pulmonary venous systems respectively, leading to systemic and pulmonary oedema. In the case of systemic oedema this tends to be dependent (legs if walking, sacrum if bed-bound) but liver congestion and ascites may also occur.

HINTS AND TIPS

Although dividing heart failure into RVF and LVF seems complicated, it is worth taking the time to learn this because it makes it much easier to work out logically the cause of a given set of signs and symptoms.

Symptoms

Dyspnoea (shortness of breath), fatigue and weakness, nocturia, cough, epigastric discomfort and anorexia are common in cardiac failure. The New York Heart Association (NYHA) classification is commonly used (Fig. 19.4).

Dyspnoea results from pulmonary oedema, impaired skeletal muscle function, depressed respiratory muscle function and reduced lung function. It can present in a number of ways:

- Exertional dyspnoea – as cardiac failure worsens, the level of exertion required to cause dyspnoea decreases until the patient is breathless at minimal exertion (e.g. when dressing or even when speaking).
- Orthopnoea – the increased central blood volume when the patient lies flat is often too much for the failing heart to pump resulting in the development of pulmonary oedema. Patients who have severe LVF often sleep with several pillows to prop them up.
- Paroxysmal nocturnal dyspnoea – after being asleep for some time the patient is awakened by severe breathlessness, which is relieved only after standing or sitting upright. It is thought that this is due to pulmonary oedema due to gradual resorption of interstitial fluid overnight and nocturnal depression of respiratory function.

Fig. 19.4 The New York Heart Association (NYHA) classification of heart failure

NYHA class	Symptoms	3-year survival
I	Asymptomatic during normal activity	50%
II	Mild symptoms during normal activity	
III	Marked limitation to normal activity, comfortable only at rest	33%
IV	Symptoms at rest	0%

Fatigue and weakness result from reduced perfusion of skeletal muscles, and nocturia is due to the increased renal perfusion in the recumbent position.

Cough may be:

- A nocturnal dry cough due to bronchial oedema or cardiac asthma (bronchospasm secondary to oedema).
- Productive of pink frothy sputum due to pulmonary oedema.

Epigastric discomfort occurs in cases of hepatic congestion. Anorexia (which may be caused by oedema of the gut), ankle swelling (due to peripheral oedema) and shortness of breath (due to inadequate pulmonary perfusion) may occur in a patient who has predominantly right-sided heart failure.

EXAMINATION OF PATIENTS WHO HAVE HEART FAILURE

On observation the patient may be short of breath and cyanosed. Alternatively if the heart failure is relatively mild there may be no obvious abnormality at rest, but the dyspnoea may become apparent on exertion (e.g. when undressing before the examination).

Cardiac cachexia is a term used to describe cachexia seen in patients who have heart failure; this is due to:

- Gut and liver congestion leading to anorexia.
- Increased metabolism due to increased work of breathing and increased cardiac oxygen consumption.
- Cytokine and renin-angiotensin-aldosterone system activation (hence dramatically reduced by ACE inhibitors).

Cardiovascular system

On examination of the cardiovascular system (Fig. 19.5) note:

- Pulse – may be rapid, weak and thready if there is considerable forward failure. Watch out for arrhythmias and pulsus alternans (alternate strong and weak beats), which is a sign of LVF.
- Blood pressure – this may be normal, low in forward failure, or high in the hypertensive patient (remember that, worldwide, hypertension is a very common cause of heart failure).

- Jugular venous pressure (JVP) – this is elevated in CCF and pure right-sided failure (the normal jugular venous pressure is 2–3 cm above the sternal angle).
- Carotid pulse – look for abnormal pulse character because it may reveal a possible aetiology for the cardiac failure (e.g. aortic stenosis or regurgitation).
- Apex beat – may be displaced downward and laterally in a patient who has an enlarged left ventricle. A diffuse apex beat is a sign of severe left-ventricular dysfunction.
- Heart sounds – on auscultation there may be a third heart sound. Tachycardia combined with a third (or fourth heart sound) is referred to as a gallop rhythm.
- Murmurs – these may signify a possible cause of heart failure (e.g. aortic valve murmurs and mitral valve murmurs). Remember: mitral regurgitation can occur as a result of left-ventricular dilatation (which leads to stretching of the mitral valve ring) and will, therefore, be caused by heart failure, and not a cause of it, in some cases. This is called functional mitral regurgitation.
- Peripheral oedema – this may be elicited over the sacrum or over the ankle. Take care because oedema may be tender. The extent to which the oedema extends up the legs is an indication of the extent of the fluid overload.

Respiratory system

In addition to dyspnoea and possible cyanosis, the patient might have bilateral basal fine end-inspiratory crepitations extending from the bases upwards. This is classic of pulmonary oedema. There might also be pleural effusions and expiratory wheeze (secondary to cardiac asthma). Sleep apnoea is common in heart failure, this may be central, obstructive or mixed. Look for obesity and a large neck circumference suggesting obstructive sleep apnoea. Central sleep apnoea may progress in severity until patients have pauses in breathing while awake (Cheyne-Stokes breathing).

Fig. 19.5A Consequences of left and right ventricular failure

	LV failure	RV failure
Symptoms	Dyspnoea secondary to pulmonary oedema and lactic acidosis	Dyspnoea secondary to poor pulmonary perfusion
	Fatigue due to poor cardiac output and lactic acidosis	Fatigue due to poor LV filling (and therefore poor cardiac output and lactic acidosis)
Signs	Hypotension, cold peripheries and renal impairment – all due to poor LV output	Hypotension and cold peripheries due to poor LV filling (and therefore poor LV output)
	LV third heart sound – heard best at the apex	RV third heart sound – very soft and best heard at the left lower sternal edge
	Bilateral basal crepitations	Elevated JVP
	Signs of CCF – severe chronic LV failure leads to fluid retention	Ascites, hepatic enlargement and peripheral oedema

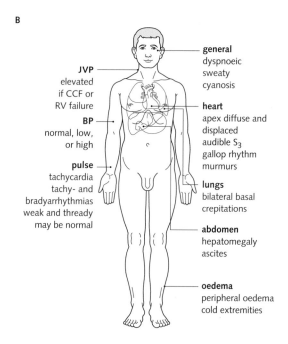

Fig. 19.5 (A) Consequences of left and right ventricular failure. One or the other will be dominant and the clinical picture varies accordingly. Often there are signs of both. CCF, congestive cardiac failure; JVP, jugular venous pressure; LV, left ventricular; RV, right ventricular. (B) Clinical findings in a patient who has heart failure. BP, blood pressure; CCF, congestive cardiac failure; RV, right ventricular.

Gastrointestinal system

Patients with CCF or pure RVF might show signs of hepatomegaly and ascites.

> **HINTS AND TIPS**
>
> Take care when palpating the liver or attempting to elicit hepatojugular reflux, because CCF can result in tender hepatomegaly.

INVESTIGATION OF HEART FAILURE

Blood tests

Electrolytes and renal function

Hypokalaemia and hyponatraemia are common findings in patients who are on diuretic therapy. There may also be renal impairment due to hypoperfusion r diuretic therapy. Hyponatraemia is common in heart failure and is due to high circulating vasopressin levels (dilutional hyponatraemia).

Hyperkalaemia may be seen in patients who are being treated with potassium-sparing diuretics (e.g. amiloride or spironolactone), angiotensin-converting enzyme (ACE) inhibitors (e.g. ramipril or perindopril) or angiotensin II receptor blockers (ARBs), such as losartan or candesartan.

Full blood count

Severe anaemia may lead to heart failure. There may be a leucocytosis secondary to infection, which may exacerbate failure. Conversely, chronic heart failure (irrespective of aetiology) frequently leads to mild anaemia.

Liver function tests

Liver congestion may lead to impaired hepatic function, resulting in elevated hepatic enzymes and bilirubin.

Brain natriuretic peptide

Assays of BNP are increasingly used as a screening test for heart failure in the community, with serum levels elevated in heart failure (see also Neurohumoral factors, p. 140).

Arterial blood gases

These show hypoxia, hypocapnoea and metabolic acidosis. Patients who are profoundly hypoxic might require artificial ventilation.

Electrocardiography

This may be normal or may show ischaemic or hypertensive changes. Look out for evidence of arrhythmias. If these are suspected, a 24-h ECG should be performed.

Chest radiography

There may be cardiomegaly indicating a dilated left ventricle. Pulmonary oedema may be seen with prominent pulmonary veins, upper lobe blood diversion and Kerley B lines (horizontal lines of fluid-filled fissures at the costophrenic angle). The stages of oedema on a chest X-ray are:

1. Pulmonary venous congestion.
2. Interstitial oedema (pleural effusion, Kerley B lines).
3. Frank alveolar oedema.

Echocardiography

This is an essential test in heart failure; it is non-invasive and can be performed on and off the ward. It can help to determine:

- Left and right ventricular dimensions and function.
- Abnormalities of regional wall motion usually indicating coronary artery disease.
- Any structural or functional abnormalities for all valves.
- Pressure differences across narrowed valves and also estimation of pulmonary artery pressure.
- Intracardiac thrombus (although transoesophageal echocardiography is more sensitive for that purpose).
- Exclusion of intracardiac shunt.

Cardiac catheterization

It is important to evaluate underlying coronary artery disease as a cause of heart failure as coronary revascularization (where necessary) may improve the pumping ability of the heart. This is usually performed when heart failure symptoms have been stabilized with medical therapy, unless there is objective evidence of acute ischaemia.

MANAGEMENT OF HEART FAILURE

The most common clinical presentation seen in the outpatients department and on the ward is the patient who has chronic LVF or CCF (heart failure with fluid retention).

Before discussing this, two clinical situations will be covered because they are both emergencies and make good viva questions to ask in finals. These are:

1. Management of acute LVF.
2. Management of acute RVF.

Management of acute left ventricular failure

HINTS AND TIPS

Acute LVF is a very common condition and is also a medical emergency. Rapid venodilatation is required. It is, therefore, important that you know all the management steps in Fig. 19.6, including drugs and doses, before finals. If the patient is extremely unwell and may need endotracheal intubation, an anaesthetist should be called immediately.

This is a medical emergency that you will almost certainly encounter in your first year as an FY1. You will be expected to administer first-line treatment by yourself so it is important to know not only the drugs to use, but also all the doses and routes of administration. This tends to be a pass/fail question in vivas.

The patient in acute LVF has pulmonary oedema and is very breathless and distressed. He or she will be hypoxic and may cough up pink frothy sputum. Low cardiac output may lead to hypotension.

Your aim is to relieve the pulmonary oedema rapidly.

If the patient has cardiogenic shock and is very hypotensive, inotropic agents may be needed and you should call your senior immediately because in this situation the blood pressure should be improved first.

Learn the management guide given in Fig. 19.6.

Management of acute right ventricular failure

Patients with an inferior or posterior myocardial infarction (MI) may present with predominantly RVF. This is not common, but it is important to recognize the signs and to know how to treat it.

Remember Starling's law of the heart, where the force of contraction is proportional to the stretch applied to the muscle. It is often possible to improve function by increasing heart volume (unless the ventricle is severely dysfunctional, in which case this makes no difference).

HINTS AND TIPS

Treatment of acute RVF is opposite to that of acute LVF: fluid may be beneficial whereas in LVF it must be removed. Remember that isolated acute RVF is rare, whereas CCF and LVF are common.

In the post-MI patient, dehydration, diuretic use and the use of nitrates are all common. All of these conspire to reduce heart volume.

If right-ventricular function is impaired a reduced heart volume has the effect of reducing function further resulting in poor left-ventricular filling and hypotension. In fact, an impaired right ventricle requires greater than normal filling in order to maintain normal output.

Therefore, a patient who has an inferior MI and hypotension should be assessed carefully.

Fig. 19.6 Management of acute left ventricular failure (LVF)

Management (in order)	Notes
1. Sit the patient up	To reduce venous return to the heart
2. Administer 100% oxygen via a facial mask	Improvement of arterial oxygen tension will reduce myocardial oxygen debt and improve myocardial function
3. Establish peripheral intravenous access and administer:	
IV morphine 5–10 mg or diamorphine 2.5–5 mg	Morphine is a good anxiolytic and has pulmonary vasodilating and venodilating effects. Diamorphine is more potent, but there has been a shortage in the UK since 2005, and in many hospitals it will not be readily available
IV metoclopramide 10 mg	Metoclopramide prevents vomiting secondary to opiates. Metoclopramide is preferred to cyclizine as the latter causes tachycardia, but should not be given to women under 20 due to increased risk of oculogyric crisis
IV furosemide (frusemide) 80–100 mg	Furosemide (frusemide) is a venodilator so its initial effect is to reduce load; it is also a powerful diuretic and will cause salt and water excretion, so reducing fluid retention
	By reducing load these drugs reduce the backpressure on the pulmonary circulation and hence relieve pulmonary oedema by allowing resorption of fluid back from the extracellular to the intracellular space
4. Insert a urinary catheter	The patient will have a diuresis and is too ill to use a bedpan; it is important to monitor fluid output to detect renal impairment early
5. Intravenous nitrates	Given as a continuous infusion; help by vasodilating both veins and arterioles and so reducing load; the dose is titrated to prevent hypotension (a common side effect of nitrates). GTN can be given by a spray while it is drawn up.
6. CPAP	Very effective – it literally pushes fluid out of the alveoli back into the circulation; specialist equipment is required
	When the patient is stable, continue management as for chronic left ventricular failure

CPAP, continuous positive airway pressure; IV, intravenous.

You must be aware that hypotension after inferior MI might be secondary to the combination of RVF and relative underfilling of the right ventricle, and that treatment is careful fluid challenge with central venous pressure monitoring.

Provided that there is no evidence of pulmonary oedema (suggesting the presence of significant left-ventricular impairment), the correct management is a fluid challenge.

Management of chronic heart failure

The main agents used in the treatment of heart cardiac failure are:

- ACE inhibitors (angiotensin II receptor blockers if patients are intolerant of ACE inhibitors).
- β-Blockers.
- Diuretics.
- Spironolactone.
- Nitrates.
- Digoxin.
- Hydralazine.

A dilated heart generally means chronic rather than acute heart failure.

Angiotensin-converting enzyme inhibitors

The role of the renin-angiotensin system in heart failure is discussed on pp. 139–40. It is not difficult to see that inhibition of formation of angiotensin II could be beneficial by reducing systemic vasoconstriction and the sodium and water retention caused by aldosterone.

Angiotensin II increases efferent arteriolar tone and, therefore, increases glomerular filtration. Because ACE inhibitors remove this ability to regulate efferent arteriolar tone, the glomerular filtration rate declines and renal failure ensues in patients who have renal artery stenosis or any other condition in which renal blood flow is reduced (e.g. marked hypotension).

The ACE inhibitors have been shown to reduce the mortality rate in patients who have heart failure. They are first-line drugs for all patients unless there is a specific contraindication (e.g. renal artery stenosis or profound hypotension).

Clinical use of angiotensin-converting enzyme inhibitors

ACE inhibitors are usually started at low doses because they can cause first-dose hypotension. Patients most likely to suffer from this are:

- The elderly.
- Patients who are on high doses of diuretics.

Once the dose has been established, renal function and electrolytes should be checked one week later to ensure no deterioration has taken place in renal function. Hyperkalaemia is another complication that is due to a reduction in aldosterone activity (aldosterone causes sodium absorption in exchange for potassium in the distal convoluted tubule). Other side effects of ACE inhibitors are:

- Cough – occurs in 5% patients on these agents. It is caused by inhibition of the metabolism of bradykinin (another function of ACE). Cough usually appears in the first few weeks of treatment. This is a side effect of all drugs in this class and treatment needs to be stopped in some cases.
- Loss of taste (or a metallic taste) may occur.
- Rashes and angioedema.

Once the drug has been introduced the dose should be increased to the recommended dose if possible (e.g. ramipril 10 mg daily or perindopril 8 mg daily).

Angiotensin II receptor blockers

There are two types of angiotensin II receptor: AT1 and AT2. Losartan is a selective AT1 blocker and was the first of these drugs to be established for use as an antihypertensive. Candesartan has been shown to benefit patients with heart failure; however, other agents are emerging and are being evaluated for similar benefit.

The spectrum of activity is the same as that of ACE inhibitors, but the main advantage is that these drugs do not prevent the breakdown of bradykinin, so cough does not occur as a side effect.

β-Blockers

Patients with heart failure have an abnormally high level of circulating catecholamines. There is also a down-regulation of β-receptors in response to this. The realisation that catecholamines damage the heart by increasing myocardial work, rather than being an adaptive response to heart failure, led to a reversal of traditional thinking. Trial evidence has shown the β-blockers bisoprolol, carvedilol and metoprolol are effective therapy in chronic heart failure, reducing mortality by as much as 30%. This could be for a number of reasons:

- Reduction in myocardial oxygen demand and ischaemia.
- Decreased incidence of arrhythmias.
- Peripheral vasodilatation with non-selective β-blockers that have some α-blockade as well.
- Antioxidant effects (carvedilol).

They do cause myocardial depression and therefore should be introduced by specialists while the patient is stable. The strategy is 'start low and go slow'. If the patient's heart failure symptoms deteriorate then the dose can be reduced or the drug can be temporarily withheld, but all patients without a firm contraindication should receive a β-blocker.

Diuretics

Loop diuretics, such as furosemide and thiazide diuretics such as bendrofluazide or metolazone (Fig. 19.7) have an important role in salt and water excretion. They provide symptomatic relief, but have no effect on mortality in heart failure.

Aldosterone antagonists

Spironolactone is a weak diuretic that acts by blocking aldosterone receptors in the distal convoluted tubule. Aldosterone promotes sodium retention and potassium excretion; it also has a number of unfavourable extrarenal effects, including sympathetic stimulation, parasympathetic inhibition, vascular damage and impairment of arterial compliance, all of which adversely affect cardiac function. It promotes fibrosis and adverse remodelling of the heart. It is thought that spironolactone potentiates the action of ACE inhibitors by suppressing aldosterone activity and its adverse effects. Patients with severe heart failure receiving both drugs have a 30% lower mortality rate than patients receiving placebo. Caution is needed, however, as both medications cause potassium retention, which can reach dangerous levels. It is, therefore, crucial to measure serum electrolytes regularly. Other side effects of spironolactone include gynaecomastia and breast pain in men.

Eplerenone is licensed in patients post myocardial infarction who have clinical signs of heart failure and LV systolic impairment, and has been shown to confer a mortality benefit in this group. Unlike spironolactone, it does not have oestrogenic effects.

COMMUNICATION

Patients with heart failure should be advised to monitor their weight at home, in conjunction with their degree of breathlessness on exertion. If these parameters increase, the dose of diuretic can be adjusted by the patient. If the opposite occurs and the patient is more dehydrated than usual (weight loss) then diuretic dose can be reduced as necessary. This is especially important if the patient has diarrhoea, as renal failure can ensue, if combined treatment with several drugs (for example, furosemide, spironolactone and ACE inhibitor) is continued in this setting.

Nitrates

The nitrates (e.g. isosorbide mononitrate and isosorbide dinitrate) are veno- and arteriolar dilators and therefore, act by reducing load. Intravenous nitrates are useful in the treatment of the acutely sick patient with cardiac failure. Oral nitrates may provide some

Fig. 19.7 Site of action and side effects of different diuretics

Examples	Site of action	Side effects
Loop diuretics: furosemide (frusemide), bumetanide, ethacrynic acid	Thick ascending loop of Henle	Ototoxicity with ethacrynic acid; hypokalaemia; exacerbation of gout
Thiazide diuretics: bendroflumethiazide (bendrofluazide), hydrochlorthiazide, metolazone	Distal convoluted tubule	Hyperglycaemia, gout, elevated triglycerides/LDL, hypokalaemia, hyponatraemia
Potassium-sparing diuretics: amiloride, spironolactone	Collecting duct and distal convoluted tubule	Hyperkalaemia – use with caution with ACE inhibitors

ACE, angiotensin-converting enzyme; LDL, low-density lipoprotein.

symptomatic relief in chronic cardiac failure. The combination of nitrates and hydralazine has been shown to reduce mortality in heart failure.

Digoxin

Digoxin is a cardiac glycoside. It inhibits the sodium/potassium pump on the sarcolemmal and cell membranes. This adenosine triphosphate (ATP)-dependent pump plays a role in transporting calcium out of the cell. Its inhibition, therefore, prevents this, resulting in increased intracellular calcium concentration, which in cardiac muscle results in a positive inotropic effect.

In AV node tissue the effect of an increased calcium concentration is to prolong the refractory period and decrease AV node conduction velocity, so slowing AV node conduction of the cardiac impulse – a negative chronotropic effect.

It is generally accepted that digoxin is an extremely useful drug in patients with atrial fibrillation and heart failure; it does not reduce mortality in sinus rhythm but there is evidence that it may reduce the frequency of admissions. Retrospective analysis showed that patients with low therapeutic digoxin levels saw a mortality benefit; those with high levels saw an increase in sudden cardiac death, so this strategy is probably best used with monitoring of drug levels.

Pharmacokinetics

Digoxin has a half-life of 24–36 h and it takes 3–4 weeks to reach a steady plasma level after oral loading. Intravenous loading speeds this up slightly because the time taken for absorption in the gut is bypassed; 40% of digoxin in the blood is protein bound.

Excretion is predominantly renal (10% excreted in the stools) and digoxin should not be used in renal failure. In mild renal impairment the dose is reduced.

Side effects

Plasma levels of digoxin should be measured where there is suspicion of toxicity. Patients can still experience toxicity with plasma levels in the normal range. Blood is taken 6 h after an oral dose. Digoxin toxicity is more likely in patients who:

- Have renal failure.
- Are hypokalaemic – digoxin competes with potassium for binding to the sodium/potassium ATPase.
- Are taking amiodarone or verapamil (which displace digoxin from protein binding sites), erythromycin (which prevents inactivation of digoxin by gut bacteria) or captopril (which reduces renal clearance of digoxin).

Signs of digoxin toxicity are:

- Bradycardia, AV block and sinus arrest.
- Nausea and vomiting.
- Xanthopsia (yellow discolouration of visualized objects).

Hydralazine

Hydralazine is a potent vasodilator, predominantly of arterioles; therefore, it reduces after load, which acts to improve cardiac function. Side effects include flushing and a lupus-like syndrome. It is prescribed in combination with a nitrate such as ISDN in patients who cannot tolerate an ACE inhibitor or ARB, and also as an additional therapy in severe heart failure, especially where there is pulmonary hypertension. In a subgroup analysis, it appears that Afro-Caribbean and African American patients particularly benefit from this approach, while this group is believed to benefit less than others from ACE inhibitors.

Cardiac resynchronization therapy

Approximately one-third of patients with heart failure have an abnormality in the conduction pathway. This manifests as prolongation of the QRS duration (>120 ms) and results in parts of the ventricle being activated in an dyssynchronous manner. Consequently, relaxation in diastole is also dyssynchronous with parts of the ventricle relaxing while other parts are still contracting. In normal hearts, the effects of this are generally not noticed. However, in dilated, poorly functioning hearts it has a significant effect in reducing stroke volume and cardiac output and can lead to mitral regurgitation. Resynchronization treatment involves implanting a pacemaker to activate the ventricles in a synchronous manner to improve contraction and filling, and subsequently stroke volume and cardiac output. Such pacemakers are called biventricular devices as three pacing leads are used: in the right atrium, the right ventricle and left ventricle (via the coronary sinus). This closer simulates normal physiological activation of the ventricles. Clinical trials have shown that the use of such devices significantly improves patients' quality of life, the amount of exercise they are able to perform, and reduces both hospitalisations for heart failure and mortality. Current NICE guidance recommends CRT in patients who experience severe symptoms (NYHA class III–IV) with an ejection fraction <35% and prolonged QRS duration in sinus rhythm. Some patients may also benefit from a device with defibrillator function (known as a CRT-D), though the indications are relatively complex (See NICE guidance TA95).

Further reading

ACC/AHA Committee and task force members, 2005. Guidelines for the evaluation and management of chronic heart failure in the adult: executive summary. Circulation 112, e154–e235.

Cleland, J., Daubert, J.C., Erdmann, E., et al., 2005. The effect of Cardiac Resynchronization on Morbidity and Mortality in Heart Failure (CARE-HF). N. Engl. J. Med. 352, 1539–1549.

Foody, J.M., Farrell, M.H., Krumholz, H.M., 2002. Beta-blocker therapy in heart failure: scientific review. JAMA 287, 883–889.

Gibbs, C.R., Jackson, G., Lip, G.Y.H., 2000. ABC of heart failure. Non-drug management. BMJ 320, 366–369.

Heart Outcomes Prevention Evaluation Study Investigators (HOPE), 2000. Effects of ramipril on cardiovascular and microvascular outcomes in people with diabetes mellitus. Lancet 355, 253–259.

Jackson, G., Gibbs, C.R., Davies, M.K., Lip, G.Y.H., 2000. ABC of heart failure. Pathophysiology. BMJ 320, 167–170.

Millane, T., Jackson, G., Gibbs, C.R., Lip, G.Y.H., 2000. ABC of heart failure. Acute and chronic management strategies. BMJ 320, 559–562.

Pitt, B., Zannad, F., Remme, W.J., et al., 1999. The effect of spironolactone on morbidity and mortality in patients with severe heart failure. N. Engl. J. Med. 341, 709–717.

Cardiomyopathy 20

DEFINITION OF CARDIOMYOPATHY

Cardiomyopathy is heart muscle disease, often of unknown cause. Ischaemic cardiomyopathy is heart failure due to underlying coronary artery disease and is discussed elsewhere. There are several types (Fig. 20.1):

- Dilated cardiomyopathy.
- Hypertrophic cardiomyopathy.
- Restrictive cardiomyopathy.
- Arrhythmogenic right-ventricular cardiomyopathy.
- Takotsubo cardiomyopathy.
- Others including left ventricular non-compaction.

DILATED CARDIOMYOPATHY

The heart is dilated and has impaired function. The coronary arteries are normal. Causes of dilated cardiomyopathy include:

- Genetics (familial DCM) – approximately 40%.
- Alcohol.
- Viral infection (parvovirus, echovirus, coxsackievirus, and enteroviruses most likely).
- Untreated hypertension.
- Autoimmune disease.
- Thyrotoxicosis.
- Drugs and toxins (e.g. cocaine, doxorubicin, cyclophosphamide, trastuzumab (herceptin), lead).
- Haemochromatosis.
- Acquired immune deficiency syndrome (AIDS).
- Tachycardiomyopathy (chronic tachyarrhythmia causing heart failure).

Clinical features

Progressive biventricular cardiac failure leads to:

- Fatigue.
- Dyspnoea.
- Peripheral oedema.
- Ascites.

Other complications secondary to the progressive dilatation of the ventricles include:

- Mural thrombi with systemic or pulmonary embolization.
- Dilatation of the tricuspid and mitral valve rings leading to functional valve regurgitation.
- Atrial fibrillation.
- Ventricular tachyarrhythmias and sudden death.

Investigation

Investigations to aid diagnosis are listed below.

Chest radiography

This may show:

- Enlarged cardiac shadow.
- Signs of pulmonary oedema (upper lobe blood diversion or interstitial shadowing at the bases).
- Pleural effusions.

Electrocardiography

Electrocardiography may highlight:

- Tachycardia.
- Poor R wave progression across the chest leads.
- Conduction delay such as left bundle branch block.

Echocardiography

Points to consider with echocardiography include:

- Can the dilated ventricles be easily visualized?
- Can the regurgitant valves be seen?

Fig. 20.1 Different types of cardiomyopathy. AV, aortic valve; HCM, hypertrophic cardiomyopathy; LA, left atrium; LV, left ventricle; MR, mitral regurgitation; MV, mitral valve.

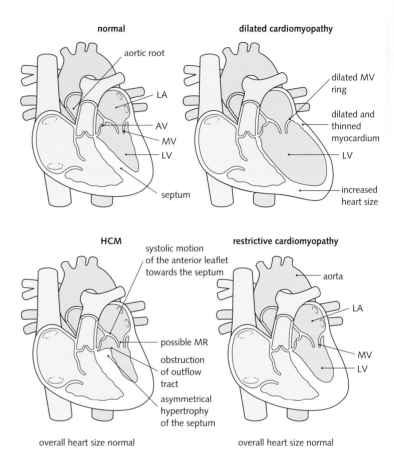

Occasionally, intracardiac thrombus may be seen. Transthoracic echocardiography is not a reliable method for diagnosing this, but it can be accurately diagnosed by transoesophageal echocardiography.

Cardiac catheterization

This is important to exclude coronary artery disease (the most common cause of ventricular dysfunction).

Magnetic resonance imaging

This is an excellent non-invasive tool for assessment of patients with cardiomyopathy, and late enhancement with gadolinium can provide useful information about the aetiology and prognosis.

Blood tests

Thyroid function tests, CK (to look for primary muscle diseases), a full blood count (anaemia), and autoimmune screen. Viral titres may be useful.

Management

The management plan follows four basic steps (the same applies for any other case of cardiac failure):

1. Search for and treat any underlying cause (e.g. stop alcohol).
2. Treat cardiac failure (diuretics, ACE inhibitors or β-blockers).
3. Treat any arrhythmias (β-blockers, digoxin or amiodarone for atrial fibrillation, or amiodarone for ventricular arrhythmias).
4. Consider anticoagulation with warfarin to prevent mural thrombi.

After optimization of medical therapy, device therapy should be considered (see pp. 122, 149). Cardiac transplantation may also be a treatment option.

HYPERTROPHIC CARDIOMYOPATHY

This disorder is characterized by unexplained LVH (>15 mm, or >12 mm if a known gene carrier or has a known first-degree relative). The most common pattern disproportionately affects the septum, but LVH may be concentric or disproportionately affect other parts of the heart (e.g. the apex). The majority of mutations resulting in HCM affect genes encoding sarcomere proteins.

The myocytes of the left ventricle are abnormally thick when examined microscopically and their layout is disorganized (myocardial disarray). This makes left-ventricular filling more difficult than normal and grossly disordered. There is dynamic left-ventricular outflow tract obstruction in around 40% of cases, most commonly due to systolic anterior motion of the mitral valve into the thickened septum, but sometimes the cavity can become occluded. This condition is often called hypertrophic obstructive cardiomyopathy (HOCM).

Clinical features

There are four main symptoms:

1. Angina (even in the absence of coronary artery disease) – due to the increased oxygen demands of the hypertrophied muscle.
2. Palpitations – there is an increased incidence of atrial fibrillation and ventricular arrhythmias in this condition.
3. Syncope and sudden death – which may be due to left-ventricular outflow tract obstruction by the hypertrophied septum or to a ventricular arrhythmia. Syncope may often result from inappropriate vasodilatation on exercise.
4. Dyspnoea – due to the stiff left ventricle, which leads to a reduced cardiac output and to pulmonary venous congestion.

The signs (Fig. 20.2) to watch for are:

- Jerky peripheral pulse – the second rise palpable in the pulse is due to the rise in left-ventricular pressure as the left ventricle attempts to overcome the outflow tract obstruction.
- Double apical beat – the stiff left ventricle causes raised left ventricular end-diastolic pressure. The atrial contraction is, therefore, very forceful to fill the left ventricle. It is this atrial impulse that can be felt in addition to the left-ventricular contraction that gives this classical sign.
- Systolic thrill – felt at the left lower sternal edge.

- Systolic murmur – crescendo and decrescendo in nature, and best heard between the apex and the left lower sternal edge.

It can be difficult to differentiate between HCM and aortic stenosis on examination. Use the following features to help:

- Pulse – slow rising in aortic stenosis, jerky or with a normal upstroke in HCM.
- Second heart sound – reduced in intensity in significant aortic stenosis.
- Thrill and murmur – both found in the second right intercostal space in aortic stenosis and at the left lower sternal edge in HCM.
- Variation of the murmur with Valsalva manoeuvre or with standing from squatting – the murmur of HCM (but not AS) is increased because the volume of the left ventricle is reduced by these manoeuvres and, therefore, the outflow gradient worsens.

Diagnosis and investigations

Electrocardiography

This is usually abnormal in HCM. The most common abnormalities are T wave and ST segment abnormalities; the signs of left-ventricular hypertrophy may also be present. Q waves due to the hypertrophied septum may mimic old MI.

Continuous ambulatory electrocardiography

The presence of non-sustained ventricular tachycardia is common in patients who have HCM and is risk factor sudden death. Sustained VT is relatively uncommon. These tests are usually performed as part of a yearly screening programme for these patients.

Echocardiography

This is the most useful investigation because it confirms the diagnosis and can be used to assess the degree of outflow tract obstruction.

Characteristic echocardiography findings include:

- Unexplained hypertrophy – the distribution can be identified.
- Abnormal systolic anterior motion of the anterior leaflet of the mitral valve.
- Left-ventricular outflow tract obstruction.

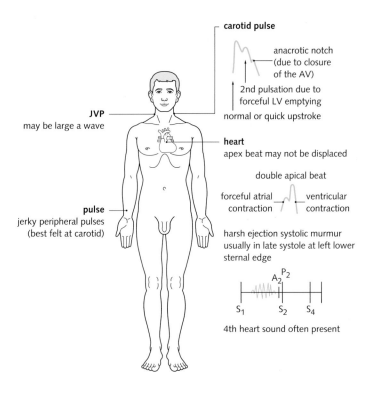

Fig. 20.2 Important clinical signs in hypertrophic obstructive cardiomyopathy. AV, aortic valve; JVP, jugular venous pressure; LV, left ventricle.

carotid pulse

anacrotic notch (due to closure of the AV)

2nd pulsation due to forceful LV emptying

normal or quick upstroke

JVP
may be large a wave

heart
apex beat may not be displaced

double apical beat

forceful atrial contraction — ventricular contraction

pulse
jerky peripheral pulses (best felt at carotid)

harsh ejection systolic murmur usually in late systole at left lower sternal edge

$A_2 P_2$

S_1 S_2 S_4

4th heart sound often present

Exercise testing

Lack of the normal rise or a fall in blood pressure on exercise is a risk factor for sudden death in HCM. All patients with HCM should have an exercise test to look for this, and it should be repeated periodically.

Prognosis

Children who are diagnosed when they are under 14 years of age have a poor prognosis and a high incidence of sudden death. Adults have a better prognosis, but they also have a higher sudden cardiac death rate than the general population. Another outcome is progressive cardiac failure with cardiac dilatation. Atrial fibrillation is common and often tolerated poorly.

Management

Drug management
   As with aortic stenosis, vasodilators should be avoided because they worsen the gradient across the obstruction. Therefore, patients who have HCM should not receive nitrates.
   β-Blockers (β-adrenoceptor antagonists) are used because their negative inotropic effect acts to decrease the contractility of the hypertrophied septum and reduces the outflow tract obstruction. Disopyramide may be used in combination or alone to treat obstruction. Verapamil or diltiazem may be given in symptomatic HCM in the absence of obstruction. Antiarrhythmic agents are important in patients with documented arrhythmias. Amiodarone or sotalol may be used for AF (along with anticoagulation).

COMMUNICATION

Patients should be advised that first-degree relatives should be screened with a transthoracic echocardiogram and undergo gene testing in cases of dilated or hypertrophic cardiomyopathy as these are often hereditary.

Device therapy

Dual chamber pacing to reduce the outflow gradient may be considered in selected patients, though evidence for benefit is lacking.
   An implantable cardioverter defibrillator (ICD) should be considered in patients at high risk of sudden cardiac death (see box below).

Percutaneous treatment (alcohol septal ablation)

In suitable cases, alcohol can be injected down the septal branch of the left anterior descending coronary artery, causing necrosis of the myocardial tissue that gives rise to the obstruction.

Surgery

A myomectomy is performed on the abnormal septum. This is the treatment of choice if other cardiac structural abnormalities need surgical correction.

RESTRICTIVE CARDIOMYOPATHY

This is an uncommon cause of cardiomyopathy in developed countries. In the West most cases are a variant of HCM – first-degree relatives may have classical HCM. The ventricular walls are excessively stiff and impede ventricular filling; therefore, end-diastolic pressure is increased. The systolic function of the ventricle is often normal.

Presentation is identical to that of constrictive pericarditis, but the two must be differentiated because pericardial constriction can be treated with surgery.

Possible causes of restrictive cardiomyopathy include:
• Storage diseases (e.g. glycogen storage diseases).
• Infiltrative diseases (e.g. amyloidosis, sarcoidosis).
• Scleroderma.
• Endomyocardial diseases (e.g. endomyocardial fibrosis, hypereosinophilic syndrome or carcinoid)

Clinical features

The main features are:
• Dyspnoea and fatigue due to poor cardiac output.
• Peripheral oedema and ascites.

• Elevated jugular venous pressure with a positive Kussmaul sign (increase in jugular venous pressure during inspiration).

Management

There is no specific treatment and the condition usually progresses towards death relatively quickly; most patients do not survive beyond 10 years after diagnosis.

ARRHYTHMOGENIC RIGHT-VENTRICULAR CARDIOMYOPATHY

This condition is a probably under-diagnosed cause of sudden death. It is characterised by fibrofatty replacement of the myocardium, particularly in the right ventricular free wall (though bilateral and left ventricular variants have been described). The main problem that this causes is heart rhythm disturbance ranging from ectopic beats to sustained ventricular arrhythmias and even sudden cardiac death. There may also be impairment of right-ventricular function. Patients present with palpitation, syncope, heart failure or sudden death. The diagnosis is best made with cardiac MRI if clinical suspicion arises.

There is no curative treatment, so management is aimed at preventing complications. This includes the use of ACE inhibitors and diuretics for the treatment of heart failure, antiarrhythmic agents and consideration of ICD implantation in patients at high risk of sudden cardiac death.

TAKOTSUBO CARDIOMYOPATHY

Takotsubo cardiomyopathy is named for a type of Japanese octopus pot, which resembles the characteristic shape of the left ventricle in this condition. Typically, the apex dilates ('ballooning'), with the rest of the ventricle spared, though mid- and basal versions have been described. The cardiomyopathy presents after a stressful event, most commonly in a post-menopausal woman, and patients may complain of chest pain or shortness of breath, with ischaemic ECG changes. After the initial presentation (which may be life-threatening) the prognosis is usually good, with full resolution of the cardiomyopathy in weeks or months. A small proportion die acutely of arrhythmia (generally Torsades de pointes due to QT prolongation) or cardiogenic shock. The disease may recur.

Further reading

Kushwaha, S.S., Fallon, J.T., Fuster, V., 1997. Restrictive cardiomyopathy. N. Engl. J. Med. 336, 267–276.

Oakley, C., Dec 1997. Aetiology, diagnosis, investigation, and management of the cardiomyopathies. BMJ 315, 1520–1524.

Pennell, D.J., 2002. Arrhythmogenic right ventricular cardiomyopathy. www.escardio.org/knowledge/cardiology_practice/ejournal_vol1/Vol1_no7.htm.

Spirito, P., Seidman, C.E., McKenna, W.J., Maron, B.J., 1997. The management of hypertrophic cardiomyopathy. N. Engl. J. Med. 336, 775–785.

Wynne, S., Braunwald, E., 2001. The cardiomyopathies and myocarditides. In: Braunwald, E., Zipes, D.P. (Eds.), Heart disease: a textbook of cardiovascular medicine. sixth ed. W B Saunders & Co, Elsevier.

Pericarditis and pericardial effusion

Objectives

By the end of this chapter you should:
- Be able to outline the clinical features of acute pericarditis.
- Be able to describe the ECG features of acute pericarditis.
- Be able to recognize the physical signs of cardiac tamponade.

The pericardium forms a strong protective sac around the heart. It is composed of an outer fibrous and an inner serosal layer with approximately 50 mL of pericardial fluid between these in the healthy state.

ACUTE PERICARDITIS

Acute pericarditis is caused by inflammation of the pericardium (Fig. 21.1).

Clinical features

History

The chest pain of acute pericarditis is usually central or left-sided pain that is sharp in nature and classically relieved by sitting forwards. Aggravating factors include lying supine, coughing or swallowing.

Dyspnoea may be caused by the pain of deep inspiration or the haemodynamic effects of an associated pericardial effusion.

Examination

The patient may have a fever and tachycardia.

A pericardial friction rub may be heard on auscultation of the heart. This is a high-pitched scratching sound (therefore, heard best with the diaphragm). It characteristically varies with time and may appear and disappear from one examination to the next. It sounds closer to the ears than a murmur and occurs in both systole and diastole.

Investigation

Blood tests

These will provide evidence of active inflammation – raised white cell count, erythrocyte sedimentation rate (ESR) and C-reactive protein (CRP), and also clues about the underlying cause. The following blood tests are appropriate:

- Full blood count.
- ESR and CRP.
- Urea, creatinine and electrolytes.
- Viral titres in the acute and convalescent phase (3 weeks later); also urine and faecal samples for viral studies and a Monospot test may be useful.
- Blood cultures.
- Autoantibody titres (e.g. antinuclear antibodies and rheumatoid factor).
- Cardiac enzymes and cardiac troponin T/ troponin I – these may be elevated, suggesting that the inflammatory process involves the myocardium (myopericarditis).

Electrocardiography

Superficial myocardial injury caused by pericarditis results in characteristic ECG changes (Fig. 21.2):

- Concave ST segment elevation is often present in all leads, except AVR and V1. PR segment depression is more specific for acute pericarditis.
- Subsequently, the ST segments return to normal and T wave flattening occurs, these may become inverted.
- Finally, all of the changes resolve and the ECG trace returns to normal (this may take several weeks or, if the inflammation persists, months).

Chest radiography

This is normal in most cases of uncomplicated acute pericarditis; however, a number of changes are possible:

- A pericardial effusion may develop and if large will result in enlargement of the cardiac shadow, which assumes a globular shape.
- Pleural effusions may also be seen.

Fig. 21.1 Causes of acute pericarditis

Cause	Examples/comment
Viral infection	Coxsackie virus A and B, echovirus, Epstein-Barr virus, HIV
Bacterial infection	Pneumococci, staphylococci, Gram-negative organisms, *Neisseria meningitidis*, *N. gonorrhoeae*
Fungal infection	Histoplasmosis, candidal infection
Other infections	Tuberculosis
Acute MI	Occurs in up to 25% of patients between 12 h and 6 days after infarction
Uraemia	Usually a haemorrhagic pericarditis, which can rapidly lead to cardiac tamponade; uraemic pericarditis is an indication for haemodialysis
Autoimmune disease	Acute rheumatic fever, SLE, rheumatoid arthritis, scleroderma
Other causes	Neoplastic disease, other inflammatory diseases, e.g. sarcoidosis, Whipple disease, Behçet syndrome, Dressler syndrome

A dissecting thoracic aortic aneurysm may occasionally present as acute pericarditis or a pericardial effusion. Therefore, be careful to look for a widened mediastinum on the chest radiograph and if this is suspicious a computed tomography scan of the chest or trans-oesophageal echo (TOE) should be performed to avoid missing this diagnosis.

Echocardiography

This is the best investigation for confirming the presence of a pericardial effusion. In uncomplicated acute pericarditis, however, the echocardiogram may be normal.

Management

Any treatable underlying cause should of course be sought and treated appropriately. Most cases of pericarditis are viral or idiopathic. The main aims of management are, therefore, analgesia and bed rest. Non-steroidal anti-inflammatory agents are the most effective for this condition. Colchicine may be useful and occasionally a short course of oral corticosteroids is required.

Fig. 21.2 ECG changes of pericarditis. Note the concave or saddle-shaped ST elevation seen in all leads except AVR.

A pericardial effusion may be present. If large or causing tamponade this can be drained. Analysis of the effusion may provide clues about the underlying cause of the pericarditis. Recurrence is rare but, if it does recur, colchicine or steroids will generally abort the episode.

DRESSLER SYNDROME

Dressler syndrome is a syndrome of fever, pericarditis and pleurisy occurring more than 1 week after a cardiac operation or myocardial infarction (MI). It can occur only if the pericardium has been exposed to the blood. Antibodies form against the pericardial antigens and then attack the pericardium in a type III autoimmune reaction.

Patients present with fever, malaise and chest pain. They exhibit the classic signs of acute pericarditis; they may also have arthritis. Cardiac tamponade is not uncommon.

Chest radiography shows pleural effusions. Echocardiography may reveal a pericardial effusion.

Initial management consists of non-steroidal antiinflammatory agents and aspirin; corticosteroids may be added if the symptoms persist.

CONSTRICTIVE PERICARDITIS

Constrictive pericarditis occurs when the pericardium becomes fibrosed and thickened and eventually restricts the filling of the heart during diastole. Causes are listed in Fig. 21.3.

Clinical features

The restricted filling of all four chambers of the heart results in low-output failure.

Initially, the right-sided component is more marked, resulting in a high venous pressure and hepatic congestion.

Later, left-ventricular failure (LVF) becomes apparent with dyspnoea and orthopnoea.

Examination

On examination, the signs of RVF and LVF are evident, but the ventricles are not enlarged.

Fig. 21.3   Causes of chronic constrictive pericarditis

Viral infection
Tuberculosis
Mediastinal radiotherapy
Mediastinal malignancy
Autoimmune disease

Note that any cause of acute pericarditis can persist and lead to chronic constrictive pericarditis. The diseases listed here, however, are the most common causes.

The single most important feature in the examination of such a patient is the jugular venous pressure (JVP), which is elevated. Kussmaul sign – an increase in the JVP during inspiration – may be evident.

Another important feature of the JVP is a rapid x and y descent, the presence of which (quite difficult sign) excludes cardiac tamponade.

The heart sounds are often soft. Atrial fibrillation is common.

Investigation

Blood tests are carried out to exclude a possible underlying cause (e.g. leucocytosis in infection, viral titres).

On chest radiography the heart size is normal. There may be signs of a neoplasm or tuberculosis. Pleural effusions are not uncommon. Tuberculous pericarditis may be associated with radiographically visible calcification.

Echocardiography shows good left-ventricular function. CT or MRI may be helpful.

Cardiac catheterization is usually diagnostic because it shows the classic pattern of raised and equal left and right end-diastolic pressures with normal left-ventricular function on the ventriculogram.

Management

The only definitive treatment is pericardectomy.

Antituberculous therapy may be required if the underlying cause is tuberculosis and should be continued for 1 year.

PERICARDIAL EFFUSION

A pericardial effusion is an accumulation of fluid in the pericardial space.

Cardiac tamponade describes the condition where a pericardial effusion increases the intrapericardial pressure such that it leads to haemodynamic compromise.

Causes

Causes of pericardial effusion (Fig. 21.4) include:

- Acute pericarditis (see Fig. 21.1).
- MI with ventricular wall rupture.
- Chest trauma.
- Cardiac surgery.
- Aortic dissection.
- Neoplasia.

Clinical features

A pericardial effusion may remain asymptomatic, even if very large, if it accumulates gradually. As much as 2 L of fluid can be accommodated without an increase in intrapericardial pressure if it accumulates slowly, but as little as 100 mL can cause tamponade if it appears suddenly.

Fig. 21.4 Causes of a pericardial effusion

Type of effusion	Examples
Transudate (<30 g/L protein)	Congestive cardiac failure, hypoalbuminaemia
Exudate (>30 g/L protein)	Infection (viral, bacterial or fungal), postmyocardial infarction, malignancy (e.g. local invasion of lung tumour), systemic lupus erythematosus, Dressler syndrome
Haemorrhagic	Uraemia, aortic dissection, trauma and postcardiac surgery

History

The only symptoms produced by a large chronic effusion may be a dull ache in the chest or dysphagia from compression of the oesophagus.

If cardiac tamponade is present, however, the patient may complain of dyspnoea, abdominal swelling (due to ascites) and peripheral oedema.

Examination

The important examination findings in a patient who has tamponade are:

- Low blood pressure.
- Pulse – tachycardia with low volume pulse, and may be pulsus paradoxus (where there is an exaggerated reduction of the pulse >10 mmHg during inspiration).
- Soft heart sounds
- Low urine output.
- Raised jugular venous pressure.

Possible mechanisms for pulsus paradoxus

These are:

- Increased venous return during inspiration filling the right heart and restricting left-ventricular filling, because the pericardium forms a rigid sac with only limited space within it.

- Downward movement of the diaphragm causing traction on the pericardium and tightening it further (this theory is not widely supported).

Investigation

Electrocardiography

A pericardial effusion results in the production of small voltage complexes with variable axis (electrical alternans is caused by the movement of the heart within the fluid).

On chest radiography the heart may appear large and globular.

Echocardiography reveals the pericardial effusion. Right-ventricular diastolic collapse is a classical echocardiographic sign of tamponade.

Management

The pericardial effusion should be drained if causing haemodynamic compromise or if there is doubt about the underlying cause. If the patient is in cardiogenic shock due to tamponade an emergency pericardial needle aspiration may be performed followed by formal drainage once the patient has been resuscitated.

Both techniques involve insertion of the drain or needle just below the xiphisternum and advancing it at 45° to the skin in the direction of the patient's left shoulder. The fluid should be sent for cytology, microscopy, culture and biochemical analysis of protein content.

Long-term treatment depends upon the underlying cause; a surgical 'window' may be required.

COMMUNICATION

Following drainage of pericardial effusion and discharge from hospital, patients should be made aware of the symptoms they will experience should the effusion reaccumulate, in order that they should seek medical help. These symptoms include lethargy, shortness of breath, abdominal swelling and peripheral oedema.

Further reading

Spodick, D.H., 2003. Acute cardiac tamponade. N. Engl. J. Med. 349, 684–690.

Sagristà-Sauleda, J., Angel, J., Permanyer-Miralda, G., Soler-Soler, J., 1999. Long-term follow-up of idiopathic chronic pericardial effusion. N. Engl. J. Med. 341, 2054–2059.

Sagristà-Sauleda, J., Angel, J., Sánchez, A., et al., 2004. Effusive constrictive pericarditis. N. Engl. J. Med. 350, 469–475.

Objectives

By the end of this chapter you should:
- Understand the natural history, diagnosis and consequences of rheumatic fever.
- Be able to list the causes of mitral and aortic valve disease.
- Be able to recognize the clinical signs and evaluate the severity of heart valve disease.
- Appreciate the effects on normal physiology of mitral and aortic valve stenosis and regurgitation.
- Be able to remember the treatment modalities for different valve lesions.
- Be aware of different types of heart valve prosthesis.

This topic is touched on in Chs 10 and 2, but it is covered here in more detail.

Valve lesions are a common short-case question both in finals and in the membership examination. It is possible to learn valve disease parrot fashion – once you know it you will not forget it again so it will be time well spent (Fig. 22.1). Alternatively, familiarity with the physiology (see *Crash course: Cardiovascular system*) will enable you to understand the features of valve disease from first principles.

RHEUMATIC FEVER

As mentioned in Chs 12 and 23, rheumatic fever is much less common in the developed world than in developing countries due to better social conditions and antibiotic therapy, and also because of a reduction in the virulence of β-haemolytic streptococcus. It is still a major problem in the developing world, where it is the most common cause of acquired valve disease.

Causes

Rheumatic fever is caused by a group A streptococcal pharyngeal infection. It occurs 2–3 weeks later in a small percentage of children aged 5–15 years. It is an antibody-mediated autoimmune response (type II hypersensitivity) and occurs where antibodies directed against bacterial cell membrane antigens cross-react and cause multiorgan disease.

Clinical features

Diagnosis is entirely clinical. Diagnosis based on the Duckett-Jones criteria requires evidence of preceding β-haemolytic streptococcal infection (e.g. increased antistreptolysin O titres) plus one major criterion or two minor criteria. Major criteria are:

- Carditis – involves all layers (pancarditis) and is usually asymptomatic.
- Arthritis – a migrating polyarthritis affecting the larger joints.
- Sydenham's chorea – usually occurs months after the initial disease and characterized by involuntary movements of the face and mouth due to inflammation of the caudate nucleus.
- Erythema marginatum – seen mainly on the trunk; the rash has raised red edges and a clear centre and the shape of the lesions changes with time.
- Nodules – pea-sized subcutaneous nodules on the extensor surfaces (painless).

Minor criteria are:

- Fever.
- Previous rheumatic fever.
- Raised erythrocyte sedimentation rate (ESR) or C-reactive protein (CRP).
- Long PR interval.
- Arthralgia.

Investigations

Blood tests reveal raised inflammatory markers (ESR and CRP) and rising antistreptolysin O (ASO) titres when taken 2 weeks apart. The throat swab may be positive.

Management

Treatment with high-dose benzylpenicillin is started immediately to eradicate the causative organism. Anti-inflammatory agents are given to suppress the autoimmune response. Salicylates are effective. Corticosteroids are used if there is any carditis. Long-term antibiotics

Valve disease

Fig. 22.1	Valve lesions and their abbreviations	
Valve involved	**Lesion**	**Abbreviation**
Mitral valve	Mitral stenosis	MS
	Mitral regurgitation	MR
	Floppy (prolapsing) mitral valve	MVP
Aortic valve	Aortic stenosis	AS
	Aortic regurgitation	AR
Tricuspid valve	Tricuspid regurgitation	TR
	Tricuspid stenosis	TS
Pulmonary valve	Pulmonary stenosis	PS
	Pulmonary regurgitation	PR

(usually penicillin) are recommended for a minimum of 5 years (or until the patient is 21) to prevent recurrent rheumatic fever. Long-term follow-up is needed to identify any valve disease.

HINTS AND TIPS

Acute rheumatic fever is not common in the developed world, but it is a good idea to have knowledge of this disease because there are still many elderly people suffering the after-effects of a childhood infection. It is also important to recognize and treat acute rheumatic fever promptly.

Fig. 22.2 Pathophysiology of mitral stenosis. AF, atrial fibrillation; LA, left atrium; LV, left ventricle; JVP, jugular venous pressure; MV, mitral valve; RA, right atrium; RV, right ventricle; TR, tricuspid regurgitation.

MITRAL STENOSIS

Causes

The most common cause of mitral stenosis (MS) is rheumatic fever (Fig. 22.2). Other causes are rare:

- Congenital.
- Malignant – lung carcinoid (systemic carcinoid causes right-sided valve disease).
- Systemic lupus erythematosus.
- Mucopolysaccharidoses, e.g. Hurler syndrome (causing glycoprotein deposition on the mitral leaflets).
- Endocardial fibroelastosis spreading onto the valve
- Lutembacher syndrome is actually a coincidental ASD associated with rheumatic MS

Other conditions may mimic mitral stenosis by causing obstruction of inflow to the left ventricle. These include left atrial myxoma, left atrial thrombus and hypertrophic cardiomyopathy.

Rheumatic fever causes fusion of the cusps and commissures, and thickening of the cusps, which then become immobile and stenosed in a fish-mouth configuration. An immobile valve cannot close properly and is, therefore, often regurgitant as well.

Clinical features

The main presenting features of mitral stenosis are:

- Dyspnoea – this may be due to pulmonary hypertension or pulmonary oedema. Patients who have mitral stenosis have an increased incidence of chest infections, which may cause dyspnoea.

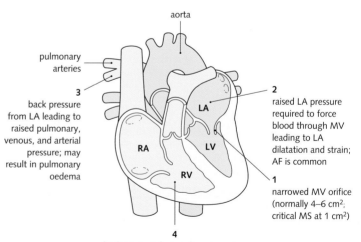

aorta

pulmonary arteries

3 back pressure from LA leading to raised pulmonary, venous, and arterial pressure; may result in pulmonary oedema

LA

RA

LV

RV

2 raised LA pressure required to force blood through MV leading to LA dilatation and strain; AF is common

1 narrowed MV orifice (normally 4–6 cm²; critical MS at 1 cm²)

4 back pressure from pulmonary artery causes RV strain and hypertrophy and eventually RV failure with raised JVP, ascites, hepatomegaly, and peripheral oedema; dilatation of RV may lead to dilatation of tricuspid valve ring and TR

Haemoptysis – there is an increased incidence of pulmonary vein and alveolar capillary rupture.

Palpitations – atrial fibrillation is common in this condition (due to enlargement of the left atrium) and may cause palpitations, which are often accompanied by a sudden worsening in the dyspnoea because the loss of the atrial contraction (upon which the heart has become dependent) causes a considerable reduction in cardiac output.

Systemic emboli – a recognized complication of atrial fibrillation.

Symptoms that are secondary to effects of left atrial enlargement include:

Hoarseness due to stretching of the recurrent laryngeal nerve.

Dysphagia due to oesophageal compression.

Left lung collapse due to compression of the left main bronchus.

Examination

The principal clinical findings (Fig. 22.3) are:

Loud first heart sound (S_1) because of slow diastolic filling.

A tapping apex beat that is not displaced (a palpable S_1).

An opening snap after the second heart sound (S_2) followed by a low rumbling mid-diastolic murmur, heard best at the apex with the patient on his or her left side and in expiration. If you have not listened in exactly this way you cannot exclude MS. Both the opening snap and loud S_1 may be absent of the valve is heavily calcified.

A presystolic accentuation of the mid-diastolic murmur, if the patient is in sinus rhythm; this is absent if the patient has atrial fibrillation. Severity is related to the duration, not the intensity, of the mid-diastolic murmur.

Loud and palpable pulmonary component of the second heart sound (P_2), if pulmonary hypertension has developed, and there may be a right ventricular heave. Tricuspid regurgitation may be present.

HINTS AND TIPS

Mitral stenosis is a difficult murmur to hear. It is, therefore, vital to listen for the murmur correctly (i.e. with the patient on his or her left side in full expiration).

Investigations

Investigations that may aid diagnosis include the following.

Electrocardiography

Atrial fibrillation may be seen. P mitrale is another feature and is only seen in sinus rhythm. The P wave in lead II is abnormally long (0.12 s) and may have an 'M' shape.

Chest radiography

This shows the enlarged left atrium, resulting in a horizontal left main bronchus. The mitral valve itself may be calcified and, therefore, visible. There may be prominent pulmonary vessels.

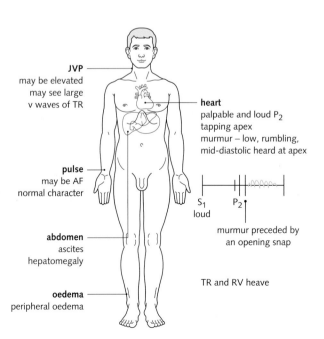

Fig. 22.3 Clinical findings in patients who have mitral stenosis. AF, atrial fibrillation; S_1, first heart sound; P_2, pulmonary component of second heart sound; RV, right ventricle; TR, tricuspid regurgitation.

Echocardiography

The mitral valve can be visualized and the cross-sectional area measured. This can also be estimated using Doppler measurements. Pulmonary hypertension can also be evaluated.

Cardiac catheterization

This is performed on most patients before valve replacement to exclude any coexistent coronary artery disease and evaluate any mitral regurgitation that may be present.

Management

Medical management

Medical treatment of MS may consist of:

- Digoxin or a small dose of β-blocker – may be used to treat atrial fibrillation, and by prolonging diastole allow the left ventricle more time to fill. A β-blocker may be lifesaving in pregnancy (MS is often previously undiagnosed).
- Direct current (DC) cardioversion – may be successful in patients who have atrial fibrillation of recent onset, but only if they have been fully anticoagulated for at least 4 weeks.
- Anticoagulation – recommended in all patients who have MS and atrial fibrillation.
- Diuretics – used to treat the pulmonary and peripheral oedema.

Mitral valvuloplasty

Mitral valvuloplasty involves the passage of a balloon across the mitral valve and its inflation, so stretching the stenosed valve. This procedure is carried out via a percutaneous route and only requires a local anaesthetic and light sedation. The following features make a patient unsuitable for this procedure:

- Marked mitral regurgitation.
- A history of systemic emboli.
- Calcified or thickened rigid mitral valve leaflets.

Surgical management

This is indicated in patients who have a mitral valve area of 1 cm^2 or less. Note that restenosis may occur after any valvuloplasty or valvotomy. In carefully selected patients this does not occur for many years; early restenosis within 5 years may occur in those who have thickened or rigid valves.

Open mitral valvotomy

Open mitral valvotomy is performed under general anaesthetic using a median sternotomy incision and requires cardiopulmonary bypass. It is used in patient who have already had a mitral valvuloplasty or who have mild mitral regurgitation.

Closed mitral valvotomy

This has now been superseded by mitral valvuloplasty. It does not require cardiopulmonary bypass; a curved incision is made under the left breast. It is worth knowing this because patients in finals examinations may have this scar.

Mitral valve replacement

This is used for calcified or very rigid valves unsuitable for valvuloplasty or valvotomy.

MITRAL REGURGITATION

The mitral valve may become incompetent for four reasons (Fig. 22.4):

1. Abnormal mitral valve annulus.
2. Abnormal mitral valve leaflets.
3. Abnormal chordae tendineae.
4. Abnormal papillary muscle function.

HINTS AND TIPS

When considering the causes of regurgitation of any valve it is useful to divide the causes into:
- Abnormalities of the valve ring.
- Abnormalities of the valve cusps and leaflets.
- Abnormalities of the supporting structures.

Pathophysiology

In mitral regurgitation (MR) the regurgitant jet of blood flows back into the left atrium and with time the left atrium dilates and accommodates the increased volume and pressure. There is, however, also increased back pressure in the pulmonary veins and as the MR worsens pulmonary hypertension develops, which may eventually cause RVF.

The left ventricle is dilated, because the blood entering from the left atrium with each beat is increased; over time this results in LVF. Therefore, severe chronic MR is left untreated will result in biventricular failure. (Mitral stenosis differs because it does not cause LVF.)

Fig. 22.4   Causes of mitral regurgitation

Site of pathology	Pathology
Mitral annulus	Senile calcification Left ventricular dilatation and enlargement of the annulus Abscess formation during infective endocarditis
Mitral valve leaflets	Infective endocarditis Rheumatic fever Mitral valve prolapse Congenital malformation Connective tissue disorders – Marfan syndrome, Ehlers-Danlos syndrome, osteogenesis imperfecta, pseudoxanthoma elasticum
Chordae tendineae	Idiopathic rupture Myxomatous degeneration Infective endocarditis Connective tissue disorders
Papillary muscle	Myocardial infarction Infiltration – sarcoid, amyloid Myocarditis

Clinical features

These vary depending upon whether the MR is chronic or acute:

- Chronic mitral regurgitation develops slowly so allowing the heart to compensate and usually presents with a history of fatigue and dyspnoea.
- Acute MR presents with severe dyspnoea due to pulmonary oedema. The left atrium has not had time to dilate to accommodate the increased volume due to regurgitation of blood back through the mitral valve. The pressure increase is, therefore, transmitted directly to the pulmonary veins, resulting in pulmonary oedema.

Acute MR can be rapidly fatal and needs to be looked for in patients following myocardial infarction (MI) (papillary muscle rupture occurs at days 4–7 after MI, but papillary muscle dysfunction may occur earlier) and in patients who have infective endocarditis.

Examination

Features that may be seen are illustrated in Fig. 22.5 and include the following:

- Atrial fibrillation – an irregularly irregular pulse is common, especially in patients who have chronic MR and a dilated left atrium.
- Jugular venous pressure may be elevated – if the patient has developed pulmonary hypertension and right-heart failure, or fluid retention.

- The apex is displaced downward and laterally as the left ventricle dilates – eventually LVF may result. (Note that in MS the apex is not displaced because the left ventricle is protected by the stenosed mitral valve.)
- The murmur of MR is pansystolic and typically best heard at the apex – the murmur radiates to the axilla. Note that the loudness of the murmur is not an indicator of the severity of the MR.
- Signs of congestive cardiac failure – i.e. third heart sound, bilateral basal inspiratory crepitations, ascites and peripheral oedema.
- P_2 may be loud and there may be a right ventricular heave – if pulmonary hypertension has developed.

Mitral valve prolapse

This is also known as floppy mitral valve or click-murmur syndrome. Factors to consider are:

- This is a common disorder affecting approximately 4% of the population and more females than males.
- The mitral valve may merely prolapse minimally into the left atrium or cause varying degrees of MR.
- Most cases are idiopathic, but floppy mitral valve is seen with greater frequency in certain conditions (e.g. Marfan syndrome and other connective tissue disorders).
- Most patients are asymptomatic, the disorder being diagnosed at routine medical examination. Some patients present with fatigue, atypical chest pain and palpitations.
- Examination reveals a mid-systolic click at the apex. This may or may not be followed by a systolic murmur of mitral regurgitation. The murmur may be best heard at the left sternal edge or round the patient's back.
- Prophylaxis against infective endocarditis is only indicated in those patients who have MR.
- Most patients require no further treatment other than reassurance.

Investigations

The following investigations may aid diagnosis.

Electrocardiography

There may be atrial fibrillation and left-ventricular hypertrophy.

Chest radiography

An enlarged left ventricle may be seen as an increase in the cardiothoracic ratio. The mitral valve may be calcified and, therefore, visible.

Fig. 22.5 Clinical findings in patients who have mitral regurgitation. A$_2$, aortic component of second heart sound; AF, atrial fibrillation; CCF, congestive cardiac failure; P$_2$, pulmonary component of second heart sound.

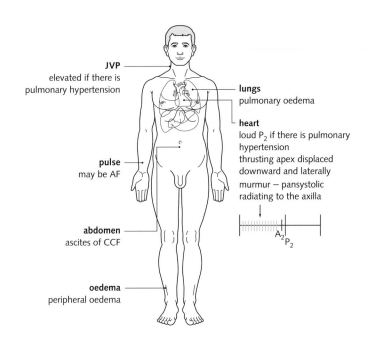

JVP
elevated if there is
pulmonary hypertension

lungs
pulmonary oedema

heart
loud P$_2$ if there is pulmonary hypertension
thrusting apex displaced downward and laterally
murmur – pansystolic radiating to the axilla

pulse
may be AF

A$_2$
P$_2$

abdomen
ascites of CCF

oedema
peripheral oedema

Echocardiography

The mitral valve can be clearly seen and the regurgitant jet visualized. The left atrial size and left-ventricular size and function can be assessed. Suitability for mitral valve repair is better evaluated with TOE.

Cardiac catheterization

Most patients have minimal MR on echocardiography and do not require catheterization. This is performed to assess the severity of the MR and to exclude other valve lesions and coronary artery disease.

Management

Medical management

This may consist of diuretics and ACE inhibitors to treat the congestive cardiac failure.

Surgical management

Patients are considered for surgery if the MR is severe at echocardiography and cardiac catheterization. It is important to act before irreversible left ventricular damage and severe pulmonary hypertension have occurred.

Mitral valve repair

This may take the form of mitral annuloplasty, repair of a ruptured chorda or repair of a mitral valve leaflet. These procedures are performed on patients who have mobile non-calcified and non-thickened valves.

Mitral valve replacement

This is performed if mitral valve repair is not possible. Both repair and replacement of the mitral valve require a median sternotomy incision and cardiopulmonary bypass.

AORTIC STENOSIS

The most common form of aortic stenosis (AS) is valvular AS; however, aortic stenosis may also occur at the sub- or supravalvular level (Fig. 22.6).

Pathophysiology

The left-ventricular outflow obstruction results in an increased left-ventricular pressure. The left-ventricle undergoes hypertrophy and more vigorous and prolonged contraction to overcome the obstruction and maintain an adequate cardiac output. Myocardial oxygen demand is increased and, because systole is prolonged, diastole is shortened and, therefore, myocardial blood supply from the coronary arteries is reduced (coronary artery flow occurs during diastole; see *Crash course: Cardiovascular system*).

Clinical features

Although patients are often asymptomatic, a number of symptoms are characteristic of AS, including:

Fig. 22.6 Causes of aortic stenosis	
Type of AS	**Cause**
Valvular AS	Congenital most common, males > females (deformed valve can be uni-, bi-, or tricuspid) Senile calcification Rheumatic fever Severe atherosclerosis
Subvalvular AS	Fibromuscular ring HOCM
Supravalvular AS	Associated with hypercalcaemia in Williams syndrome, a syndrome associated with elfin facies, mental retardation, strabismus, hypervitaminosis D and hypercalcaemia; the inheritance is autosomal dominant

HOCM, hypertrophic obstructive cardiomyopathy.

- Dyspnoea – may lead to orthopnoea and paroxysmal nocturnal dyspnoea as the left ventricle fails.
- Angina – due to the increased myocardial work and reduced blood supply (the coronary arteries may be normal).
- Dizziness and syncope – especially on exertion.
- Sudden death.
- Systemic emboli.

Patients who have aortic stenosis may present with angina, but an exercise test is absolutely contraindicated in patients who have severe aortic stenosis, because even the mildest exertion can cause syncope or sudden death. It is, therefore, crucial to examine every patient carefully before recommending an exercise ECC.

Examination

The following findings are common in valvular AS (Fig. 22.7):

- A slow rising, small volume pulse – best felt at the carotid pulse.
- A low blood pressure.
- Heaving apex beat – rarely displaced.
- Ejection systolic murmur at the aortic area radiating to the carotids accompanied by a palpable thrill.
- Obscured or absent aortic component of the second heart sound (A_2).
- Signs of LVF.

Investigations

Electrocardiography

This usually shows sinus rhythm and a picture of left-ventricular hypertrophy with strain – a tall R wave in lead V5 with a deep S wave in lead V2 and T wave inversion in the lateral leads.

Fig. 22.7 Clinical findings in patients who have aortic stenosis.

BP low with narrow pulse pressure

carotid pulse slow rising

heart

lungs bilateral basal crepitations due to left ventricular failure

S_1 A_2 P_2 S_1

pulse low volume

- ejection systolic murmur in aortic area radiating to carotid arteries
- palpable thrill
- apex may not be displaced
- heaving apex
- obscured aortic second sound

Chest radiography

An enlarged cardiac shadow may occur due to left-ventricular hypertrophy. The valve may be calcified and, therefore, visible. There may also be evidence of pulmonary oedema.

Echocardiography

This will show the valve in great detail including the number of cusps and their mobility, and the presence of calcification. It will also show left-ventricular hypertrophy or failure, and the aortic valve gradient can be measured using Doppler echocardiography.

Cardiac catheterization

This may provide information on the valve gradient and on left-ventricular failure, if not available from echocardiography. The coronary arteries are also assessed to rule out coronary artery disease that will require bypass grafting.

Management

Medical management

Apart from the use of diuretics to treat LVF, many anti-anginal drugs and ACE inhibitors are avoided in AS because they might:

- Have a negative inotropic effect and result in acute pulmonary oedema (if LV function is impaired).
- Cause vasodilatation, resulting in worsening of the gradient across the aortic valve.

Percutaneous and trans-apical valves

Recently, devices have been developed that can be deployed either through percutaneous catheters or using a trocar through the apex of the heart (trans-apical aortic valve insertion or TAVI). These devices may be considered in those that are too sick for valve surgery and, as the technologies develop further, may replace much traditional surgery in the future.

Surgical management

This is considered in all symptomatic patients who have marked stenosis (aortic valve gradient >50 mmHg). Without operation the outcome for these patients is very poor (50% 2-year survival in severe aortic stenosis).

Aortic valve replacement is usually performed using a median sternotomy incision and requires cardiopulmonary bypass. In some young patients a Ross procedure may be performed. In this case the patient's own pulmonary valve is moved to the aortic position, and is replaced by a porcine or cadaveric graft, which will then last much longer as it is not exposed to systolic pressure.

Aortic valvuloplasty is performed in children and rarely in the very elderly.

AORTIC REGURGITATION

Aortic regurgitation (AR) may be due to an abnormality of the valve cusps themselves or dilatation of the aortic root and, therefore, the valve ring (Fig. 22.8).

Pathophysiology

The regurgitation of blood back into the left ventricle after each systole results in an increased end-diastolic volume and an increased stroke volume. The left ventricle works harder and becomes hypertrophied. If the AR worsens the left ventricle may no longer be able to compensate and LVF will result. If the situation deteriorates any further, then congestion results. The backpressure from the left ventricle may also cause pulmonary hypertension and RVF, but this is uncommon.

Clinical features

Moderate and mild AR is often asymptomatic. Dyspnoea is the main presenting feature (Fig. 22.9).

Examination

Characteristic findings in aortic regurgitation are:

- A collapsing high-volume pulse (waterhammer pulse) – due to the increased stroke volume and the rapid run-off of blood back into the left ventricle after systole. This is better felt at the carotid pulse, but it can also be felt at the radial pulse by lifting the arm and feeling the pulse with the fingers across it. The tapping quality is felt between the examiner's middle and distal interphalangeal joints.
- A wide pulse pressure on measuring blood pressure.

Fig. 22.8	Causes of aortic regurgitation
Type of disease	**Cause**
Valve disease	Congenital Rheumatic fever Infective endocarditis Rheumatoid arthritis SLE Connective tissue disease (e.g. Marfan syndrome, pseudoxanthoma elasticum)
Aortic root disease	Marfan syndrome Osteogenesis imperfecta Type A aortic dissection Ankylosing spondylitis Reiter syndrome Psoriatic arthritis

SLE, systemic lupus erythematosus.

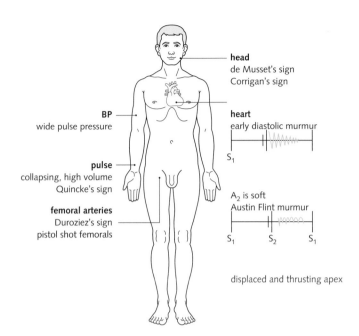

Fig. 22.9 Clinical findings in patients who have aortic regurgitation. A_2, aortic component of second heart sound; S_1, first heart sound; S_2, second heart sound.

- Downward and laterally displaced apex, which has a thrusting nature.
- Murmur best heard at the left lower sternal edge with the patient sitting forward and in full expiration – it is a soft high-pitched early diastolic murmur, which is sometimes difficult to hear, so be sure to listen for it properly with a diaphragm.
- Increased flow across the aortic valve may produce an ejection systolic murmur.
- May be signs of left-ventricular or congestive failure.
- Other signs include de Musset sign (head bobbing with each beat), Corrigan sign (prominent pulsation in the neck), Quincke sign (visible capillary pulsation in the nailbed), pistol shot femoral pulses (an audible femoral sound) and Duroziez sign (another audible murmur over the femoral arteries – a to-and-fro sound).
- The Austin Flint murmur – heard when the regurgitant jet causes vibration of the anterior mitral valve leaflet. The murmur is similar to that of MS, but with no opening snap.

Investigations

Electrocardiography

This shows left-ventricular hypertrophy.

Chest radiography

The left ventricle may be enlarged and there may be pulmonary oedema.

Echocardiography

The structure of the aortic valve and the size of the regurgitant jet may be seen. Aortic root size and left-ventricular function can be assessed.

Cardiac catheterization

This enables assessment of aortic root size, severity of aortic regurgitation, left-ventricular function and co-existent coronary artery disease.

Management

Medical management

The use of diuretics and ACE inhibitors is valuable to treat cardiac failure in these patients. It is, however, important to make the diagnosis and surgically treat this condition before the left ventricle dilates and fails.

Surgical management

Aortic valve replacement is considered if the patient is symptomatic or if there are signs of progressive left-ventricular dilatation. The aortic root may also need to be replaced if it is grossly dilated.

ASSESSING THE SEVERITY OF A VALVE LESION

Once a valve lesion has been diagnosed it is useful to be able to comment on its severity. This is judged by clinical, echocardiographic and angiographic means in most cases (Fig. 22.10).

TRICUSPID REGURGITATION

Causes

Most cases of tricuspid regurgitation (TR) are due to dilatation of the tricuspid annulus resulting from dilatation of the right ventricle. This may be due to any cause of RVF or pulmonary hypertension.

Occasionally, the tricuspid valve is affected by infective endocarditis (usually in intravenous drug abusers). Rarer causes include congenital malformations and the carcinoid syndrome.

Ebstein anomaly

This congenital malformation is caused by downward displacement of the tricuspid valve into the body of the right ventricle. The valve is regurgitant and malformed. The condition is associated with other structural cardiac abnormalities and there is a high incidence of both supraventricular and ventricular tachyarrhythmias.

Clinical features

The symptoms and signs are due to the backpressure effects of the regurgitant jet into the right atrium, which are transmitted to the venous system causing a prominent v wave in the jugular venous waveform (Fig. 22.11).

Fig. 22.10   Features indicating severity of valve disease

Valve disease	Features
MS	Proximity of opening snap to second heart sound and duration of murmur Valve area assessed on echocardiography Evidence of pulmonary hypertension on echocardiography and cardiac catheterization
MR	Symptoms and signs of pulmonary oedema Size of regurgitant jet and poor left ventricular function on echocardiography Evidence of pulmonary hypertension on echocardiography and cardiac catheterization
AS	Presence of symptoms Low-volume pulse and BP, obscured or absent aortic second sound Severity of aortic gradient and poor left ventricular function on echocardiography or cardiac catheterization
AR	Signs of LVF Left ventricular function and size of regurgitant jet on echocardiography or cardiac catheterization

AS, aortic stenosis; AR, aortic regurgitation; BP, blood pressure; LVF, left ventricular failure; MS, mitral stenosis; MR, mitral regurgitation.

Fig. 22.11   Clinical findings in patients who have tricuspid regurgitation. Look out for signs of the underlying cause of right-heart failure such as mitral valve disease or pulmonary disease. JVP, jugular venous pressure; P$_2$, pulmonary component of second heart sound; S$_1$, first heart sound; S$_2$, second heart sound.

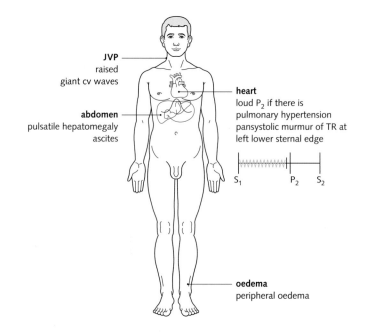

JVP
raised
giant cv waves

heart
loud P$_2$ if there is pulmonary hypertension
pansystolic murmur of TR at left lower sternal edge

abdomen
pulsatile hepatomegaly
ascites

S$_1$ P$_2$ S$_2$

oedema
peripheral oedema

Fatigue and discomfort, owing to ascites or hepatic congestion, are the commonest features. Patients usually present with symptoms of the disease causing the underlying RVF; the TR is often an incidental finding.

Management

The mainstay of management is medical with diuretics and angiotensin-converting enzyme inhibitors to treat the RVF and fluid overload. Tricuspid valve replacement is considered in very severe cases.

OTHER VALVE LESIONS

These are summarized in Fig. 22.12.

PROSTHETIC HEART VALVES

Examples of mechanical and biological heart valves are shown in Figs 22.13 and 22.14. You should aim to be especially familiar with artificial valve sounds as they very commonly pop up in exams. Mechanical valves

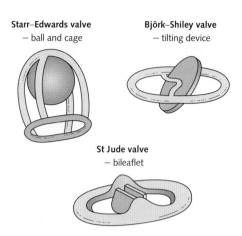

Fig. 22.13 Types of mechanical heart valve. Note that all patients must be anticoagulated for life and the international normalized ratio (INR) must be kept at approximately 3:4 – this lowers the risk of thromboembolism. They last for about 15 years. All patients who have prosthetic valves require antibiotic prophylaxis against infective endocarditis.

impart a metallic quality to the first (mitral) or second (aortic) heart sound. Some patients may have both types of valve. All patients with prosthetic aortic valves (even tissue valves) will have a systolic flow murmur. Patients with mitral valves may have a quiet pansystolic murmur due to turbulent blood flow in the left ventricle, but loud pansystolic murmurs require investigation. Diastolic murmurs are generally a worrying sign and require investigation for endocarditis, paravalvular leak or valve failure. A short, quiet diastolic murmur in a mitral prosthesis may be innocent but it is better to err on the side of caution.

Fig. 22.12 Overview of other valve lesions

Valve lesion	Cause	Clinical features	Management
Tricuspid stenosis	Rheumatic fever, carcinoid syndrome; rare	Venous congestion – JVP raised, large a waves, ascites, hepatomegaly, peripheral oedema, soft diastolic murmur at left lower sternal edge	Treat pulmonary hypertension, valve replacement
Pulmonary stenosis	Congenital malformation – Noonan syndrome, tetralogy of Fallot, maternal rubella syndrome, carcinoid syndrome	If mild asymptomatic, if severe – RVF and cyanosis, ejection systolic murmur in the pulmonary area (second left ICS), wide splitting of second heart sound	Pulmonary valvuloplasty or pulmonary valve replacement
Pulmonary regurgitation (PR)	Dilatation of the valve ring secondary to pulmonary hypertension, infective endocarditis	RVF in severe cases, low-pitched diastolic murmur in pulmonary area, Graham Steell murmur – in severe PR the murmur is high pitched due to the forceful jet and best heard at the left parasternal edge (i.e. similar to that in aortic regurgitation but with signs of severe pulmonary hypertension and RVF)	Treat underlying disease

ICS, intercostal space; JVP, jugular venous pressure; RVF, right ventricular failure.

Fig. 22.14 Types of biological heart valve

Type of valve	Features
Xenograft	Manufactured from porcine valve or pericardium and mounted on a frame (on chest X-ray only the mounting ring can be seen)
	Lasts for about 10 years
Homograft	Cadaveric valve graft
	More durable than a xenograft
Anticoagulation is necessary only if the patient has atrial fibrillation.	

Further reading

ACC/AHA, 2006. Guidelines for the management of patients with valvular heart disease. Circulation 114, e84–e231.

Braunwald, E., 2001. Valvular heart disease. In: Braunwald, E., Zipes, D.P. (Eds.), Heart Disease: A Textbook of Cardiovascular Medicine, sixth ed. W B Saunders & Co, Elsevier.

Carabello, B.A., Crawford, F.A., 1997. Valvular heart disease. N. Engl. J. Med. 337, 32–41.

By the end of this chapter you should:
- Understand the criteria necessary for a diagnosis of infective endocarditis.
- Be able to list the cardiac conditions that predispose to endocarditis.
- Be aware of the complications of infective endocarditis.
- Be able to recognize the clinical signs of endocarditis.
- Understand the principles of antibiotic therapy in infective endocarditis.
- Be able to define the indications for surgery in infective endocarditis.

DEFINITION OF INFECTIVE ENDOCARDITIS

Infective endocarditis describes the condition where there is infection of the endothelial surface of the heart by a microorganism. Heart valves are most commonly affected, but any area causing a high-pressure jet through a narrow orifice may be involved (e.g. ventricular septal defect).

The Duke criteria are used in the diagnosis of infective endocarditis (Fig. 23.1)

EPIDEMIOLOGY OF INFECTIVE ENDOCARDITIS

Infective endocarditis is an evolving disease. Traditionally, the main predisposing condition was rheumatic fever; however, the incidence of rheumatic fever in developed countries has dropped significantly because of improved social conditions and antibiotic therapy. Now, in developed countries different groups of patients are presenting with infective endocarditis for the following reasons:

- Increased number of prosthetic valve insertions.
- Increased number of patients who have congenital heart disease surviving to adulthood.
- Increasing elderly population.
- Increasing intravenous drug abuse.
- Antibiotic resistance.

With this change in the population affected by infective endocarditis, the organisms are also changing; for example, coagulase-negative staphylococci, which used to be uncommon, are now the most common organisms seen on prosthetic valves (Fig. 23.2).

People with the conditions listed in Fig. 23.3 are at an increased risk of developing infective endocarditis. It used to be that such patients were routinely given antibiotic prophylaxis before a variety of procedures. Since 2008, NICE has recommended instead that infections are treated promptly in those at risk; and that they receive prophylactic antibiotics (chosen to cover common organisms that cause endocarditis) only when they undergo gastrointestinal or genitourinary procedures where there is already suspected infection. This change was made due to lack of evidence of benefit and a known risk of harm (including anaphylaxis and the development of antibiotic resistance), but the new guidelines have caused controversy.

PATHOPHYSIOLOGY OF INFECTIVE ENDOCARDITIS

The development of endocarditis depends on a number of factors:

- Presence of anatomical abnormalities in the heart surface.
- Haemodynamic abnormalities within the heart.
- Host immune response.
- Virulence of the organism.
- Presence of bacteraemia.

Transient bacteraemia is a common occurrence, but infective endocarditis is rare so a healthy individual who has normal cardiac anatomy is well protected (Fig. 23.4). Transient bacteraemia is associated with both dental and non-dental procedures, but also day-to-day activities such as teeth brushing. However, there is no association between these procedures and the development of infective endocarditis, which is why antibiotic prophylaxis is no longer recommended for most

Fig. 23.1 Duke criteria for the diagnosis of infective endocarditis (IE)

Criteria	Description
Major	
A	Positive blood culture for IE
	1 – Typical microorganism consistent with IE from 2 separate blood cultures, as noted below: - viridans streptococci, *Streptococcus bovis*, or HACEK* group, or - community-acquired *Staphylococcus aureus* or enterococci, in the absence of a primary focus or
	2 – Microorganisms consistent with IE from persistently positive blood cultures defined as: - two positive cultures of blood samples drawn >12 h apart, or - all of three or a majority of four separate cultures of blood (with first and last sample drawn 1 h apart)
B	Evidence of endocardial involvement
	1 – Positive echocardiogram for IE defined as: oscillating intracardiac mass on valve or supporting structures, in the path of regurgitant jets, or on implanted material in the absence of an alternative anatomic explanation, or abscess, or new partial dehiscence of prosthetic valve or
	2 – New valvular regurgitation (worsening or changing of preexisting murmur not sufficient)
Minor	
	Predisposition: predisposing heart condition or intravenous drug use Fever: temperature >38.0 °C (100.4 °F) Vascular phenomena: major arterial emboli, septic pulmonary infarcts, mycotic aneurysm, intracranial haemorrhage, conjunctival haemorrhages, and Janeway lesions Immunologic phenomena: glomerulonephritis, Osler nodes, Roth spots, and rheumatoid factor Microbiological evidence: positive blood culture but does not meet a major criterion as noted above or serological evidence of active infection with organism consistent with IE

Clinical criteria for infective endocarditis requires:

Two major criteria, or
One major and three minor criteria, or
Five minor criteria

HACEK group: Haemophilus sp., Actinobacillus actinomycetemcomitans, Cardiobacterium hominis, Eikenella corrodens, Kingella kingae.

patients. The exception is for the highest risk dental procedures in the highest risk patients, where prophylaxis is recommended.

The complications of infective endocarditis are potentially fatal and are as follows:

- Local destructive effects – valve incompetence, paravalvular abscesses, prosthetic valve dehiscence and myocardial rupture. If they progress, these local effects can result in congestive cardiac failure and cardiogenic shock; sometimes this is very rapid.
- Embolization of infected or non-infected fragments – these can result in stroke, mycotic aneurysm or cerebral abscess, ischaemic bowel, digital infarcts, renal and hepatic abscesses, and renal infarcts (hepatic infarcts are rare because the liver is supplied by the hepatic artery and the hepatic portal system).
- Type III autoimmune reaction to the organism – resulting in the deposition of immune complexes (antibody plus antigen) and a subsequent inflammatory response. A diffuse or focal glomerulonephritis, cerebral vasculitis, or arthritis may occur.

If you remember these three classes of complications of infective endocarditis it is easy to fit actual symptoms and signs into each category. To classify signs according to the pathophysiology shows that you have a full understanding of the disease process and is bound to impress examiners.

CLINICAL FEATURES OF INFECTIVE ENDOCARDITIS

History

The duration of the symptoms is variable, from a few days to several months. This tends to reflect the virulence of the organism – *Staphylococcus aureus* causes

Fig. 23.2 Common causative organisms in infective endocarditis

Organism	Comments
Streptococcus viridans group (i.e. *S. milleri*, *S. mutans*, *S. mitis*)	Still the most common causative organism; predominantly found on rheumatic heart valves or congenitally abnormal valves; can be found on prosthetic valves and in IVDAs
Staphylococcus aureus	Most common cause in IVDAs; causes rapid destruction of the valve and there is a high mortality rate
Coagulase-negative staphylococci (*Staphylococcus epidermidis*)	Most common cause in patients who have prosthetic heart valves within 2 months of operation (the high-risk time for these patients); after 2 months the risk is much lower and other organisms may be involved
Enterococci	Can cause endocarditis in any situation and are probably the second most common causative organisms in developed countries
Gram-negative bacteria, diphtheroids	Predominantly after valve surgery
Fungi	IVDAs (*Candida* spp.) and after valve surgery
Fastidious organisms (Gram-negative organisms requiring prolonged culture)	
Coxiella burnetii	

Note that a significant number of cases are culture negative (i.e. grow no organism). IVDAs, intravenous drug abusers.

apid valvular destruction and presents early whereas a *Staphylococcus epidermidis* infection of a prosthetic valve may take a few months to present. The following symptoms are common:

- Fever.
- Sweats.
- Anorexia and weight loss.
- General malaise.

Stroke is also seen as a presenting complaint, or myalgia and arthralgia. Important information to obtain from the patient for clues about the causative organism includes:

- A detailed history of any dental work, operations or infections.
- Any history of rheumatic fever.
- Any history of intravenous drug abuse.

Fig. 23.3 Conditions predisposing to infective endocarditis

Acquired valvular heart disease (stenosis or regurgitation)
Valve replacement
Congenital heart disease (excluding isolated ASD or fully repaired VSD or PDA)
Previous infective endocarditis
Hypertrophic cardiomyopathy

It is also important to find out about any drug allergies, because long-term intravenous antibiotics may be needed.

Examination

A thorough examination is vital, because it is sometimes possible to make the diagnosis on examination alone, which allows therapy to be started promptly. Failure to make the diagnosis early can have disastrous consequences, because it is not uncommon to see this disease causing rapid valve destruction and cardiogenic shock.

A full examination is required because the signs occur in all systems (Fig. 23.4).

The following signs are characteristic of infective endocarditis:

- A murmur – the heart murmur is usually that of an incompetent valve because the infection often prevents the valve from closing due to either perforation of the valve leaflets or vegetations and adhesions impeding valve movement. It is important to perform daily cardiac auscultation because the murmur may change due to progressive valve damage; this warns of imminent valve failure and an urgent echocardiogram is then necessary to evaluate the degree of valvular incompetence. The murmur of mitral regurgitation may become louder as the regurgitation gets worse. The murmur of aortic regurgitation also gets louder.
- Splenomegaly – a common finding especially if the history is long.

Fig. 23.4 Important clinical findings in patients who have infective endocarditis.

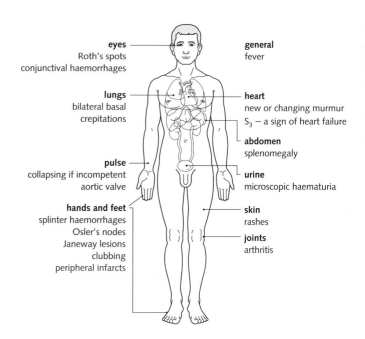

eyes
Roth's spots
conjunctival haemorrhages

general
fever

lungs
bilateral basal
crepitations

heart
new or changing murmur
S_3 – a sign of heart failure

abdomen
splenomegaly

pulse
collapsing if incompetent
aortic valve

urine
microscopic haematuria

hands and feet
splinter haemorrhages
Osler's nodes
Janeway lesions
clubbing
peripheral infarcts

skin
rashes

joints
arthritis

- Clubbing – develops after a few weeks of infective endocarditis. Other causes of clubbing include cyanotic congenital heart disease, suppurative lung disease, squamous cell carcinoma of the lung and inflammatory bowel disease.
- Splinter haemorrhages – more than four is pathological (remember that the most common cause of these is trauma).
- Osler nodes and Janeway lesions – represent peripheral emboli (possibly septic).
- Roth spots – retinal haemorrhages with a pale centre.
- Evidence of congestive cardiac failure.
- Microscopic haematuria on urine dipstick – always ask to dipstick the urine if you suspect infective endocarditis. This is a very sensitive test and easily carried out.
- Also peripheral emboli, features of a cerebrovascular event, inflamed joints.

INVESTIGATION OF A PATIENT WHO HAS INFECTIVE ENDOCARDITIS

Blood tests

Blood cultures

These are the most important investigations. Note the plural has been used because at least three sets of cultures must be performed. If possible, at least three sets should be taken at least 1 h apart *before* commencing antibiotic therapy. (If the patient is very ill and ther is a high index of suspicion of infective endocarditi it is appropriate to start antibiotics after the first se has been obtained, otherwise it is preferable to isolat the causative organism first.)

Positive blood cultures are usually obtained in a least 95% cases of bacterial endocarditis if taken befor antibiotic therapy. This allows therapy to be specificall directed according to the sensitivity of the organism.

Full blood count

Anaemia of chronic disease is common in patients wh have less acute presentations. Other findings ca include:

- Leucocytosis – may be seen as a sign of inflamma tion (usually a neutrophilia).
- Thrombocytopenia – may be an indication of dis seminated intravascular coagulopathy.
- Thrombophilia – may be seen as part of the acut phase response.

Erythrocyte sedimentation rate and C-reactive protein

These are elevated as signs of inflammation. They are valuable markers of disease activity and repeated measurements every few days provide information on the patient's response to treatment.

Renal function

This may be impaired due to infarction or immune complex-mediated glomerulonephritis. This also needs repeating every few days during treatment as both aminoglycoside antibiotics and disease progression may cause renal impairment.

Liver function tests

These may be deranged due to septic microemboli.

Electrocardiography

ECGs should be taken daily due to the high risk of developing heart block in patients with infective endocarditis affecting the aortic root.

Urinanalysis

As well as the bedside urine dipstick, formal urine microscopy should be performed to look for casts as seen in glomerulonephritis.

Chest radiography

This may be clear or may show signs of pulmonary oedema.

Echocardiography

Transthoracic echocardiography will reveal any valve incompetence and may also identify vegetations on the valve. This test is not very sensitive and cannot be used to exclude small vegetations.

Transoesophageal echocardiography is over 90% sensitive in diagnosing vegetations.

Remember that echocardiography is not a diagnostic test in infective endocarditis. It may help confirm the diagnosis and give information about the severity of the valve damage, but blood cultures are the only specific diagnostic test of infective endocarditis.

MANAGEMENT OF INFECTIVE ENDOCARDITIS

There are two main aims in the management of infective endocarditis:

1. To treat the infection effectively with appropriate antibiotics with the minimum of drug-related complications.

2. To diagnose and treat complications of the endocarditis (i.e. congestive cardiac failure, severe valve incompetence, peripheral abscesses, renal failure, etc.).

Antibiotic therapy

If infective endocarditis is suspected and the patient is unwell, antibiotic therapy is started as soon as the blood cultures have been taken. The choice of agent can then be modified once the organism is known. Intravenous therapy is used initially in all cases. This may be via the central or peripheral route.

Choice of antibiotic regimen

A microbiologist is the best person to decide what the antibiotic regimen should be and all cases of infective endocarditis should be reported to the microbiologist as soon as possible, even if blood cultures are negative.

Duration of antibiotic therapy

This depends upon the organism and the clinical response to treatment. Most bacterial infections require at least 6 weeks of intravenous therapy, although some centres change to oral therapy after 2 weeks if the response is good. The most important thing to remember is that the patient must be closely monitored after changing to oral therapy and after stopping therapy. If there is any evidence of recurrent disease activity intravenous therapy should be recommenced.

Monitoring antibiotic therapy

Blood should be taken for:
- Antibiotic levels (gentamicin, vancomycin).
- To calculate the minimum inhibitory concentration (MIC) – the MIC gives an indication of the sensitivity of the organism to the antibiotics used. If it is not satisfactory another antimicrobial may be added.

In addition to antibiotic therapy the source of infection should be sought – the patient needs a thorough dental examination and any infected teeth removed because this is a common cause of recurrent bacteraemia.

COMPLICATIONS OF INFECTIVE ENDOCARDITIS

The following complications may occur:
- Congestive cardiac failure – the use of diuretics and ACE inhibitors may be necessary. If cardiac failure remains severe due to profound valvular incompetence, surgery to replace the valve is required.

- Thromboembolic complications – the use of anticoagulants is controversial; however, anticoagulation is used for patients who have thrombotic phenomena, such as pulmonary embolus or deep venous thrombosis. Patients who have metal prosthetic valves should remain on anticoagulation, although it is often preferable to change from warfarin to heparin as this is more easily reversed. Patients who have cerebral or peripheral arterial emboli are not anticoagulated, because there is a risk of haemorrhage into the infarct.

MONITORING OF PATIENTS WHO HAVE INFECTIVE ENDOCARDITIS

This should include:

- Daily examination – this is the most important. Look for worsening valvular incompetence, cardiac failure, new splinter haemorrhages, Roth spots, Osler nodes and so on, all of which are suggestive of ongoing active disease.
- Temperature chart – an increase in temperature after the patient has been apyrexial for some time can represent reactivation of the infection and blood cultures should be sent immediately.
- Daily urine dipstick for microscopic haematuria – this is representative of disease activity
- Twice-weekly blood tests for full blood count, renal function, erythrocyte sedimentation rate, C-reactive protein and liver function.

Fig. 23.5 Indications for valve replacement in infective endocarditis.

Heart failure
Uncontrolled infection
Prevention of embolism from large vegetations

- Daily ECG – look for lengthening of the PR interval. If an abscess develops around the aortic root or in the septum this affects the atrioventricular node and may lead to complete heart block.
- Weekly echocardiography – to assess vegetation size if they are visible, but more importantly to assess left-ventricular function and the severity of the valve incompetence. However, a repeat echocardiogram should be considered sooner if the patient's condition deteriorates.

Operative intervention in active infective endocarditis carries a high mortality rate and marked morbidity. Indications for replacement of the infected valve are listed in Fig. 23.5. The patient should complete a full course of intravenous antibiotic treatment (at least 6 weeks) postoperatively.

HINTS AND TIPS

Close monitoring of patients who have infective endocarditis is crucial, because any deterioration can lead to catastrophic valve incompetence if missed.

Further reading

Habib, G., Hoen, B., Tornos, P., et al., 2009. Guidelines on the prevention, diagnosis, and treatment of infective endocarditis (new version 2009): the Task Force on the Prevention, Diagnosis, and Treatment of Infective Endocarditis of the European Society of Cardiology (ESC). Endorsed by the European Society of Clinical Microbiology and Infectious Disease (ESCMID) and the International Society of Chemotherapy ISC) for Infection and Cancer. Eu Heart J. 30 (19), 2369–2413.

National Institute for Health and Clinical Excellence (NICE), 2008. Clinical guideline 64. Prophylaxis against infective endocarditis. http://www.nice.org.uk/CG064.

Hypertension 24

Objectives

By the end of this chapter you should:
- Know the criteria for the diagnosis of hypertension.
- Be able to describe the non-pharmacological measures to treat hypertension.
- Be able to list the major drug classes used in treatment of hypertension and outline their adverse effects.
- Be able to recognize phaeochromocytoma as a cause of hypertension and understand the investigations and management steps involved.

Hypertension is a major risk factor for cerebrovascular disease, myocardial infarction (MI), cardiac failure, peripheral vascular disease and renal failure. To reduce the risk of these it is important to diagnose and adequately treat hypertensive patients.

DEFINITION OF HYPERTENSION

Normal blood pressure increases with age and varies throughout the day according to factors such as stress and exertion. There is also an underlying diurnal variation, with the lowest blood pressure occurring at around 4 a.m.

The definition of hypertension, therefore, is that level of blood pressure associated with an increased risk of complications. This equates to a level above 140/90 mmHg in adults. Revise the categories of hypertension (stage 1, stage 2, severe – see Ch. 11). In some patients, diastolic blood pressure may be normal whilst systolic blood pressure is raised. This is known as isolated systolic hypertension (ISH).

CAUSES OF HYPERTENSION

Over 95% cases of hypertension are idiopathic and this is termed primary hypertension.

Secondary causes of hypertension are important to exclude because they may be curable and are more common than previously thought.

CLINICAL FEATURES OF HYPERTENSION

These are described in Ch. 11 and will not be repeated word for word here. The following is a summary of the clinical features of hypertension.

History

Most patients are entirely asymptomatic, but the presenting complaint may be headache, dizziness, fainting or visual disturbance.

HINTS AND TIPS

There is no correlation between symptoms and severity of hypertension in the vast majority of patients.

When checking the past medical history, ask about other risk factors for ischaemic heart disease such as:
- Smoking.
- Diabetes mellitus.
- Hypercholesterolaemia.
- Family history of heart disease.

Also be aware of the following:
- Evidence of cerebrovascular disease (cerebrovascular accident) or MI in the past.
- If the patient is young think about possible secondary causes (e.g. recurrent urinary tract infections).

When checking the drug history, ask about all current medications including proprietary analgesics and the oral contraceptive pill.

With regard to the family history:
- Ask about family history of hypertension.
- If the patient is young, think about possible secondary causes (e.g. family history of renal problems or cerebrovascular disease in polycystic kidney disease).

An assessment of social history should take into account:
- Smoking.
- Alcohol intake.
- Level of stress at work.
- Likelihood of non-compliance with medication.

Examination

Hypertension is diagnosed after a clinic blood pressure of $\geq 140/90$ mmHg is confirmed by ABPM or HBPM (see Ch. 11). Severe hypertension (>180/110 mmHg) diagnosed in clinic does not require ABPM or HBPM for confirmation.

Fig. 24.1 shows the important features to note on examination of a patient who has hypertension. Remember to look for signs of end-organ damage and signs of possible underlying causes of secondary hypertension.

The following are examples of end-organ damage secondary to hypertension:

- Ischaemic heart disease.
- Cardiac failure.
- Left-ventricular hypertrophy.
- Cerebrovascular disease.
- Peripheral vascular disease.
- Renal impairment.
- Hypertensive retinopathy.

INVESTIGATION OF A PATIENT WHO HAS HYPERTENSION

Investigations, as listed in Fig. 24.2, should be performed at presentation and repeated on a yearly basis as a measure of how well the hypertension is responding to treatment. For example, left-ventricular hypertrophy should gradually regress once hypertension has been successfully controlled.

These investigations are also directed towards looking for evidence of end-organ damage and possible causes of secondary hypertension.

If the patient is at high risk of having secondary hypertension then further investigations are indicated. The criteria for excluding secondary hypertension are as follows:

- Under 35 years of age.
- Symptoms and signs of malignant (also known as accelerated or severe) hypertension (i.e. blood pressure >180/110 mmHg, grade 3 or 4 hypertensive retinopathy or cardiac failure at a young age).
- Symptoms of an underlying cause (e.g. phaeochromocytoma – sweating, dizzy spells, tachycardia).
- Signs of an underlying cause (e.g. differential blood pressure in both arms, hyperkalaemia or Cushingoid appearance).

INVESTIGATION OF SECONDARY HYPERTENSION

All patients should have the investigations listed in Fig. 24.2. For those patients at high risk of secondary hypertension the following screening tests should exclude most causative conditions:

- 24-h urine protein and creatinine clearance to exclude marked renal pathology.
- 24-h urine catecholamines or vanillylmandelic acid (VMA) and 5-hydroxy indole acetic acid

Fig. 24.1 Important clinical findings in hypertensive patients. Look for signs of end-organ damage and signs of the underlying cause of hypertension. It is essential to keep an open mind. This illustration is only a guide and there are many other possible findings (e.g. signs of thyroid disease or Cushing disease). CCF, congestive cardiac failure; JVP, jugular venous pressure.

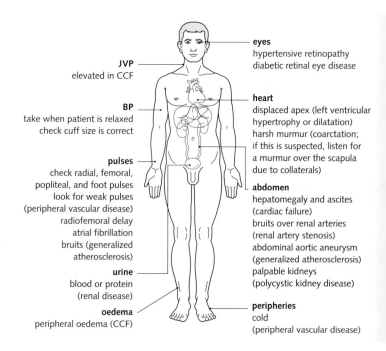

Fig. 24.2 Investigations for hypertension

Blood tests	Renal function and electrolytes, blood lipid profile, blood glucose
ECG	Can provide evidence of LVH (i.e. R wave in V5 > 25 mm, deep S wave in V2 or R wave in V5 added to S wave in V2 > 35 mm, R wave in AVL > 11 mm, lateral T wave inversion)
Echocardiogram	LVH, usually concentric in nature (i.e. left ventricular wall thickness > 1.1 cm); performed routinely at some centres because LVH is thought to be a valuable indicator of prognosis
Urine dipstick	Microscopic haematoma or proteinuria

LVH, left ventricular hypertrophy.

(5HIAA) to exclude phaeochromocytoma and carcinoid syndrome, respectively (three sets of urinary catecholamines should be tested).
- 24-h urine cortisol excretion and dexamethasone suppression test to exclude Cushing disease.
- Renal ultrasound to reveal any overt structural abnormality (e.g. phaeochromocytoma, small kidney or polycystic kidneys).
- CT or MR angiogram to exclude renal artery stenosis. The kidney in renal artery stenosis depends heavily upon increased levels of angiotensin II to provide adequate blood pressure for renal perfusion. This is abruptly stopped by the administration of an ACE inhibitor and the reduction in renal blood flow that results can be detected by the scan.

MANAGEMENT OF HYPERTENSION

Importance of treating hypertension

Hypertension is a common disorder that, if left untreated, damages a number of systems. Complications of hypertension include:
- Cardiac failure.
- Renal failure.
- Stroke.
- Ischaemic heart disease.
- Peripheral vascular disease.

This end-organ damage can largely be prevented by adequate blood pressure control.

However, hypertension is difficult to diagnose because patients are often asymptomatic. Treatment is, therefore, difficult because patients are less likely to comply with drug regimens or follow-up visits to their doctor.

> **COMMUNICATION**
>
> Explain to patients that hypertension can be well treated with medications, but, untreated, hypertension can have serious complications. They may not experience symptoms even if their blood pressure is elevated, so it is important to continue with their treatment even if they feel well.

Non-pharmacological management

This is important because in patients who have mild hypertension it may result in a decrease in blood pressure sufficient to avoid the need for drug therapy. The following non-pharmacological treatments are recognized:
- Weight loss.
- Reduction in alcohol consumption (currently, the maximum recommended weekly intakes are 21 units for men and 14 units for women).
- Reduction in salt intake.
- Diet low in fat with five portions of fruit and vegetables a day.
- Regular exercise.

All other risk factors for ischaemic heart disease should be sought and treated in these patients as a matter of routine.

Pharmacological management

There are many effective agents (Fig. 24.3). The main categories are as follows:
- Diuretics.
- Antiadrenergic agents – β-blockers (β-adrenoceptor antagonists), α-blockers (α-adrenoceptor antagonists) and centrally acting agents.
- Calcium channel blockers.
- ACE inhibitors and angiotensin II receptor blockers.
- Vasodilators.

> **HINTS AND TIPS**
>
> The use of β-blockers alone for phaeochromocytoma can result in severe hypertension due to the unopposed action of noradrenaline on the α-receptors.

Fig. 24.3 Overview of drugs used to treat hypertension

Class of drug	Examples	Indications	Precautions/ contraindications	Adverse effects
Diuretics	Thiazides (e.g. bendroflumethiazide (bendrofluazide)) loop diuretics (e.g. furosemide (frusemide))	Mild hypertension or in conjunction with other agents for more severe hypertension	Thiazides exacerbate diabetes mellitus; all diuretics should be avoided in patients who have gout if possible	Hypokalaemia, dehydration, exacerbation of renal impairment, gout
Antiadrenergic agents	β-Blockers (e.g. atenolol, propranolol, metoprolol)	Moderate to severe hypertension (note that they are antianginal)	Asthma, cardiac failure, severe peripheral vascular disease	Postural hypotension, bronchospasm, fatigue, impotence, cold extremities
	α-Blockers (e.g. prazosin, doxazosin)	Moderate to severe hypertension	Postural hypotension	
	Centrally acting agents (e.g. methyldopa)	Moderate hypertension (safe during pregnancy)	Postural hypotension, galactorrhoea, gynaecomastia, haemolytic anaemia	
Calcium channel blockers	Nifedipine, amlodipine	Moderate hypertension*	Cardiac failure, heart block (second- or third-degree) – these are contraindications mainly for verapamil and diltiazem	Postural hypotension, headache, flushing, ankle oedema
ACE inhibitors	Captopril, enalapril, lisinopril	Moderate to severe hypertension, especially with cardiac failure	Renal artery stenosis, pregnancy	Postural hypotension, dry cough, loss of taste, renal failure, hyperkalaemia
Angiotensin-II receptor blockers	Losartan, valsartan	Moderate to severe hypertension, especially with cardiac failure	Renal artery stenosis, pregnancy	Postural hypotension, renal failure, hyperkalaemia
Direct renin inhibitors	Alskiren	No specific indication currently	Pregnancy, breastfeeding, renal artery stenosis	Postural hypotension, diarrhoea
Vasodilators	Hydralazine	Moderate to severe hypertension	SLE	Postural hypotension, headache, lupus-like syndrome
	Sodium nitroprusside (as an intravenous infusion)	Malignant hypertension		Weakness, cyanide toxicity if drug not protected from light

ACE, angiotensin-converting enzyme; SLE, systemic lupus erythematosus.
*Diltiazem and verapamil are less commonly used for hypertension because they have a more pronounced action on heart muscle and conductive tissue, respectively. Diltiazem is used predominantly for angina; verapamil for its antiarrythmic effects.

These agents may be used alone or in combination to achieve good blood-pressure control. Remember that patient compliance is likely to be better if:

- The disease and its complications have been fully explained.
- The treatment options have been discussed with the patient.
- The drugs used have been explained and common side effects discussed.
- Once-daily preparations are used.
- Polypharmacy is avoided (i.e. the drug regimen is kept as simple as possible by using a higher dose of a single agent before adding another drug).

Recommended treatment of hypertension

The 2011 NICE/British Hypertension Society guidelines for the treatment of hypertension suggest:

- Using non-pharmacological measures in all hypertensive and borderline hypertensive people.
- Initiating antihypertensive drug treatment in people with severe hypertension, stage 2 hypertension, or stage 1 hypertension in patients less than 80 years old who have target organ damage, diabetes, cardiovascular disease, renal disease, or a 10-year cardiovascular risk score of ≥20% (see below).
- Optimal blood pressure treatment targets are systolic blood pressure <140/90 mmHg in patients <80 years, or <150/90 mmHg in patients ≥80 years.

The choice of drug(s) to treat newly diagnosed hypertension is suggested in the NICE/BHS guidelines, and varies according to the patient's age and ethnicity, as well as co-existing disease.

These guidelines are changing constantly (for most up-to-date guidelines please refer to www.bhsoc.org) and clinical practice varies from hospital to hospital.

Follow-up of patients who have hypertension

This is every bit as important as the initial treatment. Patients should be seen on a yearly basis. The follow-up should involve:

- Examination to look for evidence of end-organ damage – especially cardiovascular system and retinas.
- Urine dipstick.
- ECG.
- Blood tests for urea, creatinine and electrolytes – these may be deranged due to renal damage secondary to hypertension or to the drug therapy or both.
- Echocardiography if the patient had left-ventricular hypertrophy at diagnosis – it is appropriate to repeat the echocardiography until the hypertrophy has resolved.
- A screen of risk factors for ischaemic heart disease (i.e. blood lipid profile and blood glucose) and lifestyle advice if necessary.

Cardiovascular risk

It is possible to estimate the risk of a patient developing cardiovascular disease (MI, stroke/transient ischaemic attack – TIA, angina and death), based on their age, sex, smoking habit, lipid levels (HDL and LDL) and blood pressure. The risk is represented as either <10%, 10–20% or >20% over a 10 year period. Cardiovascular risk has important implications for management including primary and secondary prevention. Risk calculators can be found on the internet or at the back of the British National Formulary (BNF).

PHAEOCHROMOCYTOMA

Phaeochromocytoma is a rare tumour of the chromaffin cells – 90% occur within the adrenal medulla and 10% are extramedullary; 10% are malignant and 10% are bilateral.

Clinical features

Paroxysmal catecholamine secretion results in a variety of signs and symptoms including:

- Hypertension.
- Headaches.
- Sweating attacks.
- Postural hypotension.
- Acute pulmonary oedema.

These symptoms are characteristically paroxysmal, although patients might have persistent hypertension.

Investigations

Investigations include:

- ECG-ST elevation or T wave inversion may be seen transiently.
- Echocardiography – shows left-ventricular hypertrophy or dilated cardiomyopathy
- 24-h urinary catecholamines or VMA – these are raised (at least three measurements should be taken because of the intermittent nature of the catecholamine excretion).
- Computed tomography of the adrenals or metaiodobenzylguanidine (MIBG) scan if the tumour is extra-adrenal.
- Selective venous sampling.

Management

Careful blood pressure control is vital before any invasive procedure as follows:

- Initially, α-blocker is used (phenoxybenzamine, an irreversible α-blocker, is commonly used).
- β-Blockade may then be added if required – the use of β-blockers alone may result in severe hypertension due to the unopposed action of noradrenaline on the α-receptors. The tumour is then removed surgically.

Further reading

National Institute for Health and Clinical Excellence (NICE)/British Hypertension Society (BHS) guidelines, 2011. Hypertension: Clinical management of primary hypertension in adults. www.nice.org.uk/CG127.

Congenital heart disease 25

Objectives

By the end of this chapter you should:
- Be able to list the congenital heart diseases that are associated with cyanosis.
- Be able to outline the different types of atrial septal defect.
- Be able to recognize the clinical signs of a ventricular septal defect.
- Be able to describe the pathophysiological process that occurs if a significant intracardiac shunt is untreated.
- Be able to define the four main features of tetralogy of Fallot.

DEFINITION OF CONGENITAL HEART DISEASE

Congenital heart disease refers to cardiac lesions present from birth.

CAUSES OF CONGENITAL HEART DISEASE

Many factors both genetic and environmental affect cardiac development in the uterus; therefore, not surprisingly, no single cause can explain all cases (Fig. 25.1). Causes include:

- Maternal rubella – in addition to cataracts, deafness and microcephaly, this can cause patent ductus arteriosus (PDA) and pulmonary stenosis.
- Fetal alcohol syndrome – associated with cardiac defects (as well as microcephaly, micrognathia, microphthalmia and growth retardation).
- Maternal systemic lupus erythematosus – associated with fetal complete heart block (due to transplacental passage of anti-Ro antibodies).

There are many genetic associations with congenital heart disease, including:

- Trisomy 21 – endocardial cushion defects, atrial septal defect (ASD), ventricular septal defect (VSD) and tetralogy of Fallot.
- Turner syndrome (XO) – coarctation of the aorta.
- Marfan syndrome – aortic dilatation and aortic and mitral regurgitation.
- Kartagener syndrome – dextrocardia and cilia dysmotility.

COMPLICATIONS OF CONGENITAL HEART DISEASE

Before discussing individual lesions it is important to have a grasp of the significance of congenital heart disease. Lesions have effects depending upon their size and location. These include:

- Central cyanosis – defined as the presence of more than 5 g/dL of reduced haemoglobin in arterial blood. Central cyanosis can be caused by congenital heart disease due to shunting of venous blood straight into the arterial circulation bypassing the lungs. This type of cyanosis does not, therefore, respond to increasing the concentration of inspired oxygen.
- Congestive cardiac failure – this occurs due to the inability of the heart to maintain sufficient tissue perfusion as a result of the cardiac lesion. This may occur in infancy (e.g. due to a large VSD or transposition of the great arteries), or in adulthood in less severe conditions.
- Pulmonary hypertension – this develops over time as a result of an abnormal increase in pulmonary blood flow due to a left-to-right shunt (e.g. ASD, VSD, PDA). This increased flow results in changes to the pulmonary vessels with smooth muscle hypertrophy and obliterative changes. The pulmonary vascular resistance increases causing pulmonary hypertension. Eventually pulmonary pressure exceeds systemic pressure causing reversal of the shunt, and this results in a syndrome of cyanotic heart disease called Eisenmenger syndrome.
- Infective endocarditis – congenital heart disease may result in lesions prone to bacterial colonization.

Ventricular septal defect (VSD)
Atrial septal defect (ASD)
Patent ductus arteriosus (PDA)
Pulmonary stenosis – causes cyanosis if severe
Coarctation of the aorta
Aortic stenosis
Tetralogy of Fallot – causes cyanosis
Transposition of the great arteries – causes cyanosis
Other causes of cyanotic congenital heart disease –
pulmonary atresia, hypoplastic left heart, severe
Ebstein anomaly with ASD

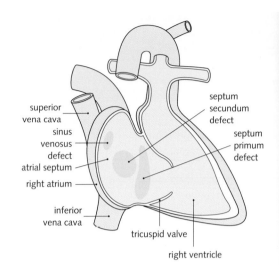

Fig. 25.2   Location of the three main types of atrial septal defect. The heart is viewed from the right side. The right atria and ventricular walls have been omitted to reveal the septum.

Appropriate antibiotic prophylaxis should be taken to prevent this.

- Sudden death – this may be due to arrhythmias (more common in these disorders) or outflow tract obstruction as seen in aortic stenosis.

HINTS AND TIPS

Notes on cyanosis:
- Central cyanosis is cyanosis of the tongue.
- Peripheral cyanosis is cyanosis of the peripheries (lips, feet, hands, etc.).
- Cyanosis caused by pulmonary disease or cardiac failure improves on increasing inspired oxygen.
- Cyanosis caused by a right-to-left shunt bypassing the lungs does not improve on increasing inspired oxygen.

ATRIAL SEPTAL DEFECT

Although a common cause of congenital heart disease, atrial septal defect (ASD) is often not diagnosed early because it can be difficult to detect clinically.

There are three main types of ASD based on the location of the defect in the atrial septum (Fig. 25.2):

1. Septum primum (also called ostium primum ASD) – this defect lies adjacent to the atrioventricular valves and these are often also abnormal and incompetent.
2. Septum secundum (also called ostium secundum ASD) – the most common form of ASD, it is mid-septal in location.
3. Sinus venosus ASD – this lies high in the septum and may be associated with anomalous pulmonary venous drainage (where one of the pulmonary veins drains into the right atrium instead of the left).

Clinical features

The magnitude of the left-to-right shunt depends upon the size of the defect and also the relative pressures on the left and right sides of the heart.

History

In early life patients are usually asymptomatic. In adult life, however, symptoms of dyspnoea, fatigue and recurrent chest infections occur. As time goes by the increased pulmonary blood flow results in pulmonary hypertension and eventually reversal of the shunt and Eisenmenger syndrome. Supraventricular arrhythmias may develop later.

Examination

The findings on examination of a patient who has an ASD (Fig. 25.3) depend upon the following factors:

- Size of the ASD.
- Presence or absence of pulmonary hypertension.
- Presence of shunt reversal.

The second heart sound is widely split because closure of the pulmonary valve is delayed due to increased pulmonary blood flow. The splitting is fixed in relation to respiration because the communication between the atria prevents the normal pressure differential between right and left sides that occurs during respiration. This is referred to as fixed splitting of the second heart sound.

The increased pulmonary blood flow causes a mid systolic pulmonary flow murmur.

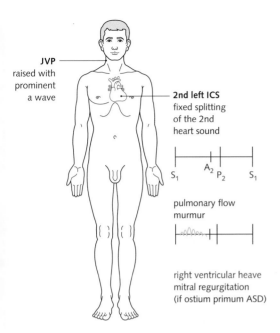

JVP
raised with
prominent
a wave

2nd left ICS
fixed splitting
of the 2nd
heart sound

S_1 A_2 P_2 S_1

pulmonary flow
murmur

right ventricular heave
mitral regurgitation
(if ostium primum ASD)

Fig. 25.3 Physical findings in all patients who have an atrial septal defect (ASD). If the ASD is large and there is pulmonary hypertension, check for loud P_2 at the second left intercostal space (ICS) and for a prominent right ventricular heave. If there is shunt reversal you will find clubbing, central cyanosis and signs of congestive cardiac failure (i.e. peripheral oedema, ascites and bilateral basal crepitations). A_2, aortic component of second heart sound; JVP, jugular venous pressure; P_2, pulmonary component of second heart sound; S_1, first heart sound.

HINTS AND TIPS

Eisenmenger syndrome can occur in any condition involving a left-to-right shunt. With worsening pulmonary hypertension the shunt eventually reverses (changes to right to left) causing blood to bypass the lungs and resulting in profound cyanosis that is not responsive to oxygen therapy. There is no treatment at this late stage.

If pulmonary hypertension has developed, there is reduction of the left-to-right shunt and the pulmonary flow murmur disappears; instead there is a loud pulmonary component to the second heart sound because the increased pressure causes the pulmonary valve to slam shut.

If Eisenmenger syndrome occurs the patient becomes centrally cyanosed and develops finger clubbing.

Investigation

Electrocardiography

Patients who have ostium secundum ASD usually have right axis deviation. Those who have an ostium primum defect have left axis deviation.

Chest radiography

The pulmonary artery appears dilated and its branches are prominent. The enlarged right atrium can be seen at the right heart border and the enlarged right ventricle causes rounding of the left heart border.

Echocardiography

The right side of the heart and the pulmonary artery are dilated. The ASD may be directly visualized and a jet of blood may be seen passing through it. Associated mitral or tricuspid valve incompetence may be seen.

Cardiac catheterization

This again reveals the ASD because the catheter can be passed across it. Serial oxygen saturation measurements are made at different levels from the superior vena cava through the atrium and the right ventricle into the pulmonary artery. At the level of the left-to-right shunt there will be a step-up increase of the oxygen saturation as blood from the left side enters the right. This measurement can be used to calculate the size of the shunt, which helps determine whether operative correction of the ASD is required.

Magnetic resonance imaging

This is increasingly used in assessment of patients with congenital heart disease. It offers excellent image quality and haemodynamic data and does not involve ionizing radiation.

Management

If there are signs of congestive cardiac failure, diuretics and angiotensin-converting enzyme inhibitors may be of benefit.

The primary aim in these patients is to diagnose the ASD early and evaluate its severity to be able to repair the defect before pulmonary hypertension occurs. Once the patient has developed pulmonary hypertension repair does not stop its deterioration. All ASDs with pulmonary to systemic flow ratios exceeding 1.5:1 should be repaired. Operative closure requires cardiopulmonary bypass and involves a median sternotomy scar.

A new technique has been developed where the ASD is closed percutaneously using a device with two deformable discs connected by a narrow waist. This is introduced via a cardiac catheter and involves only a venous puncture.

PATENT FORAMEN OVALE

Around 25% of the population have a patent foramen ovale (or PFO), which is a remnant of the fetal circulation that allows blood to bypass the lungs. In the remaining 75%, the foramen closes with the increase in left atrial pressure that occurs during the neonate's first breaths. If present, a PFO may allow blood to cross to the left atrium (shunt) at all times, or sometimes only during valsalva.

Stroke of unknown aetiology in a young patient with a PFO may be an indication to undergo percutaneous device closure to prevent further paradoxical emboli. It has also been suggested that PFO might be associated with migraine, though trials of closure have had mixed results.

VENTRICULAR SEPTAL DEFECT

This is the most common congenital cardiac abnormality.

The ventricular septum is made up of two main components:

1. The membranous septum – situated high in the septum and relatively small. This is the most common site for a VSD.
2. The muscular septum – this is lower and defects here may be multiple.

Clinical features

History

In the neonate, a small VSD will be asymptomatic but a large VSD will result in the development of left-ventricular failure. This occurs because in the neonate pulmonary pressures are very high and a right-to-left shunt occurs via the VSD; if this is very large the left ventricle cannot cope and fails. The signs of LVF in a neonate are as follows:

- Failure to thrive, feeding difficulties and sweating on feeding.
- Tachypnoea and intercostal recession.
- Hepatomegaly.

The adult who has a VSD may be asymptomatic or may present with dyspnoea due to pulmonary hypertension (which may develop over many years as a consequence of the left-to-right shunt) or Eisenmenger syndrome.

Examination

The findings on examination of a patient who has a VSD (Fig. 25.4) vary according to the following criteria:

- Size of the VSD – a small VSD causes a loud pansystolic murmur that radiates to the apex and axilla. A very large VSD causes a less loud pansystolic murmur, but may be associated with signs of left ventricular and right ventricular hypertrophy.
- Presence or absence of pulmonary hypertension.
- Presence of shunt reversal.

Investigation

Chest radiography

This may show an enlarged left ventricle with prominent pulmonary vascular markings. Pulmonary oedema may be seen in infants.

Echocardiography

This will show the VSD and its size and location, and can help to evaluate the effects on cardiac function.

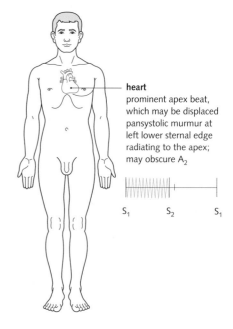

heart
prominent apex beat, which may be displaced pansystolic murmur at left lower sternal edge radiating to the apex; may obscure A$_2$

S_1 S_2 S_1

Fig. 25.4 Physical findings in all patients with a ventricular septal defect (VSD). If the VSD is large, the apex is displaced and pulmonary hypertension can develop. This results in a loud P$_2$ (pulmonary component of second heart sound) and right ventricular heave. Eisenmenger syndrome might also develop, with clubbing, cyanosis and disappearance of the pansystolic murmur. A$_2$, aortic component of second heart sound; S$_1$, first heart sound; S$_2$, second heart sound.

Magnetic resonance imaging

This can be used if further assessment is needed, or if the VSD is not well seen on echocardiography.

Management

Approximately 30% of cases close spontaneously, most of these by the time the child is 3 years of age. Some do not close until the child is 10 years old. Defects near the valve ring or near the outlet of the ventricle do not usually close.

Operative closure is the treatment of choice (if there is a significant left-to-right shunt) and is recommended for all lesions that have not undergone spontaneous closure. Some small lesions are managed conservatively; such a patient may be a case in finals and has a loud pansystolic murmur.

A VSD is a risk factor for infective endocarditis so the appropriate prophylactic measures should be taken.

PATENT DUCTUS ARTERIOSUS

In the fetus most of the output of the right ventricle bypasses the lungs via the ductus arteriosus. This vessel joins the pulmonary trunk (artery) to the descending aorta distal to the left subclavian artery (Fig. 25.5). The ductus arteriosus normally closes about 1 month after birth in full-term infants and takes longer to close in premature infants.

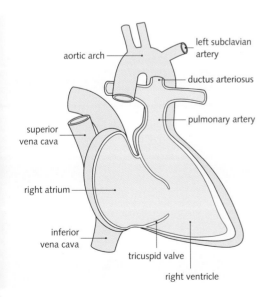

Fig. 25.5 Position of the ductus arteriosus.

Clinical features

The factors that determine the nature of the clinical features are the same as in VSD and ASD (i.e. the size of the defect, the size of the shunt, the presence of pulmonary hypertension, and the development of Eisenmenger syndrome).

A patent ductus arteriosus (PDA) is more likely in babies born at high altitude, probably due to the low atmospheric oxygen concentration. This lesion is also common in babies who have fetal rubella syndrome.

History

A small PDA is asymptomatic, but a large defect causes a large left-to-right shunt and may lead to left-ventricular failure (LVF) with pulmonary oedema causing failure to thrive and tachypnoea.

Adults who have undiagnosed PDA may develop pulmonary hypertension and present with dyspnoea.

Differential cyanosis occurs in adults with reversal of the shunt as the venous blood enters the systemic circulation below the subclavian arteries causing cyanosis and clubbing of the lower extremities whereas the arms remain pink.

Examination

The classic findings in a patient who has PDA (Fig. 25.6) are:

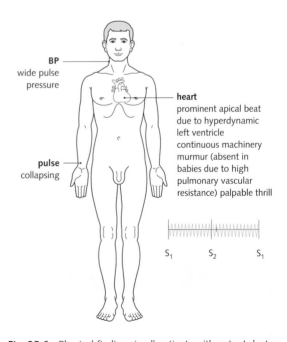

Fig. 25.6 Physical findings in all patients with patent ductus arteriosus (PDA). Patients with a large PDA have a loud pulmonary component of the second heart sound (P_2) due to pulmonary hypertension and the murmur is soft or absent. In those who have Eisenmenger syndrome there is differential cyanosis and the toes are clubbed.

- Collapsing high-volume pulses – this is due to the effect of the run-off of blood back down the ductus.
- A loud continuous machinery murmur heard in the second left intercostal space.
- A palpable thrill in the same place.

Management

The management of PDA involves two stages:

1. Pharmacological closure in neonates – indomethacin may induce closure if given early (by inhibiting prostacyclin production).
2. Operative closure of the PDA – this can be performed as an open procedure where the PDA is ligated or divided. Alternatively a percutaneous approach can be performed with introduction of an occluding device via a cardiac catheter. Antibiotic prophylaxis is required for all patients before operative correction because PDA is a risk factor for infective endocarditis.

COARCTATION OF THE AORTA

In this condition there is a congenital narrowing of the aorta, usually beyond the left subclavian artery. There are two main types:

1. Infantile type – this presents soon after birth with heart failure.
2. Adult type – the obstruction develops more gradually and presents in early adulthood. This type is associated with a high incidence of bicuspid aortic valve.

An adaptive response to the coarctation develops in those patients who do not present in infancy. This involves the development of collateral blood vessels, which divert blood from the proximal aorta to other peripheral arteries bypassing the obstruction. These collaterals are seen around the scapula as tortuous vessels that can sometimes be palpated and as prominent posterior intercostal arteries that cause rib notching visible on chest radiography. These collaterals take some years to develop and are rarely seen before 6 years of age.

Clinical features

History

Infants may present with failure to thrive and tachypnoea secondary to LVF. Alternatively coarctation may present as rapid severe cardiac failure with the infant in extremis.

Adults whose condition is not diagnosed in childhood may present with:

- Hypertension diagnosed at routine medical testing.

- Symptoms of leg claudication.
- Left ventricular failure.
- Subarachnoid haemorrhage from associated berry aneurysm.
- Angina pectoris due to premature heart disease.

Examination

Careful examination of these patients is vital because the diagnosis must not be missed. The physical findings in patients who have coarctation of the aorta are shown in Fig. 25.7. Check for:

- Blood pressure – it is always important to take blood pressure in both arms whenever performing the cardiovascular examination. Aortic dissection and coarctation where the obstruction is proximal to the left subclavian artery both cause a pressure differential between the arms. The blood pressure in the legs is also lower than in the arms.
- Radiofemoral delay and weak leg pulses – it is important to always look for radiofemoral delay because it is diagnostic of this condition.
- A heaving displaced apex beat due to left-ventricular hypertrophy.
- Murmurs – the coarctation may cause a systolic murmur (or a continuous murmur if the narrowing is very tight). This is located below the left clavicle. The collaterals cause an ejection systolic murmur

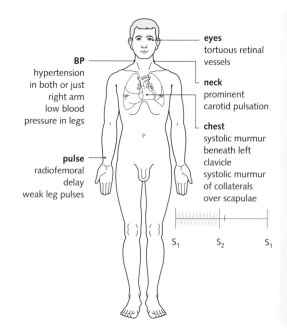

Fig. 25.7 Physical findings in patients with coarctation of the aorta. If the coarctation is severe there is a continuous murmur beneath the left clavicle and signs of left-ventricular failure (bilateral basal crepitations and audible third heart sound).

that can be heard over the scapulae. There may be a murmur associated with a bicuspid aortic valve, which is ejection systolic in nature and is located over the aortic area.

Investigation

Electrocardiography

This reveals left ventricular hypertrophy and often right bundle branch block.

Chest radiography

Rib notching might be seen in children over 6 years of age. (Because the first and second intercostal arteries arise from the vertebral arteries there is no rib notching on these ribs.) The aortic knuckle is absent and a double knuckle is seen (made up of the dilated subclavian artery above and the poststenotic dilatation of the aorta below).

Echocardiography

The coarctation and any associated lesion may be visualized, but imaging the thoracic aorta can be difficult. Coarctation is associated with a number of other congenital abnormalities (e.g. bicuspid aortic valve, transposition of the great arteries, septum primum ASD and mitral valve disease).

Cardiac catheterization

This localizes the coarctation accurately and also provides more information on associated lesions.

Magnetic resonance imaging

This provides very good three-dimensional reconstruction of the coarctation and is a useful tool prior to treatment in order to correct the coarctation.

Management

The most popular first-line treatment is an operation to relieve the obstruction. Without correction the prognosis is extremely poor and most patients die by 40 years of age. Balloon angioplasty has emerged as an alternative first-line treatment and avoids the need for sternotomy and cardiopulmonary bypass.

Coarctation may be complicated by infective endocarditis so antibiotic prophylaxis should be used.

OTHER LESIONS IN CONGENITAL HEART DISEASE

The conditions discussed above are those most likely to be seen in the examination situation. There are, however, a number of less common congenital cardiac abnormalities and these are discussed in Fig. 25.8.

Fig. 25.8 Uncommon causes of congenital cardiac abnormalities

Congenital cardiac defect	Anatomical abnormality	Clinical features	Treatment
Congenital aortic stenosis (acyanotic)	Stenosis may be valvular (most common), subvalvular, or supravalvular; note Williams syndrome – autosomal dominant condition with hypercalcaemia and supravalvular aortic stenosis	More common in males; child may be hypotensive, dyspnoeic and sweaty; increased incidence of angina and sudden death, especially on exertion; ejection systolic murmur heard in the second right ICS; may be signs of left ventricular strain (heaving apex) and failure (S_3, tachycardia and bilateral basal crackles)	Operative correction of the stenosis is the treatment of choice; in very small infants valvuloplasty is preferred in the first instance
Hypoplastic left heart (cyanotic)	Underdevelopment of all or part of the left side of the heart	Heart failure occurs in the first week of life; echocardiography is diagnostic	Surgical treatment is the only option and the mortality rate is extremely high
Pulmonary artery stenosis (cyanotic	Stenosis at one or many points along the pulmonary arteries; associated with tetralogy of Fallot in some cases;	If mild the patient may be asymptomatic with signs of RVH (i.e. left parasternal heave) and a pulmonary ejection	Diagnosis is confirmed by echocardiography; pulmonary angioplasty may provide a definitive cure; if there is a

Continued

Fig. 25.8 Uncommon causes of congenital cardiac abnormalities—cont'd

Congenital cardiac defect	Anatomical abnormality	Clinical features	Treatment
only if severe)	complication of maternal rubella infection	systolic murmur; if severe blood flows from the right side to the left through the foramen ovale and the child is cyanosed and dyspnoeic	recurrence or the lesion is not suitable for pulmonary angioplasty the obstruction may be removed surgically
Tetralogy of Fallot (cyanotic)	Four components: (1) VSD; (2) pulmonary stenosis; (3) overriding aorta; (4) RVH – blood flow therefore passes from the right ventricle through the VSD and through the aorta, resulting in a right-to-left shunt	Most children present with cyanosis within the first year of life; patients may have 'spells' of intense cyanosis from time to time due to a sudden increase in the right to left shunt – these attacks can be terminated by squatting, which increases systemic resistance and therefore reduces the right-to-left shunt	Total surgical correction is the treatment of first choice; in very young infants who have severe pulmonary atresia a palliative operation to reduce the pulmonary obstruction usually provides relief and a definitive procedure can be carried out later, when the risk is lower
Complete transposition of the great arteries (cyanotic)	The aorta arises from the right ventricle and the pulmonary artery arises from the left ventricle – the two circulations are therefore parallel; death is rapid if there is no communication between them so it is also common to see an ASD, VSD or PDA in these infants	Early cardiac failure and cyanosis are the most common presenting features; symptoms are less severe in those infants who have a large communication between the two sides; diagnosis is made by echocardiography and cardiac catheterization	Medical treatment of cardiac failure and the use of prostaglandin E1 to prevent postnatal closure of the ductus can help; operative procedures to create a large ASD might also help in the short term; surgical correction of the transposition is the definitive treatment

ASD, atrial septal defect; ICS, intercostal space; PDA, patent ductus arteriosus; RVH, right ventricular hypertrophy; S₃, third heart sound; VSD, ventricular septal defect.

NOTES ON PULMONARY HYPERTENSION AND EISENMENGER SYNDROME

Pulmonary hypertension

This causes mild dyspnoea when the shunt is from left to right and severe dyspnoea with the progression of pulmonary hypertension. Signs on examination include:

- Dominant a wave in the jugular venous pulse.
- Palpable and loud pulmonary component of second heart sound.
- Ejection systolic murmur in pulmonary area due to increased flow.
- Right ventricular heave.
- Tricuspid regurgitation if the right ventricle dilates.

Echocardiography allows assessment of the pulmonary pressures. This is vital because the shunt should be corrected before significant pulmonary hypertension develops.

Eisenmenger syndrome

This refers to the situation where a congenital cardiac abnormality initially causes acyanotic heart disease but cyanotic heart disease develops as a consequence of raised pulmonary pressure and shunt reversal.

These clinical features are also seen in patients who have cyanotic congenital heart disease (i.e. where the lesion results in a right-to-left shunt from the outset). Cyanosis develops when the level of reduced haemoglobin is over 5 g/dL.

Dyspnoea is usually relatively mild considering the profound hypoxia these patients have (oxygen saturations of 50% are not uncommon).

Complications include:

- Clubbing – develops in the fingers and toes.
- Polycythaemia and hyperviscosity – with resulting complications of stroke and venous thrombosis. Regular venesection or anticoagulation may be necessary.
- Cerebral abscesses – especially in children.

Paradoxical emboli – emboli from venous thrombosis may pass across the shunt and give rise to systemic infarcts.

Further reading

Brickner, M.E., Hillis, L.D., Lange, R.A., 2000. Congenital heart disease in adults. Part I N. Engl. J. Med. 342, 256–263, Part II N. Engl. J. Med. 342, 334–342.

Gatzoulis, M.A., Webb, G.D. (Eds.), 2003. Diagnosis and Management of Adult Congenital Heart Disease, first ed. Churchill Livingstone, Edinburgh.

Task Force of the ESC, 2003. Management of grown up congenital heart disease. Eur. Heart J. 24 (11), 1035–1084.

SELF-ASSESSMENT

Best of fives (BOFs)

1. A 65-year-old man is found to have right ventricular failure. Which clinical sign is most likely to be elicited on examination?
   A. Hypertension
   B. Hepatomegaly
   C. Cyanosis
   D. Bilateral basal crepitations
   E. Mid-diastolic murmur

2. A 35-year-old male presents with fever, clubbing, haematuria and a murmur. What is the most likely diagnosis?
   A. Infectious mononucleosis
   B. Rheumatic fever
   C. Infective endocarditis
   D. Haemolytic-uraemic syndrome
   E. Tetralogy of Fallot

3. A 28-year-old female presents to the emergency department following a faint. Which of the following is the most classic feature of cardiac syncope?
   A. Gradual onset
   B. Warning symptoms
   C. Rapid recovery
   D. Residual neurological deficit
   E. Precipitated by sudden turning of the head

4. A 45-year-old female is found to have a pansystolic murmur. Which of the following causes this?
   A. Mitral regurgitation
   B. Aortic regurgitation
   C. Tricuspid stenosis
   D. Atrial septal defect
   E. Aortic stenosis

5. Which of the following is correct regarding adenosine?
   A. It blocks conduction through the sinoatrial node
   B. It has a half-life of approximately 20 s
   C. It causes slowing of the ventricular rate in ventricular tachycardia
   D. It is administered initially as a dose of 12 mg
   E. It is contraindicated in asthma

6. Which of the following is correct regarding ventricular tachycardia?
   A. It is a narrow complex tachycardia
   B. It classically occurs at a rate of 300/s
   C. It should be treated with atropine
   D. It is a life-threatening condition
   E. It may be caused by hyponatraemia

7. An 81-year-old lady is prescribed digoxin. Which of the following is correct regarding digoxin?
   A. It acts to slow conduction of the sinoatrial node
   B. It is contraindicated in Wolff–Parkinson–White syndrome
   C. Its main route of excretion is by the liver
   D. It has a very short half-life
   E. Its effects are enhanced by hyperkalaemia

8. Which is correct regarding infective endocarditis?
   A. The most common causative organisms in Western countries are the Streptococcus viridians group
   B. Fungal infections are commonly seen on the aortic valve
   C. Enterococci are very rare
   D. Staphylococcus aureus is associated with a benign progressive disease
   E. A negative blood culture rules out infective endocarditis

9. A 74-year-old male is admitted with shortness of breath. On examination, crepitations are heard up to the mid-zones. A diagnosis of acute left ventricular failure is made. Which of the following treatments would not be used in the acute setting?
   A. β-Blockers
   B. Diuretics
   C. Oxygen
   D. Morphine
   E. Continuous positive airway pressure

10. A 42-year-old man is admitted with central crushing chest pain radiating to the left arm. Which of the following treatments would not be administered immediately?
    A. Morphine
    B. GTN spray
    C. Oxygen
    D. Thrombolysis
    E. Aspirin

11. A 28-year-old male is admitted with sharp chest pain that is eased by lying down. An ECG showed ST elevation in all leads. What is the most likely diagnosis?
    A. ST elevation myocardial infarction
    B. Pleurisy
    C. Pericarditis
    D. Pneumothorax
    E. Migraine

12. Which is correct with respect to Q waves on a 12-lead ECG?
    A. They are always pathological
    B. They suggest transmural myocardial infarction
    C. In leads I and aVL, they suggest old inferior myocardial infarction

D. They are due to depolarization current towards the lead
E. They are usually transient

13. Which clinical sign is most closely associated with pericarditis?
A. Janeway lesions
B. Clubbing
C. Pericardial rub
D. Conjunctival haemorrhages
E. Parasternal heave

14. Which ECG feature is most consistent with left ventricular hypertrophy?
A. Deep S wave in lead V6 = 25 mV
B. R wave in V5 and S wave in V2 = 35 mV
C. Broad QRS complexes = 12 mm
D. T wave inversion in leads II, III, aVF, V5 and V6
E. P pulmonale

15. Which clinical feature allows differentiation between atrial fibrillation and SVT?
A. Palpitations are less severe and frequent
B. Precipitation by excessive coffee drinking
C. Association with chest pain
D. Normal resting ECG
E. Irregularly irregular pulse

16. Which of the following is the most common cardiac malformation?
A. Atrial septal defect
B. Ventricular septal defect
C. Patent ductus arteriosus
D. Tetralogy of Fallot
E. Ebstein anomaly

17. A 63-year-old smoker presents with chest pain, nausea and sweating. His ECG shows ST elevation in leads II, III and aVF. Which coronary artery is most likely to be affected?
A. Left main stem
B. Left anterior descending
C. Circumflex
D. Right coronary artery
E. Obtuse marginal artery

18. What is the mode of inheritance of hypertrophic cardiomyopathy?
A. Autosomal dominant
B. Autosomal recessive
C. X-linked dominant
D. X-linked recessive
E. Non-mendelian

19. A keen medical student examining a patient on the ward palpates a tapping apex beat. What is the cause?
A. Left ventricular hypertrophy
B. Surgical emphysema
C. Mitral stenosis
D. Pericardial effusion
E. Left ventricular aneurysm

20. A worried mother takes her 6-month old baby to the GP as she is worried he looks blue. The GP suspects cyanotic congenital heart disease. Which of the following is not a feature of tetralogy of Fallot?
A. Mitral stenosis
B. Overriding aorta
C. Ventricular septal defect
D. Right ventricular hypertrophy
E. Pulmonary stenosis

21. A radiologist reports a chest X-ray as 'consistent with cardiac failure'. Which of the following radiological signs would you not expect to find?
A. Kerley B lines
B. Oligaemic lung fields
C. Cardiomegaly
D. Pleural effusion
E. Alveolar shadowing

22. A 72-year-old lady is found to have left bundle branch block on her ECG. Which of the following are true of the condition?
A. QRS complexes are wider than 0.2 s
B. Is characterised by M shaped complexes in V1
C. It may respond to atropine
D. New LBBB is an indication for thrombolysis
E. May cause syncope

23. A 78-year-old male presents with a fever. On auscultation of the heart a 'plop' is heard. What is the most likely diagnosis?
A. Infective endocarditis
B. Rheumatic fever
C. Mitral valve prolapse
D. Pericarditis
E. Atrial myxoma

24. A 45-year-old male presents acutely unwell to the emergency department. He is pale and sweaty. He complains of chest pain going through to between the shoulder blades. On checking his blood pressure he is found to have a difference of 50/30 mmHg between left and right arms. What is the most likely diagnosis?
A. Acute myocardial infarction
B. Pulmonary embolus
C. Aortic dissection
D. Acute aortic regurgitation
E. Tension pneumothorax

25. A 32-year-old basketball player is admitted with sudden onset shortness of breath. On examination there is air entry throughout the chest but there is an early diastolic murmur. What is the most likely cause?
A. Pneumothorax
B. Aortic regurgitation
C. Mitral stenosis
D. Pneumonia
E. Aortic dissection

26. A patient suffers a cardiac arrest whilst on the cardiology ward. Which of the following are true regarding advanced life support?
    A. Pulseless VT requires an immediate synchronised DC shock
    B. Adrenaline (1 μg) is administered every 3–5 min
    C. Atropine is given in cases of PEA/asystole
    D. VT/VF cardiac arrest has a better prognosis than asystole
    E. ALS and not BLS is the resuscitation protocol used in hospitals

27. Which of the following is not a reversible cause of cardiac arrest?
    A. Hypothermia
    B. Myocardial infarction
    C. Pulmonary embolus
    D. Pneumothorax
    E. Hypercapnia

28. A 40-year-old male collapses on the ward. He is not breathing and has no pulse. What is the most important initial action?
    A. Start CPR
    B. Check the airway
    C. Administer a precordial thump
    D. Attempt unsynchronised DC cardioversion
    E. Give high flow oxygen

29. Which of the following is true regarding tetralogy of Fallot?
    A. Pulmonary hypertension is a prominent feature
    B. Squatting helps ease symptoms
    C. It includes patent ductus arteriosus
    D. Requires antibiotic prophylaxis
    E. Cyanosis persists after total surgical correction

30. A 63-year-old male presents to the emergency department with chest pain one week after presenting with a STEMI. He complains of a sharp pain that is worse when sitting forward. ECG shows ST elevation in all leads. What is the most likely diagnosis?
    A. Dressler syndrome
    B. Pneumothorax
    C. Further ST elevation myocardial infarction
    D. Aortic dissection
    E. Unstable angina

31. Which of the following are true with regards to AV nodal disorders?
    A. An ischaemic cause is due to circumflex artery disease in 40% of cases
    B. They are usually reversible due to anterior myocardial infarction
    C. May be associated with aortic valve endocarditis
    D. May respond to adenosine
    E. Third-degree AV block is always associated with syncope

32. A 28-year-old IV drug user is thought to have endocarditis. Which of the following is a minor criterion for the diagnosis of infective endocarditis?
    A. Prolonged QRS duration
    B. Raised antistreptolysin titre
    C. Growth of Staphylococcus aureus in sputum culture
    D. Erythema multiforme
    E. Vegetations visualised on echocardiography

33. A 45-year-old woman is admitted with chest pain and ST elevation in all leads of her ECG, one week after a viral illness. What is the most appropriate treatment?
    A. Thrombolysis
    B. Primary percutaneous coronary intervention
    C. Aspirin 300 mg and clopidogrel 300 mg
    D. Paracetamol
    E. Ibuprofen

34. A 74-year-old man is prescribed a β-blocker after a non-ST elevation myocardial infarction. Which of the following is a recognised side effect?
    A. Flushing
    B. Ankle swelling
    C. Raynaud's phenomenon
    D. Renal impairment
    E. Tachycardia

35. A 74-year-old lady is admitted with fever and microscopic haematuria. She had a prosthetic aortic valve replacement 4 years ago. Which clinical sign is least likely to be found on examination?
    A. Roth spots
    B. Splenomegaly
    C. First-degree heart block
    D. Early diastolic murmur
    E. Pericardial rub

36. A 32-year-old male is found to have a blood pressure of 165/76 mmHg. He is thought to have secondary hypertension. Which of the following would not cause this?
    A. Cushing disease
    B. Addison disease
    C. Hypothyroidism
    D. Conn syndrome
    E. Phaeochromocytoma

37. Which of the following clinical features does not suggest end organ damage in hypertension?
    A. Dysarthria
    B. High creatinine
    C. Early diastolic murmur
    D. Cotton-wool spots
    E. Voltage criteria for LVH

38. A 62-year-old woman is reviewed in clinic. She is known to have previous rheumatic fever. Which of the following is a feature of the disease?
    A. It affects mitral and aortic valves only

B. It is caused by valve infection with group B streptococci
C. Results in cusp and commissural fusion
D. Requires antibiotic prophylaxis to prevent endocarditis
E. Is the most common cause of mitral regurgitation

39. A 67-year-old male is admitted in extremis to the emergency department. His ECG shows a broad complex tachycardia. The staff are unsure whether this represents VT or SVT with aberrancy. Which of the following features/treatments are correct?
A. Concordance is present in VT
B. Capture beats are present in SVT with aberrancy
C. Fusion beats are seen in SVT with aberrancy
D. Intravenous verapamil can help to differentiate between the two
E. If in doubt treat as SVT

40. A 68-year-old lady is admitted with a massive anterior ST elevation MI. There is no primary PCI immediately available. The decision is taken to thrombolyse her. Which of the following is a contraindication to thrombolysis?
A. A history of intracranial bleed
B. Diabetes mellitus
C. Blood pressure of 180/100 mmHg
D. Thrombolysis within the last 6 months
E. COPD

41. Which of the following are correct with respect to the character of the arterial pulse?
A. Slow rising pulse is a feature of aortic regurgitation
B. Collapsing pulse can be a feature of mitral regurgitation
C. Bisferiens pulse is associated with heart failure
D. Pulsus alternans is a feature of atrial fibrillation
E. Radiofemoral delay occurs in coarctation of the aorta

42. A 75-year-old woman complains of palpitations. The junior doctor reviewing her ECG reports that there are no P waves visible. Which of the following conditions is associated with this ECG finding?
A. Atrial flutter
B. Ventricular tachycardia
C. Third-degree atrioventricular block
D. Sick sinus syndrome
E. Atrial fibrillation

43. An 82-year-old male is found to have significant aortic stenosis. Which of the following is not a feature of this?
A. Sudden death
B. Dyspnoea
C. Syncope
D. Angina
E. Valve gradient of 35 mmHg

44. A 45-year-old woman is found to have mitral stenosis on echocardiography. Which of the following is a feature of the condition?

A. A displaced apex beat
B. Malar flush
C. A pansystolic murmur heard best at the apex
D. An early diastolic murmur best heard with the diaphragm of the stethoscope
E. An end-diastolic murmur best heard with the bell of the stethoscope

45. Which of the following drugs are not used to treat hypertension?
A. Atenolol
B. Doxazosin
C. Enalapril
D. Bendroflumethiazide
E. Nicorandil

46. A 63-year-old man is reviewed in the cardiology clinic. On examination he has a median sternotomy scar. Which of the following operations has he had?
A. Aortic valve replacement
B. Implantable cardiac defibrillator (ICD) insertion
C. Temporary pacemaker insertion
D. Mitral valvuloplasty
E. Closed mitral valvotomy

47. Which of the following does not suggest syncope of cardiac origin?
A. Ejection systolic murmur
B. History of exertional chest pain
C. History of long distance travel
D. Prolonged QT interval on ECG
E. History of heavy alcohol intake

48. A 55-year-old female is found to have a blood pressure of 198/100 mmHg on routine testing. Which of the following would not be a useful investigation?
A. 12-lead ECG
B. Transthoracic echocardiography
C. Urinary catecholamines
D. 24-h protein excretion
E. Abdominal X-ray

49. Eisenmenger syndrome may be associated with which of the following?
A. Left-to-right shunt
B. Anaemia
C. Paradoxical emboli
D. Splinter haemorrhages
E. Preserved systolic function

50. Which of the following is true regarding permanent pacemakers?
A. DDD pacing is a form of single-chamber pacing
B. DDD pacing is useful in atrial fibrillation
C. AAI pacing may be indicated in SA node disorder
D. Pacemaker syndrome may occur in patients with DDD pacing
E. The suffix R denotes rhythm responsiveness

51. A 52-year-old male is referred to a cardiologist with complaint of chest tightness on walking up slopes and

after meals. It subsides at rest. Which of the following would not form part of his assessment?
A. Full blood count
B. Exercise ECG
C. Stress echocardiography
D. Coronary angiography
E. Myocardial perfusion imaging

52. A 26-year-old male arrives in the emergency department complaining of palpitation. He has a heart rate of 180 beats/min and an ECG confirms supraventricular tachycardia. Which treatment method would be inappropriate in this situation?
A. Carotid sinus massage
B. Asking the patient to blow the plunger out of a 50-mL syringe
C. Ocular pressure
D. Intravenous adenosine
E. Intravenous verapamil

53. About a quarter of the population have a patent foramen ovale. Which of the following may be associated?
A. LBBB
B. Right axis deviation
C. Endocarditis
D. Migraine
E. Mitral prolapse

54. At a neonatal check, the paediatrician hears a loud systolic murmur at the left sternal edge. Which of the following is most likely to be the cause?
A. Hypertrophic cardiomyopathy
B. Large VSD
C. Congenital aortic stenosis
D. Acute mitral regurgitation
E. Small VSD

55. An elderly retired businessman is found wandering the streets near his house. His family report that his memory has been failing over months and a diagnosis of dementia is made. Which physical sign may point to the underlying cause?
A. Pulsatile uvula
B. Pansystolic murmur
C. Tumour 'plop'
D. Splinter haemorrhages
E. Peripheral cyanosis

56. Which of the following is true regarding Takotsubo cardiomyopathy?
A. It was first described in Japanese lobster fishermen
B. It carries a 30% mortality rate in the acute phase
C. It should be treated with fluid resuscitation
D. It is more common in young men
E. It may be misdiagnosed as NSTEMI

57. Which of the following does not cause Torsades de pointes?
A. Sotalol
B. Rapid ventricular pacing

C. Hypocalcaemia
D. Hypothermia
E. Metabolic acidosis

58. A 35-year-old woman with end-stage renal failure due to IgA nephropathy has missed two dialysis sessions. She attends the emergency department feeling unwell and is found to have a potassium level of 8.4 mmol/L. Which of the following is not a feature of hyperkalaemia on the ECG?
A. QRS widening
B. Small P waves
C. Tall tented T waves
D. Increased RR interval
E. Sine waves

59. A 28-year-old woman with familial DCM becomes pregnant. As planned, her ramipril was stopped several months before. Which of the following is not a known effect of ACE inhibitors on the developing fetus?
A. Polydactyly
B. VSD
C. Renal agenesis
D. Pyloric stenosis
E. Rhabdomyosarcoma

60. Which of the following statements is true of hypertrophic cardiomyopathy?
A. It does not present after the third decade
B. It may be treated with percutaneous myomectomy
C. The interventricular septum is larger than 15 mm (or 12 mm with a first-degree relative)
D. Disopyramide is contraindicated
E. Obstruction occurs in a minority of patients

61. Which of the following medications does not extend life in heart failure?
A. Furosemide
B. Digoxin
C. Spironolactone
D. Ramipril
E. Atenolol

62. Which of the following statements concerning coronary angiography is false?
A. The inferior surface of the heart is normally supplied by the right coronary artery
B. It carries a risk of death or serious complication of around 0.01%
C. The left anterior descending artery supplies the majority of the left ventricle
D. The SA node is normally supplied by the conus artery
E. The left and right coronary arteries may communicate distally

63. A 67-year-old man goes to his GP with exertional shortness of breath and chest tightness. Which of the following is not a feature of severe aortic stenosis?
A. Soft S2
B. Seagull murmur

C. Paradoxical splitting
D. Collapsing pulse
E. Narrow pulse pressure

64. Which of the following statements is true regarding mitral prolapse?
    A. Also known as murmur-click syndrome
    B. Affects 0.1% of the population
    C. More common in women
    D. Frequently leads to mitral regurgitation
    E. Typically presents in the elderly

65. A 42-year-old man is referred to a cardiologist with shortness of breath and an enlarged heart on chest X-ray. Which of the following would be least useful in his assessment?
    A. Alcohol history
    B. Iron studies
    C. Thyroid function tests
    D. Tuberculosis blood cultures
    E. Viral titres

66. A 25-year-old woman who is being investigated for exertional shortness of breath is found to have a pulmonary venous pressure of 48 mmHg on echocardiography. Which of the following is not a feature of pulmonary hypertension?
    A. Loud S2
    B. Palpable second heart sound
    C. Heaving apex beat
    D. Raised JVP
    E. Early diastolic murmur

67. On a routine ECG, a 67-year-old Brazilian man is found to have a prolonged PR interval. Which of the following is not a cause of first-degree heart block?
    A. Age-related fibrosis
    B. β-Blockers
    C. Chagas disease
    D. Wolff–Parkinson–White syndrome
    E. Aortic stenosis

68. Which of the following pathologies is least associated with pericardial effusion?
    A. Viral pericarditis
    B. Tuberculosis
    C. Systemic lupus erythematosus
    D. Myocardial infarction
    E. Hypertrophic cardiomyopathy

69. Which of the following statements is false regarding constrictive pericarditis?
    A. It may be caused by tuberculosis
    B. Equal pressures are found on right and left heart catheterisation
    C. Is a variant of hypertrophic cardiomyopathy in some cases
    D. Kussmaul sign may be positive
    E. Pericardial calcification may be visible on X-ray

70. Which of the following is the least recognised consequence of anterior MI?
    A. Acute MR
    B. VSD
    C. Cardiac rupture
    D. Aneurysm formation
    E. Temporary heart block

71. A 54-year-old woman, who has a metal mitral valve prosthesis for previous mitral stenosis, is undergoing upper GI endoscopy for investigation of dyspepsia. She is not allergic to any antibiotics. What antibiotic prophylaxis would you recommend?
    A. Amoxicillin 1 g IV
    B. Clarithromycin 500 mg PO
    C. Co-amoxiclav 625 mg PO
    D. Metronidazole 400 mg PO
    E. None of the above

72. A 42-year-old man goes to a well man clinic. On examination, he is noted to have cannon waves in the JVP. What is the most likely pathology?
    A. Congenital complete heart block
    B. Atrial fibrillation
    C. Tricuspid regurgitation
    D. Pulmonary stenosis
    E. Right heart failure

73. You are called to the resuscitation bay in the emergency department for a trauma call. A man has been involved in a road traffic accident and is brought in by ambulance with suspected cardiac tamponade. What does Beck's triad consist of?
    A. Poor capillary refill, tachycardia and decreased level of consciousness
    B. Low arterial blood pressure, jugular venous distension and impalpable apex beat
    C. Raised JVP which drops with inspiration, low arterial blood pressure and impalpable apex beat
    D. Jugular venous distension, muffled heart sounds and low arterial blood pressure
    E. Muffled heart sounds, decreased level of consciousness and impalpable apex beat

74. Which of the following is a contraindication to prasugrel therapy?
    A. Left main stem coronary disease
    B. Diabetes
    C. Age >60 years
    D. Weight <60 kg
    E. Drug-eluting stents

75. A 42-year-old man attends his GP for a new patient check. He is found to have a blood pressure of 210/115 mmHg. Which of the following is not a consequence of hypertension?
    A. Retinopathy
    B. Left ventricular hypertrophy
    C. Nodular glomerulosclerosis
    D. Haemorrhagic stroke
    E. Papilloedema

76. A patient collapses on the ward. He is not breathing and does not have a pulse. Which of the following is not an appropriate course of action?
A. Call 2222
B. Administer 2 rescue breaths
C. Start CPR
D. Obtain IV access
E. Attach defibrillator leads

77. A 69-year-old female is brought to the emergency department in asystole. Which of the following is the only recommended drug treatment?
A. Amiodarone 300 mg IV
B. Atropine 3 mg IV
C. Adrenaline 1 mg IV
D. Sodium bicarbonate 8.4% IV
E. Calcium gluconate 10 mmol IV

78. A man suffers a myocardial infarction. Which of the following is most likely to result in temporary complete heart block?
A. Lateral MI
B. Anterior MI
C. Posterior MI
D. Anterolateral MI
E. Inferior MI

79. A 78-year-old lady with known hypertension presents with a 3-day history of diarrhoea and vomiting. Her blood shows an acute kidney injury with a potassium level of 6.5 mmol/L. Which antihypertensive drug is she most likely to be on?
A. Lisinopril
B. Atenolol
C. Amlodipine
D. Furosemide
E. Methyldopa

80. A 65-year-old man with recently-diagnosed angina experiences chest pain on exertion. He takes two sprays of his GTN, which relieves the pain. However shortly after he reports feeling dizzy and then collapses. His blood pressure is recorded as 87/43 mmHg. What is the most likely cause?

A. Acute myocardial infarction
B. GTN syncope
C. Arrhythmia
D. Pulmonary embolus
E. Seizure

Extended-matching questions (EMQs)

1. Match the ECG changes below to the most likely clinical diagnosis:

A. ST elevation V1–V4
B. ST depression V1–V4
C. V2 + V5 >35 mm
D. Prolonged QT interval
E. Concave ST elevation in all leads except AVR
F. Short p waves and tall T waves
G. ST elevation in leads II, III and AVF with ST depression in V2–V4
H. Q waves in V1–V4
I. Right axis deviation
J. Small complexes with beat-to-beat variation

Instruction: For each scenario described below, choose the SINGLE most likely diagnosis from the above list of options. Each option may be used once, more than once or not at all:

1. Family history of sudden cardiac death
2. Pericarditis
3. Longstanding hypertension
4. Pericardial effusion
5. Acute inferoposterior myocardial infarction

2. The drug(s) of choice for the following arrhythmias include:

A. Sotalol
B. Digoxin
C. Verapamil
D. Flecainide
E. Atenolol
F. Amiodarone
G. C or D
H. A, C or E
I. A and F
J. Implantable cardioverter defibrillator (ICD) and drug treatment

Instruction: For each scenario described below, choose the SINGLE most likely diagnosis from the above list of options. Each option may be used once, more than once or not at all:

1. Rhythm control for AF in a patient with known angina
2. Rhythm control for AF in an asthmatic 35-year-old man
3. Prophylaxis for SVT in the absence of an accessory pathway
4. Prophylaxis for VT in a patient with poor LV function
5. First-line rate control for AF

3. Choose the drug of choice for the treatment of hypertension in the scenario below:

A. Atenolol
B. Perindopril
C. Doxazosin
D. Methyldopa
E. Bendrofluazide
F. Amlodipine
G. Losartan
H. E or F
I. A or F

Instruction: For each scenario described below, choose the SINGLE most likely diagnosis from the above list of options. Each option may be used once, more than once or not at all:

1. 70-year-old male, recent diagnosis of angina of effort
2. 50-year-old diabetic lady who describes a dry cough having been started on ramipril
3. 28-year-old female who is 20 weeks pregnant
4. 37-year-old Afro-Caribbean male
5. 88-year-old female who is troubled by urgency of micturition

4. Which is the most appropriate next choice of cardiac investigation in the scenario described below?

A. Stress echocardiogram
B. Exercise stress test
C. Magnetic resonance imaging
D. Computed tomography
E. Myocardial perfusion scan
F. Coronary angiogram

G. Echocardiogram

H. 24-h tape (Holter monitor)

I. A or E

J. No investigations are needed

Instruction: For each scenario described below, choose the SINGLE most appropriate investigation from the above list of options. Each option may be used once, more than once or not at all:

1. 60-year-old man seen in clinic with a 3-month history of chest tightness on exertion
2. 23-year-old female who reports breathlessness on exertion and has a history of a childhood heart murmur
3. 70-year-old diabetic man who has exertional chest pain and ST depression on exercise stress testing
4. 44-year-old lady who has limited mobility and on treatment for hypertension and hypercholesterolaemia; she describes a sharp left-sided chest discomfort, but which may or may not be related to exertion. Cardiovascular examination was unremarkable
5. 40-year-old female with fast palpitations occurring for a few minutes each day. Cardiovascular examination is normal

5. Select the most likely cause of syncope in each of the clinical scenarios listed below:

A. Hypertrophic cardiomyopathy

B. Long QT syndrome

C. Complete heart block

D. Aortic stenosis

E. Postural hypotension

F. Vasovagal syncope

G. Ventricular tachycardia

H. Vertebrobasilar insufficiency

I. Epileptic seizure

Instruction: For each scenario described below, choose the SINGLE most likely diagnosis from the above list of options. Each option may be used once, more than once or not at all:

1. 70-year-old male with a history of three previous myocardial infarctions and coronary artery bypass grafting who describes a feeling of fluttering in the chest before losing consciousness
2. 65-year-old female with a 10-year history of diabetes and hypertension who describes dizziness on getting out of bed in the morning
3. 70-year-old male who describes a 3-week history of lethargy and shortness of breath on exertion. His heart rate is between 30 and 40 beats/min
4. 30-year-old male with a family history of sudden cardiac death; on examination he has a jerky pulse, a double apical impulse and ejection systolic murmur
5. 35-year-old female who is previously fit and well and loses consciousness after receiving bad news

6. From the list below select the causative factor that is most closely linked to the following complication:

A. Type III autoimmune reaction

B. Prosthetic heart valve

C. *Coxiella burnetii*

D. Recent dental work

E. Splinter haemorrhages

F. Roth spots

G. Janeway lesions

H. Coagulase-negative staphylococci

I. Libman-Sacks endocarditis

J. C or I

Instruction: For each scenario described below, choose the SINGLE most likely diagnosis from the above list of options. Each option may be used once, more than once or not at all:

1. Patient with rheumatic heart disease and no previous surgical history who has developed endocarditis
2. Glomerulonephritis
3. Culture-negative endocarditis
4. Failure to eradicate the infection in endocarditis
5. Retinal haemorrhage in the setting of infective endocarditis

7. Match the diagnosis listed below with the ECG description:

A. Left bundle branch block

B. Atrial flutter

C. Accelerated idioventricular rhythm

D. Second-degree heart block

E. Complete heart block with ventricular escape rhythm

F. Right bundle branch block

G. Hypothermia

H. Accessory pathway

I. Atrial fibrillation

Instruction: For each scenario described below, choose the SINGLE most likely diagnosis from the above list of options. Each option may be used once, more than once or not at all:

1. RSR pattern in lead V1
2. P waves which have no fixed relationship with the QRS complexes. The QRS complexes are broad and the heart rate is 35 beats/min
3. J waves
4. Delta wave
5. Left bundle branch block morphology shortly after myocardial infarction, no visible p waves, heart rate 100 beats/min

8. For each of the emergency situations outlined, select the definitive management plan:

A. Insertion of a temporary pacing wire
B. Primary angioplasty (or thrombolysis if not available)
C. Urgent echocardiogram with a view to pericardial aspiration
D. Urgent CT thorax with a view to cardiothoracic surgery
E. Urgent VQ scan with administration of subcutaneous low-molecular-weight heparin
F. Urgent CXR with a view to chest aspiration/drain
G. Urgent chest aspiration/drain
H. Administration of non-invasive ventilation and IV antibiotics
I. None of the above

Instruction: For each scenario described below, choose the SINGLE most appropriate management plan from the above list of options. Each option may be used once, more than once or not at all:

1. 36-year-old male following a road traffic accident. Lacerated skin and apparent injury to ribs on the right side of the chest anteriorly. He is extremely dyspnoeic and there is mediastinal shift towards the left with hyperresonance of the right lung field
2. 60-year-old female with known metastatic breast cancer. Presents with a 2-week history of progressive shortness of breath, no history of chest pain. Noted to be hypotensive and tachycardic on examination
3. 75-year-old man who takes diltiazem for hypertension, presents with a 3-week history of progressive lethargy and shortness of breath. He is now dizzy even sitting still. The ECG shows complete heart block and his blood pressure is 80/50 mmHg
4. 38-year-old male, recent flu-like illness. He describes left-sided chest pain, which radiates to the shoulder that has been present for 3 days constantly. The ECG shows widespread concave ST elevation but no Q waves are visible
5. 25-year-old female, 28 weeks pregnant. She has been well recently, but presents with right-sided chest pain which came on suddenly, worse on deep inspiration, and shortness of breath. She is tachycardic and hypoxic on room air

9. From the list of drugs below, select the most appropriate choice for use in the clinical scenario described below:

A. Cardioselective β-blocker
B. ACE inhibitor
C. Angiotensin receptor antagonist
D. α-Blocker
E. Calcium channel antagonist
F. Spironolactone
G. Loop diuretic
H. Hydralazine and nitrate
I. Eplerenone

Instruction: For each scenario described below, choose the SINGLE most suitable selection from the above list of options. Each option may be used once, more than once or not at all:

1. 60-year-old male, 1 day following uncomplicated angioplasty following myocardial infarction. Already prescribed aspirin, clopidogrel, statin and β-blocker
2. 68-year-old female, presented with congestive cardiac failure, found to have LV systolic impairment on echocardiogram, much improved after 2 days of loop diuretics
3. 70-year-old male with chronic heart failure, seen in the clinic. He is in NYHA class III despite already taking bisoprolol, perindopril and frusemide at optimal doses
4. 72-year-old AfroCaribbean gentleman, whose heart failure symptoms have not improved with conventional first-line treatment
5. 40-year-old male day 1 post myocardial infarction who is taking ramipril, simvastatin, aspirin and clopidogrel. His heart rate is 80 beats/min, blood pressure 140/70 mmHg and there are no signs of heart failure

10. Select the most appropriate treatment option for the following conditions:

A. Thrombolysis
B. Temporary pacemaker insertion
C. Atropine
D. Central line insertion and consideration of inotropes
E. Permanent pacemaker insertion
F. Amiodarone
G. Synchronized DC shock
H. Intravenous adrenaline (epinephrine)
I. Coronary angiogram with a view to angioplasty
J. Intravenous frusemide

Instruction: For each scenario described below, choose the SINGLE most likely management step from the above list of options. Each option may be used once, more than once or not at all:

1. Unstable angina pectoris
2. Supraventricular tachycardia with systolic blood pressure 70 mmHg
3. Ventricular tachycardia with systolic blood pressure 130 mmHg
4. Complete heart block and intermittent episodes of dizziness (no rate-slowing drugs)
5. Acute pulmonary oedema

11. From the list of drugs below select which one you would consider discontinuing as a result of adverse effect described:

A. Aspirin

B. Isosorbide mononitrate

C. Atenolol

D. Amlodipine

E. Amiodarone

F. Bendrofluazide

G. Lisinopril

H. Clopidogrel

I. Choose not to discontinue any drug

Instruction: For each scenario described below, choose the SINGLE most appropriate option from the above list of options. Each option may be used once, more than once or not at all:

1. Patient troubled by ankle swelling after starting treatment for hypertension
2. Acute deterioration in renal function after starting this treatment for the first time
3. Recent coronary angioplasty, itchy rash, but constitutionally well
4. Severe headache
5. Erectile dysfunction having started new treatment from GP for hypertension

12. From the following list of congenital heart lesions, which option correlates best with the scenario described?

A. Pulmonary stenosis

B. Aortic stenosis

C. Tetralogy of Fallot

D. Coarctation of the aorta

E. Atrial septal defect

F. Patent ductus arteriosus

G. Ventricular septal defect

H. Aortic root dilatation

I. Dextrocardia

J. A or F

K. C, E, F or G

L. B, D or H

Instruction: For each scenario described below, choose the SINGLE most likely diagnosis from the above list of options. Each option may be used once, more than once or not at all:

1. Trisomy 21
2. Maternal rubella
3. Turner syndrome
4. Marfan syndrome
5. Kartagener syndrome

13. Select the diagnosis that is suggested by the clinical findings described:

A. Tricuspid regurgitation

B. Pulmonary hypertension

C. Coarctation of the aorta

D. Atrial septal defect

E. Mitral valve prolapse

F. Ventricular septal defect

G. Aortic stenosis

H. Hypertrophic cardiomyopathy

Instruction: For each scenario described below, choose the SINGLE most likely diagnosis from the above list of options. Each option may be used once, more than once or not at all:

1. Left parasternal heave
2. Double apical impulse
3. Pulsatile liver
4. Absent second heart sound
5. Mid-systolic click and late systolic murmur

14. Match the ECG changes below to the most likely clinical diagnosis:

A. ST elevation in leads II, III and AVF with ST depression in V2–V4

B. ST elevation V1–V4

C. ST depression V1–V4

D. V2 + V5 >35 mm

E. Concave ST elevation in all leads except AVR

F. Short p waves and tall T waves

G. Q waves in V1–V4 h. Right axis deviation

H. Prolonged QT interval

I. VT/VF

Instruction: For each scenario described below, choose the SINGLE most likely diagnosis from the above list of options. Each option may be used once, more than once or not at all:

1. Hyperkalaemia
2. Pericarditis
3. Longstanding hypertension
4. Old anterior myocardial infarction
5. Acute inferior myocardial infarction

5. Select the most appropriate treatment option for the following patients:

A. Cardiac transplantation
B. VVI pacemaker
C. Coronary artery bypass surgery
D. No treatment
E. DDD pacemaker
F. Propranolol
G. Biventricular pacemaker/cardiac resynchronization therapy
H. HMG coenzyme reductase inhibitor
I. Angiotensin II receptor antagonist
J. Fibrates
K. D or F

Instruction: For each scenario described below, choose the SINGLE most likely diagnosis from the above list of options. Each option may be used once, more than once or not at all:

1. 68-year-old diabetic male with unstable angina and three-vessel coronary artery disease not amenable to percutaneous coronary intervention
2. 37-year-old female with occasional ventricular ectopics but is otherwise fit and healthy
3. 88-year-old male with intermittently fast AF requiring rate-slowing drugs now presenting with symptomatic pauses
4. 70-year-old man who is breathless on walking short distances, found to have poor LV function and broad QRS complexes. He is on optimal drug therapy and has minor coronary artery disease
5. 34-year-old diabetic female with no history of coronary artery disease, who has a fasting total cholesterol of 9.2 and normal triglycerides

16. The most well-recognized side effect of the following drugs is:

A. Cold extremities
B. Leg oedema
C. Headache
D. Muscle pain
E. Angioedema
F. Dry cough
G. Gynaecomastia
H. Thrombocytopenia
I. Constipation
J. Pulmonary fibrosis

Instruction: For each scenario described below, choose the SINGLE most likely diagnosis from the above list of options. Each option may be used once, more than once or not at all:

1. Spironolactone
2. Nitrates
3. Simvastatin
4. Carvedilol
5. Tirofiban

17. Match a cause for pulmonary hypertension in the following patients:

A. Mitral regurgitation
B. Pulmonary stenosis
C. Familial pulmonary arterial hypertension
D. Mitral stenosis
E. Aortic regurgitation
F. Rheumatoid arthritis
G. Chronic bronchitis
H. Systemic sclerosis
I. Pulmonary embolism

Instruction: For each scenario described below, choose the SINGLE most likely diagnosis from the above list of options. Each option may be used once, more than once or not at all:

1. 55-year-old male with a history of rheumatic fever. He has had frequent episodes of acute pulmonary oedema. On examination his pulse is irregularly irregular, he has a loud first heart sound and rumbling mid-diastolic murmur on auscultation
2. 64-year-old male who is a heavy smoker, has a chronic cough productive of grey sputum and is breathless on moderate exertion
3. 24-year-old female with no significant past medical history who presents with gradually worsening breathlessness on exertion. The only findings of note on examination are a prominent parasternal heave, loud pulmonary second sound and a third heart sound
4. 44-year-old female with a history of dysphagia, joint pain and cold extremities. On examination it was noted that she had taut skin over her fingers, and over her nose giving rise to a pursed mouth appearance
5. 38-year-old female on the combined oral contraceptive pill who describes a sudden onset left-sided chest pain which is worse on inspiration. She was recently in plaster having fractured her ankle

18. Match a cause for heart failure in the following patients:

A. Pulmonary hypertension
B. Aortic regurgitation
C. Aortic stenosis

D. Chemotherapy

E. Mitral stenosis

F. Systemic hypertension

G. Viral myocarditis

H. Alcohol

I. Atrial septal defect

J. Mitral regurgitation secondary to mitral valve prolapse

Instruction: For each scenario described below, choose the SINGLE most likely diagnosis from the above list of options. Each option may be used once, more than once or not at all:

1. 78-year-old male with an ejection systolic murmur loudest in the aortic area, radiating to the neck and displaced apex beat
2. 56-year-old male with ankylosing spondylitis. A collapsing pulse was noted on peripheral examination
3. 65-year-old female with a mid-systolic click and a late systolic murmur
4. 19-year-old male with a recent flu-like illness. He has a third heart sound and cardiomegaly was noted on the chest radiograph
5. 44-year-old diabetic with renal impairment. Fundoscopy revealed AV nipping, silver wiring and small haemorrhages

19. From the list below choose the most appropriate management plan for the clinical scenarios described:

A. Primary percutaneous coronary intervention (primary PCI)
B. Automated internal cardioverter defibrillator implantation
C. Heart transplantation
D. Aortic valve replacement
E. Percutaneous alcohol septal ablation
F. Percutaneous mitral valvuloplasty
G. Closure of atrial septal defect
H. Coronary angiogram
I. Coronary artery bypass graft surgery
J. Permanent pacemaker implantation
K. Mitral valve replacement
L. No intervention

Instruction: For each scenario described below, choose the SINGLE best management plan from the above list of options. Each option may be used once, more than once or not at all:

1. A 24-year-old male is admitted to hospital with severe shortness of breath, orthopnoea and ankle swelling, an echocardiogram at admission showed an ejection fraction of 10%. He had been diagnosed with idiopathic dilated cardiomyopathy 9 months previously. Despite treatment with intravenous diuretics he remained in NYHA class IV heart failure
2. A 64-year-old male patient with angina on mild exertion undergoes cardiac catheterization. This shows a severe stenosis of the left main coronary artery, and a severe stenosis of the right coronary artery, with normal left ventricular function.
3. 6 h after successful thrombolysis for an acute inferior ST elevation myocardial infarction, a routine ECG shows complete heart block. The 48-year-old male patient is well, with a normal blood pressure.
4. A 78-year-old female with permanent atrial fibrillation presents with a history of syncope. A Holter recording confirms atrial fibrillation, and shows several pauses lasting up to 7 s in duration
5. A 50-year-old male is sent for a myocardial perfusion scan to investigate a history of chest pain. The report reads '...there is a large area of reversible myocardial ischaemia in the anterior left ventricular wall...'

20. Match a likely cause for each of the following patients who suffer from systemic hypertension:

A. Cushing disease
B. 'Essential' hypertension
C. Doxazosin
D. Phaeochromocytoma
E. Addison disease
F. Hyperthyroidism
G. Renal artery stenosis
H. Persistent ductus arteriosus
I. Coarctation of the aorta
J. Conn syndrome

Instruction: For each scenario described below, choose the SINGLE most likely diagnosis from the above list of options. Each option may be used once, more than once or not at all:

1. 74-year-old male with diabetes and known coronary artery disease complaining of headaches. On several visits to his physician his blood pressure is recorded as 170/95 mmHg
2. 23-year-old female with a complaint of progressive weight loss, palpitations, anxiety and frequent loose motions.
3. 54-year-old asymptomatic male. A left paraumbilical bruit was noted on examination
4. 17-year-old male with radiological appearance of rib notching on chest radiograph
5. 18-year-old female with progressive weight gain and development of bitemporal hemianopia

BOF answers

1. B – Bilateral basal crepitations are a feature of left-ventricular failure. Mid-diastolic murmur suggests mitral stenosis, which may lead to pulmonary hypertension and right ventricular failure, but is not a sign of it.

2. C – Any patient with fever and a murmur must be investigated for infective endocarditis.

3. C – Classic cardiac syncope is of sudden onset and recovery with no warning symptoms and no neurological deficit.

4. A – Aortic regurgitation is associated with an early diastolic murmur. Atrial septal defects cause fixed splitting of the second heart sounds and possibly an ejection systolic pulmonary flow murmur. Aortic stenosis is associated with an ejection systolic murmur.

5. E – Adenosine slows conduction in the AV node. It has no influence on ventricular rate in ventricular tachycardia because the impulses are generated below the AV node. It is administered initially as a dose of 6 mg.

6. D – Ventricular tachycardia is a broad-complex tachycardia. It can be caused by hypokalaemia.

7. B – Digoxin is excreted by the kidneys. The half-life of digoxin is 36-48 h. The effects of digoxin are enhanced by hypokalaemia, sometimes causing digoxin toxicity.

8. A – Fungal infections remain rare and are usually seen in IV drug abusers and after valve surgery. Staphylococcus aureus is associated with severe and destructive infection. Enterococci are the second most common cause of bacterial endocarditis.

9. A – Whilst β-blockers are well established in the treatment of heart failure, they should not be used in the acute setting.

10. D – Thrombolysis should only be considered in patients with ST elevation myocardial infarction in the absence of contraindications.

11. C – Pericarditis classically causes saddle shaped ST elevation in all leads of a 12-lead ECG.

12. B – Pathological Q waves are wider than two small squares (0.08 s) and/or >25% of the corresponding R wave. Q waves in leads I and aVL suggest a lateral infarct. The depolarization current is away from the facing lead. Pathological Q waves are permanent.

13. C – Janeway lesions, clubbing, and conjunctival haemorrhages are features of endocarditis.

Parasternal heave suggest pulmonary hypertension.

14. B – LVH is associated with a tall R wave in V6 (>25 mV); there might also be T wave inversion in leads I, aVL, V5 and V6. Broad QRS complexes are a feature of bundle branch block. P pulmonale suggests right atrial enlargement, which could result from pulmonary hypertension.

15. E – Atrial fibrillation may be similar to SVT with respect to frequency and severity of the palpitations. Excessive coffee may precipitate both and both may cause chest pain. Both may be preceded by a normal ECG (apart from SVT due to Wolff–Parkinson–White syndrome, which has characteristic resting ECG changes).

16. B – VSD is the most common congenital cardiac abnormality.

17. D – The right coronary artery supplies the inferior myocardium. The other options are all branches of the left coronary artery.

18. A – Family members of affected patients are often offered screening.

19. C – Mitral stenosis only causes a tapping apex beat.

20. A – Mitral stenosis is not a feature of tetralogy of Fallot.

21. B – Oligaemic lung fields are a feature of pulmonary embolism.

22. D – LBBB is associated with M-shaped complexes in V6. Atropine does not affect rhythm disturbances that originate below the AV node. LBBB is usually asymptomatic unless associated with AV node disease.

23. E – Atrial myxoma characteristically is associated with a 'tumour plop', and can present with fever.

24. C – Aortic dissection causes a difference in blood pressure between arms due to involvement of the left subclavian or brachiocephalic arteries. Dissection can cause acute aortic regurgitation, but regurgitation alone would not account for this presentation.

25. B – This man is likely to have Marfan syndrome, which is associated with aortic regurgitation. Tall men are more likely to have pneumothorax than the general population but here air entry is present throughout the chest so is unlikely.

26. D – For pulseless VT a non-synchronised DC shock is administered. Atropine is no longer used in a cardiac arrest situation. BLS is essential in all settings in and out of hospital.

27. E – Hypoxia, but not hypercapnia causes cardiac arrest.
28. B – Remember ABC!
29. B – Pulmonary artery pressure is usually low because pulmonary stenosis protects the pulmonary circulation. Total surgical correction includes closure of any right-to-left shunts.
30. A – Dressler syndrome is a pericarditis that usually occurs 7–14 days after acute myocardial infarction.
31. C – The AV node is supplied by the circumflex artery in 10% of patients. Following anterior myocardial infarction, AV node disorders are usually irreversible. The opposite is true following inferior myocardial infarction. Many patients with third-degree AV block are asymptomatic but they still require permanent pacing.
32. B – Endocarditis may be associated with prolonged PR interval and occasionally AV dissociation. Blood culture growth of staphylococcus aureus and vegetations seen on echo are major criteria. Erythema nodosum, and not erythema multiforme is a minor criterion.
33. E – This lady is presenting with pericarditis, which causes saddle-shaped ST elevation in all ECG leads. The treatment of choice is a non-steroidal anti-inflammatory drug such as ibuprofen.
34. C – Flushing and ankle swelling are often reported with calcium channel blockers. Renal impairment is not a direct side effect of β-blockers. β-Blockers cause bradycardia, not tachycardia.
35. E – Pericardial rub suggests pericarditis. All the other features are associated with endocarditis, which must always be excluded in any patient with a fever and a prosthetic valve.
36. B – Addison disease (primary adrenal insufficiency) is associated with low systemic blood pressure.
37. C – Early diastolic murmur suggests aortic valve incompetence, which is not usually caused by hypertension.
38. C – Rheumatic fever can affect all heart valves. Valvular pathology is an autoimmune process (Aschoff nodule) triggered by pharyngeal infection with group A β-haemolytic streptococci, and is the most common cause of mitral stenosis. Antibiotic prophylaxis is no longer recommended.
39. A – Capture and fusion beats are a feature of VT. Verapamil can be hazardous in VT and should never be used to differentiate between SVT with aberrancy and VT. If in doubt, always treat as VT.
40. A – Diabetes itself is not a contraindication to thrombolysis but the presence of diabetic proliferative retinopathy is. Blood pressure can be reduced with intravenous glyceryl trinitrate.

41. E – Collapsing pulse can be a feature of aortic regurgitation, large arteriovenous malformations/fistulas, or marked peripheral vasodilatation. Bisferiens pulse is associated with mixed aortic valve disease. Pulsus alternans is associated with heart failure. Slow rising pulse is a feature of aortic stenosis.
42. E – Although sometimes difficult to see, P waves are not absent in atrial flutter or ventricular tachycardia. P waves are independent of the QRS complexes in complete heart block and ventricular tachycardia. Intermittent P waves are seen in sick sinus syndrome. Atrial fibrillation is the only condition where P waves are not seen on the ECG.
43. E – Shortness of breath, chest pain, and syncope are all features of severe disease.
44. B – Mitral stenosis causes a mid-diastolic murmur best heard with the bell of the stethoscope.
45. E – Although nicorandil can reduce blood pressure is used primarily as an antianginal agent.
46. A – Closed mitral valvotomy is performed through left thoracotomy incision. Mitral valvuloplasty, and temporary pacemaker insertion are performed percutaneously.
47. C – Long-distance travel suggests predisposition to deep-vein thrombosis and pulmonary embolism. Heavy alcohol intake can result in alcoholic cardiomyopathy and an array of cardiac arrhythmias, which may lead to syncope.
48. E – Abdominal ultrasound to examine the size of the kidneys is more useful than a plain X-ray of the abdomen.
49. C – Eisenmenger syndrome is associated with polycythaemia and clubbing and is irreversible.
50. C – In atrial fibrillation the random electrical atrial activity cannot be sensed and therefore dual-chamber pacing is not indicated. Pacemaker syndrome occurs with single-chamber pacemakers implanted in patients with atrial activity.
51. B – Exercise ECG testing no longer forms part of the assessment of patients with chest pain of recent onset. All other tests may be appropriate.
52. C – Pressure over the eyes, while previously recommended as a vagotonic manoeuvre, carries a risk of displacing the lens.
53. D – Migraine is felt to be associated with PFO, along with TIA and stroke. The others are not believed to have a positive association.
54. E – A small VSD produces a louder murmur than a larger one. They are more likely to close spontaneously without requiring intervention.
55. A – The wide pulse pressure causes the majority of the many eponymous signs of aortic

regurgitation, including a pulsating uvula (Müller sign). Syphilis may cause both AR and dementia (which may be treatable).

6. E – Takotsubo cardiomyopathy is also known as 'broken heart syndrome'. Long-term prognosis is generally good, though there is an initial mortality of around 10%, and ECG features may mimic those of NSTEMI.

7. B – Rapid ventricular ('overdrive') pacing may be used to terminate episodes of torsades de pointes or polymorphic VT.

8. D – The ECG may show tented T waves and small p waves at mildly raised potassium levels, but widening of the QRS complex is particularly dangerous. Widening may progress until the ECG looks like sine waves. This is a peri-arrest situation.

9. E – ACE inhibitors should not be given to women who are likely to become pregnant due to many adverse effects on the growing fetus, even very early in pregnancy. This includes effects on the musculoskeletal, cardiovascular, gastrointestinal and central nervous systems, though they are not believed to be carcinogenic.

0. E – HCM has many variants: it can present at any age and does not necessarily affect the septum. Obstruction is a feature in around 40% of patients.

1. A – Diuretics give symptomatic benefit in heart failure but have not been shown to confer a mortality benefit. ACE inhibitors and β-blockers should be given in all patients with heart failure, while spironolactone and digoxin are given to selected groups.

2. B – The risk of death or serious complication is around 1:1000.

3. D – A collapsing pulse is a feature of aortic regurgitation.

4. C – Mitral prolapse affects around 4% of the population and has a female preponderance; it is sometimes called click-murmur syndrome.

5. D – Tuberculosis is not a recognised cause of dilated cardiomyopathy, however if the enlarged heart shadow on X-ray turns out to be a pericardial effusion, TB is certainly possible.

66. C – The apex beat is not affected by pulmonary hypertension

67. D – The commonest causes of first-degree heart block are age-related fibrosis and drugs. Calcific aortic stenosis can involve conduction tissue. Worldwide, Chagas disease is a common cause.

68. E – Hypertrophic cardiomyopathy does not cause pericardial effusion but could co-exist.

69. C – Restrictive cardiomyopathy is a variant of HCM in some cases, particularly in the West.

70. E – Heart block is usually permanent after anterior MI.

71. E – NICE guidelines now no longer recommend routine antibiotic prophylaxis against endocarditis in the majority of cases.

72. A – Cannon waves occur when the atrium contracts against a closed tricuspid valve. Patients with congenital complete heart block are often asymptomatic.

73. D – Beck's triad consists of heart sounds muffled by effusion, along with raised venous pressure and low blood pressure (both are signs of tamponade).

74. D – Patients weighing less than 60 kg have an increased bleeding risk on prasugrel.

75. C – Hypertensive nephropathy causes sclerosis of the small arterioles of the kidney (hyaline arteriolosclerosis); nodular glomerulosclerosis is the histological feature of diabetic nephropathy. Papilloedema may be seen in accelerated (previously called 'malignant') hypertension.

76. B – Rescue breaths are not part of the 2010 Resuscitation council ALS algorithm.

77. C – Atropine is no longer given in asystolic arrests.

78. E – Anterior MI is most likely to result in permanent complete heart block.

79. A – ACE Inhibitors are highly likely to cause a raised potassium and Acute Kidney Injury in the contact of diarrhoea and vomiting.

80. B – Light-headedness is often reported in patients using GTN, and syncope can occur in relation to GTN-induced vasodilatation.

EMQ answers

1.

. (D) Prolonged QT interval (corrected for heart rate – QTc) on the ECG may suggest long QT syndrome, which is an inheritable condition that predisposes to sudden cardiac death, as it becomes more likely that the ensuing R wave will occur at the same time as the T wave of the previous complex. This can give rise to the so-called 'R on T' phenomenon, which may lead to torsades de pointes.

. (E) Widespread concave or saddle-shaped ST elevation occurs in pericarditis. This may be confused with ST elevation from acute myocardial infarction; however, they may be distinguished by the history and examination findings and the fact that changes on the ECG due to pericarditis do not usually correspond to a coronary territory. If in doubt an echocardiogram is helpful.

. (C) Other possible voltage criteria for LVH include tall R wave >25 mm in V5–V6, tall R wave >20 mm in lead II, and there may be T wave inversion in I, AVL, V5 and V6.

. (J) Due to fluid accumulation around the heart, the voltage on the ECG is reduced, giving rise to smaller complexes. (This may also occur if the body mass index is raised.) Movement of the heart within the pericardial fluid can give rise to electrical alternans, whereby the complexes are of varying size in the same ECG lead recording.

. (G) ST elevation in the inferior leads (II, III and AVF) suggests inferior MI. The ST depression in V2–V4 suggests posterior infarction, which occasionally occurs in isolation (so-called 'true posterior MI'). Of course ST depression in V2–V4 may reflect LAD territory ischaemia involving the anterior wall of the left ventricle.

2.

. (E) Rhythm control strategy is the aim of maintaining sinus rhythm. Numerous drugs are capable of this, the chance of success depending on duration of AF, LV function, mitral valve disease and left atrial size. A standard β-blocker should be the initial treatment option. Caution should be taken with sotalol as it also has class III effects of prolonging the QT interval, so ECG monitoring is necessary. Digoxin is effective only for rate control of AF and

flecainide is to be avoided in the presence of coronary artery disease or poor LV function.

2. (D) β-Blockers are contraindicated in asthma, so both atenolol and sotalol are ruled out. Flecainide is effective, but must be avoided in heart failure or coronary artery disease. Amiodarone is an alternative but is best avoided in young patients due to long-term toxicity and side effects.

3. (G) These agents are also effective in SVT prophylaxis as they slow conduction through the AV node and by altering the refractory period of tissues can interfere with the re-entry circuit. However, digoxin and verapamil should be avoided if there is an accessory pathway; this is because blocking the AV node will then encourage conduction by the accessory pathway instead.

4. (J) Patients with VT and poor LV function should be considered for implantable cardioverter defibrillator with or without biventricular pacing (CRT). Both β-blockers and amiodarone may reduce the frequency of VT, but are inferior treatments to ICD therapy. As an adjunct to device therapy, if tolerated, β-blockers may be beneficial in heart failure and are, therefore, preferable to amiodarone.

5. (H) First-line rate control for AF should be with a β-blocker or rate-limiting calcium channel antagonist. Digoxin is less effective as it has poor control of exercise-related tachycardia.

3.

1. (I) Atenolol and amlodipine are both suitable options for the treatment of both angina and hypertension. However, atenolol has been superseded as a first-line treatment for hypertension alone.

2. (G) ACE inhibitors and ARBs are suitable options in diabetic patients with hypertension. However, this patient describes a well-recognized side effect of ACE inhibitors and should, therefore, be changed onto an ARB.

3. (D) Methyldopa is a centrally acting antihypertensive agent that is often used to treat hypertension in pregnancy. β-blockers are used in pregnancy. Pre-eclampsia should be excluded in this patient.

4. (H) The first choice antihypertensive agent in an Afro-Caribbean patient should be either a calcium channel blocker or a diuretic.

5. (F) First-line treatment in this patient would either be a calcium channel antagonist or a diuretic. However,

215

the diuretic is likely to exacerbate her urinary symptoms (urinary tract infection having been excluded) and, therefore, amlodipine is preferable; otherwise she is likely not to be compliant!

5. (F) Vasovagal syncope is most likely in a patient of th age and in this context. It should be confirmed from the history, examination and ECG that no other cause is being overlooked.

4.

1. (B) This man has a history that is compatible with angina. The first-line investigation is an exercise stress test, which will give information about his exercise capacity and symptoms, heart rate and blood pressure response to exercise, and whether any ischaemic ECG changes are seen in association with his symptoms. If this test is positive for inducible ischaemia then the next step is coronary angiography.

2. (G) The history suggests a problem regarding structural heart disease and this is best investigated in the first instance with an echocardiogram.

3. (F) This patient has a high probability of significant coronary artery disease and there is objective evidence of ischaemia. He should have coronary angiography to evaluate his coronary anatomy and establish whether revascularization is necessary, and if so by what means (i.e. angioplasty/stenting or CABG).

4. (I) This lady's symptoms are not typical of myocardial ischaemia, but this needs to be excluded given her risk factors. She is unlikely to be able to undergo exercise stress testing and, therefore, an alternative non-invasive assessment is appropriate. Either a stress echocardiogram or myocardial perfusion scan is reasonable.

5. (H) A 24-h ECG is likely to document the cause of her palpitations as her symptoms occur on a daily basis.

5.

1. (G) This man is known to have coronary artery disease and in view of his history we would expect that his left-ventricular function is reduced due to damage from previous myocardial infarctions. The scar tissue predisposes him to ventricular tachycardia, which may well cause him to lose consciousness. An ICD is indicated if this is proven.

2. (E) Dizziness on standing is suggestive of postural hypotension. This is often due to vasodilator antihypertensive drugs, but in this case may also be due to autonomic neuropathy as a result of her diabetes.

3. (C) The heart rate suggests complete heart block and his symptoms are compatible with this. An ECG will confirm the diagnosis.

4. (A) The clinical findings and family history suggest HCM. An echocardiogram and Holter monitor should be performed.

6.

1. (D) This patient has heart valve disease resulting fro previous rheumatic fever. Endocarditis is likely t have resulted from a bacteraemia, such as that resulting from dental work. Therefore, antibiotic prophylaxis is recommended prior to dental or other invasive procedures.

2. (A) Glomerulonephritis results from a type III autoimmune reaction, in which soluble immune complexes (aggregations of antigen and IgG or IgM antibodies) are deposited in tissues such as the kidney and triggers the classical pathway of complement activation.

3. (J) Libman-Sacks endocarditis is seen in patients wit systemic lupus erythematosus and is not related t infection. Microbes that cause endocarditis and negative blood cultures include *Bartonella, Coxiella, Chlamydia, Legionella* and *Brucella* species as well as fungi and the HACEK group (*Haemophilus* species, *Actinobacillus actinomycetemcomitans, Cardiobacterium hominis, Eikenella corrodens* and *Kingella kingae* Blood cultures may also be negative if antibiotics have been started before blood cultures are taken

4. (B) It is notoriously difficult to eradicate infection fro prosthetic heart valves. The fastidiousness of the organism also plays an important part. It is extremely important to work closely with the microbiology department.

5. (F) Roth spots are retinal haemorrhages that may result from infective endocarditis.

7.

1. (F) This is the typical feature of RBBB.

2. (E) Complete heart block is exemplified by P waves which 'march' through the rhythm strip with no relationship to the QRS complexes. A ventricula escape rhythm is usually 30–40 beats/min and gives rise to wide QRS complexes.

3. (G) J waves are pathognomonic of hypothermia.

4. (H) δ waves arise from the 'pre-excitation' of the ventricular myocardium. This results from antegrade conduction via the accessory pathway The accessory pathway differs from the AV node i that it does not have a regulatory 'slowing down function. Therefore, the PR interval is shortened.

5. (C) Accelerated idioventricular rhythm is a broad complex automatic ventricular rhythm, which

commonly occurs in the first 48 h following a myocardial infarction. It rarely causes compromise and often reflects successful reperfusion of the myocardium. It is distinguished from VT as the heart rate is less than 120 beats/min.

8.

. (G) The clinical findings following trauma suggest tension pneumothorax. This is a clinical diagnosis and if untreated will result in cardiovascular collapse. It is treated without performing a chest X-ray by aspiration and insertion of a chest drain.

. (C) The differential diagnosis includes pericardial effusion, pulmonary embolus, chest infection and silent MI. The lack of chest pain or cough and the history of metastatic cancer point towards pericardial effusion and this needs to be investigated and treated urgently. The JVP may be elevated and there may be Kussmaul sign (paradoxical increase in the JVP with inspiration). Pulsus paradoxus can be detected clinically by measuring the blood pressure with inspiration. It is important to exclude a pericardial effusion before giving heparin or warfarin to cover for PE, as this may make a pericardial effusion much worse!

. (A) This man is compromised with hypotension secondary to complete heart block. The offending drug(s) should be discontinued and it is likely that he will need a permanent pacemaker (if complete heart block persists once the drug has washed out). In the meantime as he is symptomatic a temporary pacing wire should be inserted.

. (I) The history suggests pericarditis caused by a viral infection. The symptoms and ECG changes are not suggestive of ischaemia. The most important complication of this is involvement of the myocardium which can lead to impairment of ventricular function, or pericardial effusion causing haemodynamic compromise. Rarely pericardial constriction may result in the long term.

. (E) This lady has had a pulmonary embolus until proven otherwise! She should receive treatment dose low-molecular-weight heparin and be investigated either with a VQ scan (perfusion only) or CTPA-after discussion with the radiologist.

9.

. (B) This gentleman should also be started on an ACE inhibitor, as long as there is no contraindication. This has been shown to reduce mortality in large randomized clinical trials (SAVE/HOPE/TRACE studies). The renal function should be monitored.

2. (B) The next step in this lady's management is the introduction of an ACE inhibitor. ACE inhibitors have been shown to reduce both morbidity and mortality in patients with heart failure (CONSENSUS/SOLVD studies). The mechanism of benefit is thought to be attenuation of the renin-angiotensin-aldosterone axis, which mediates the neurohormonal response to heart failure.

3. (F) Spironolactone should be introduced next. This is proven to be of benefit in patients with NYHA class 3 or 4 symptoms due to heart failure (RALES study). Monitoring of the renal function is necessary.

4. (H) Patients who do not benefit from conventional first line therapy may benefit from hydralazine and nitrate in combination. This was demonstrated in African Americans in the A-HeFT study.

5. (A) This patient should be started on a β-blocker with the aim of reducing his heart rate to 60 beats/min. There is good evidence that this reduces mortality after MI (ISIS-1 study).

10.

1. (I) This patient is likely to have significant coronary artery disease, which may be amenable to angioplasty and stent treatment, or alternatively may require coronary artery bypass grafting.

2. (G) If the patient is compromised then even if the rhythm is SVT they should still be managed with DC cardioversion.

3. (F) This patient is not compromised despite ventricular tachycardia. Therefore, cardioversion can be attempted with electrolyte supplementation and amiodarone via a central venous catheter. This patient will obviously require further investigation in order to exclude myocardial ischaemia as a cause and evaluate LV function with a view to consideration of device therapy.

4. (E) This patient requires a permanent pacemaker as they are at risk of syncope or even ventricular standstill.

5. (J) Management is likely to include frusemide, oxygen, intravenous nitrates and opiates if tolerated, and non-invasive ventilation (NIV) such as continuous positive airway pressure (CPAP) if necessary. Anaesthetic input may be required and is best sought early!

11.

1. (D) Amlodipine can cause ankle swelling, and if this is troublesome, an alternative antihypertensive should be used instead. Alternatively, if another treatment is needed to control the blood pressure then the addition of a diuretic may resolve the ankle swelling.

2. (G) Acute deterioration in renal function may result if the patient has renal artery stenosis. This is because the efferent renal arteriole is preferentially dilated compared to the afferent arteriole, so the perfusion pressure across the kidney falls.

3. (I) A rash may result as a reaction to the contrast agent used for the angiogram, or as a reaction to clopidogrel. If the former is responsible, symptoms will resolve. If clopidogrel is the cause of the rash this may resolve with time. The clopidogrel should not be discontinued without discussion with a consultant cardiologist, as this may predispose to acute stent thrombosis, which is potentially fatal.

4. (B) ISMN often causes headaches and if not tolerated should be discontinued, in favour of an alternative antianginal.

5. (C) Erectile dysfunction is a well-recognized side effect of β-blockers and unless essential can be discontinued − a calcium channel antagonist, such as verapamil or diltiazem, is often prescribed instead.

12.

1. (K) Trisomy 21 is associated with several congenital heart lesions and one or more of these occur in approximately 40% of cases.

2. (J) Maternal rubella can cause a patent (also called persistent) ductus arteriosus and pulmonary stenosis as well as cataracts, deafness and microcephaly.

3. (I) The two most common cardiovascular malformations are bicuspid aortic valve (which can lead to aortic stenosis) and aortic coarctation − both obstructive lesions. Partial anomalous venous drainage and aortic dilatation are recognized, but less common.

4. (H) Because of the underlying connective tissue abnormalities, aortic root dilatation is a relatively common finding and predisposes to aortic dissection. Valve regurgitation may also occur, usually affecting the aortic or mitral valves.

5. (I) Kartagener syndrome involves dextrocardia (or situs inversus-transposition of the viscera) as well as bronchiectasis and sinusitis.

13.

1. (B) A left parasternal heave indicates pulmonary hypertension. The right ventricle sits anteriorly and this is under strain against an increased pulmonary artery pressure.

2. (H) A double apical impulse suggests hypertrophic cardiomyopathy. The left ventricle is stiff and this results in raised left-ventricular end-diastolic pressure. Therefore, the left atrium has to contract forcefully and it is this impulse in additio to left-ventricular contraction that may be palpated.

3. (A) The regurgitant jet causes back pressure in the right atrium and this is transmitted to the venou system causing hepatic congestion and (if severe pulsatile hepatomegaly.

4. (G) Obscuring of the second heart sound is indicativ of severe aortic stenosis. Other clinical signs include an ejection systolic murmur, a thrill over the precordium, slow-rising or low-volume pulse and narrow pulse pressure.

5. (E) These signs are suggestive of mitral-valve prolapse. This is usually idiopathic, but may occu in association with connective-tissue disorders.

14.

1. (F) Hyperkalaemia is associated with tall T waves and short P wave amplitudes; the changes are dependent on the K^+ concentration. At higher concentrations, the PR interval becomes longer and QRS complexes become wider and eventually asystolic cardiac arrest occurs. Note that the ECG changes in hypokalaemia are the reverse with larger P wave and smaller T amplitudes leading to VT/VF as the terminal cardiac event.

2. (E) Widespread concave or saddle-shaped ST segment elevation occurs in pericarditis. Other ECH changes that may be seen include T wave inversion and atrial fibrillation.

3. (D) Long-standing hypertension leads to left-ventricular hypertrophy.

4. (G) The chest leads V1−V4 'look' at the anterior wall the left ventricle. The presence of Q waves supports the presence of old trans-mural myocardial infarction.

5. (A) The leads II, III and AVF 'look' at the inferior wall the heart, and ST elevation on the ECG is seen the acute phase of myocardial infarction.

15.

1. (C) Diabetic patients with ongoing ischaemia and three-vessel coronary artery disease will benefit prognostically and symptomatically from revascularization.

2. (D) These symptoms should be investigated, but in th absence of pre-syncope or syncope, and with a structurally normal heart it is unusual for any treatment to be required.

(B) This is a fairly common situation. He needs rate-control when his heart runs quickly, but this suppresses the rate too much at rest. He needs a single-chamber pacemaker, as there is no need for a dual-chamber device in a patient with AF.

(G) Further symptomatic and prognostic benefit could be obtained with biventricular pacing.

(H) Familial hypercholesterolaemia needs to be excluded in this lady, who would benefit from specialist referral and family counselling. There is a high risk for the development of atheromatous vascular disease and, therefore, primary prevention is indicated.

6.

(G) Other side effects include hyperkalaemia, impotence and menstrual irregularities.

(C) Other side effects include flushing and postural hypotension.

(D) Myalgia is an important side effect of all statins and should always be investigated with serial assessments of creatinine kinase levels. A fourfold increase in the CK levels suggests that the drug should be discontinued. Liver biochemistry and function tests should also be monitored.

(A) This is in common with other β-blockers. Other side effects include broncho-spasm, bradycardia and erectile dysfunction.

(H) Bleeding with or without thrombocytopenia is a major side effect associated with the use of this glycoprotein IIa/IIIb inhibitor.

7.

(D) Rheumatic fever may result in rheumatic heart disease – most commonly affecting the mitral valve and causing mitral stenosis. The clinical signs are consistent with mitral stenosis. Atrial fibrillation is commonly seen in mitral stenosis-and is often a result of left atrial dilatation.

(G) Pulmonary hypertension as a result of chronic lung disease is known as *cor pulmonale*.

(C) Pulmonary hypertension with no precipitating factor is described as *primary*. It most commonly occurs in young women.

(H) Systemic sclerosis (scleroderma) and other autoimmune rheumatic disorders and vasculitides are an important cause of pulmonary hypertension.

5. (I) This is a clinical scenario of pulmonary embolism, recent immobilization and typical symptoms.

18.

1. (C) These signs are consistent with aortic stenosis. Displacement of the apex beat suggests that there may be left-ventricular dilatation.

2. (B) The signs are of aortic regurgitation.

3. (J) The murmur described is that of mitral valve prolapse – in this instance surgical treatment may be warranted.

4. (G) Other causes of dilated cardiomyopathy include idiopathic, excess alcohol and post-partum.

5. (F) Systemic hypertension is an important cause of heart failure.

19.

1. (C) A young patient with severe LV dysfunction and stage IV heart failure, despite maximal medical therapy. This patient should be referred for consideration of heart transplantation.

2. (I) In patients with left main stem stenosis, current evidence supports CABG surgery as the treatment of choice.

3. (I) Cardiac arrhythmia is a common complication of myocardial infarction. In the absence of cardio-vascular instability (hypotension, collapse), it is safe to observe such arrhythmias for several days, in the assumption that they will resolve without treatment.

4. (J) This is an absolute indication for permanent pacemaker implantation.

5. (H) A coronary angiogram should be performed to determine the coronary artery anatomy, and help guide revascularization.

20.

1. (B) Over 90% of hypertension is 'essential', i.e. there is no treatable cause found.

2. (D) These symptoms are all consistent with a diagnosis of phaeochromocytoma. Hyperthyroidism is not normally associated with hypertension.

3. (G) The presence of a bruit in this area may suggest the presence of renal artery stenosis.

4. (I) Rib notching is a 'pathognomonic' sign of aortic co-arctation.

5. (A) Cushing disease is caused by a primary pituitary adenoma, which may cause bitemporal hemianopia.

Glossary

Abscess a collection of pus within a cavity.

ABPM ambulatory blood pressure monitoring.

Accessory pathway an abnormal connection between atrium and ventricle that is capable of propagating a cardiac impulse.

Afterload the pressure that the left ventricle must produce to eject blood out of the heart.

Anticoagulation treatment intended to prevent blood clotting.

Angina pectoris commonly known as **angina**, is chest pain due to ischaemia (a lack of blood and hence oxygen supply) of the heart muscle, generally due to obstruction of one or more coronary artery.

Angiogram is a medical imaging technique in which an X-ray picture is taken to visualize the inner opening of blood filled structures, including arteries, veins and the heart chambers.

Angioplasty see Percutaneous coronary intervention.

Apex beat the most downward and lateral position on the chest wall where the cardiac impulse can be felt.

Arrhythmia cardiac rhythm disturbanee.

Asystole absence of contraction. Asystole is when the heart has stopped beating and is different from ventricular fibrillation where the heart is still contracting, but not in a co-ordinated manner.

Atheroma is an accumulation and swelling in artery walls that is made up of cells, or cell debris, that contain lipids (cholesterol and fatty acids), calcium and a variable amount of fibrous connective tissue.

Atrial fibrillation (AF) irregular contraction of the atria resulting from disorganized electrical activity, typically results in an irregularly irregular pulse.

Atrioventricular (AV) node region of specialized conducting tissue between the atria and ventricles that functions to regulate the electrical conduction.

Atrium one of the two (upper) collecting chambers of the heart.

Bradycardia a heart rate <60 beats/min.

Bundle branch block This is failure of conduction in either the left (LBBB) or right (RBBB) bundle branches.

Cardiac catheterization is a minimally invasive procedure to access the coronary circulation and blood filled chambers of the heart using a catheter. It can be used both for diagnosis and treatment.

Cardiac failure also called heart failure, this is a reduction in cardiac pump function such that there is inadequate perfusion to metabolizing tissues.

Cardiac output the amount of blood pumped out by the heart every minute, calculated as stroke volume (SV) × heart rate (HR).

Cardiac tamponade compression of the heart as a result of accumulation of fluid in the pericardial space. This results in reduced cardiac output and can be fatal if untreated.

Cardiomyopathy heart muscle disease.

Cardioversion reverting the heart to a normal rhythm, this can be done electrically (with a DC shock), or using drugs (pharmacological or chemical cardioversion).

Central venous pressure (CVP) the pressure of blood in the great veins as they enter the right atrium.

Contractility the strength with which the myocardium contracts.

Cyanosis bluish discoloration of the skin due to the presence of deoxygenated haemoglobin in the blood vessels.

Defibrillation is the definitive treatment for the life-threatening cardiac arrhythmias ventricular fibrillation and pulseless ventricular tachycardia. Defibrillation consists of delivering a therapeutic dose of electrical energy to the affected heart with a device called a **defibrillator**

Defibrillator can be external, transvenous, or implanted, depending on the type of device used.

Dehiscence reopening at the site of a surgical closure or apposition.

Diastole part of the cardiac cycle where the ventricles are relaxed and filling.

Echocardiogram is an ultrasound of the heart. Also known as a cardiac ultrasound, it uses standard ultrasound techniques to image two-dimensional slices of the heart.

Ectopic an event occurring at a place other than its normal location, for example ventricular ectopic beats originate from the ventricles, not the sinoatrial node.

Electrocardiogram (ECG) graphic representation of the electrical activity of the heart over time.

Electrophysiological (EP) study an invasive test used for accurate diagnosis of arrhythmia and assessment of the function of the heart's electrical pathways.

End-diastolic pressure (EDP) the amount of pressure in the ventricle at the end of diastole.

End-diastolic volume (EDV) the amount of blood in the ventricle at the end of diastole; the greatest amount found in the ventricle throughout the whole cardiac cycle.

Ejection fraction the proportion of EDV which is ejected by contraction.

GTN glyceryl trinitrate – a vasodilator often used in patients with angina.

HBPM home blood pressure monitoring.

Heart block also called AV block – this is abnormal slowing or failure of conduction from the atria to the ventricles.

Holter monitor ambulatory ECG, usually attached to the patient for 24–48 h.

Hypertension high blood pressure.

Hypertrophy increase in the size of a tissue or organ resulting from an increase in cell size.

HCM hypertrophic cardiomyopathy.

Hypotension low blood pressure.

Hypoxia low oxygen levels.

ICD implantable cardiac defibrillator – a device that is set up to detect an arrhythmia, delivering a shock to the patient as necessary.

Infective endocarditis infection of the endothelial surface of the heart by a microorganism.

Ischaemia lack of blood supply to a tissue.

Infarction tissue death caused by inadequate perfusion.

Laplace relationship a relationship between the tension, pressure and diameter of a container (implied blood vessel), as Tension = Diameter × Pressure.

Left ventricular failure is a condition that can result from any structural or functional cardiac disorder that impairs the ability of the heart to fill with or pump a sufficient amount of blood through the body.

Mean arterial pressure the average pressure in the system at any point in time, approximated as the diastolic pressure + (1/3 × pulse pressure).

Myocardial infarction a medical condition that occurs when the blood supply to a part of the heart is interrupted, most commonly due to rupture of a vulnerable plaque.

Ohm's Law a relationship between resistance, pressure and flow inside a container (implied blood vessel), as Pressure = Flow × Resistance.

Pacemaker an area that leads to cardiac electrical activation; this may be natural (intrinsic, such as the SA node) or artificial, e.g. a permanent pacemaker.

Percutaneous coronary intervention (PCI) commonly known as **coronary angioplasty** or simply **angioplasty**, is a therapeutic procedure to treat the stenotic (narrowed) coronary arteries of the heart found in coronary heart disease.

Perfusion movement of blood through an organ or tissue.

Pericarditis is an inflammation of the pericardium (the fibrous sac surrounding the heart).

Precordium the surface of the lower anterior chest wall.

Preload the pressure and volume experienced by the heart before contraction.

Radio frequency ablation (RFA) the use of radiofrequency energy to create a therapeutic burn, intended to treat cardiac arrhythmia.

Shunt flow of blood through an abnormal communication between chambers or blood vessels. This may allow blood to flow between the pulmonary and systemic circulations.

Shock a situation where insufficient blood flow is reaching the body's tissues, causes commonly described as hypovolaemic, cardiogenic or septic.

Sinoatrial (SA) node the impulse-generating (pacemaker) tissue located in the right atrium.

Sinus rhythm a rhythm under direct control from the sinoatrial node.

Sphygmomanometer a device used for measuring blood pressure.

Starlings law a phenomenon whereby the heart increases its output by increasing its strength of contraction when the fibres of the myocardium are stretched.

Stent is a tube that is inserted into a natural conduit of the body to prevent or counteract a disease-induced localized flow constriction. Often used in PCI (see above).

Stroke volume (SV) the amount of blood ejected from the left ventricle with each beat.

Stroke work (SW) the amount of external energy expended in one ventricular contraction. SW is the arterial pressure (AP) multiplied by the SV.

Supraventricular literally 'above the ventricle', i.e. originating from the atria or AV node.

Syncope temporary loss of consciousness from reduced blood flow to the brain.

Systemic vascular resistance (SVR) the resistance to blood flow offered by all of the systemic vasculature excluding the pulmonary vasculature. It is calculated as (MAP – Right Atrial Pressure)/CO.

Systole part of the cardiac cycle where the ventricles are contracting.

Tachycardia a heart rate >100 beats/min.

Torsades de pointes literally meaning 'twisting of the points', this is a form of ventricular tachycardia in which the complexes are polymorphic (i.e. have variable shape).

Total peripheral resistance (TPR) the resistance to the flow of blood in the whole system. It is calculated as arterial pressure/cardiac output.

Troponin is a complex of three proteins that is integral to muscle contraction in skeletal and cardiac muscle but not smooth muscle, damage to myocardial cells leads to an elevation in the plasma troponin level.

Vasodilatation increase in the calibre of a blood vessel.

Ventricular relating to the heart's ventricles (pumping chambers).

Ventricular fibrillation (VF) irregular uncoordinated contraction of the ventricles, fatal if untreated.

Index

223